Case Studies on Corporations and Global Health Governance

Case Studies on Corporations and Global Health Governance

Impacts, Influence and Accountability

Nora Kenworthy, Ross MacKenzie and
Kelley Lee

ROWMAN &
LITTLEFIELD
─────── INTERNATIONAL
London • New York

Published by Rowman & Littlefield International, Ltd.
Unit A, Whitacre Mews, 26-34 Stannary Street, London SE11 4AB
www.rowmaninternational.com

Rowman & Littlefield International, Ltd. is an affiliate of Rowman & Littlefield
4501 Forbes Boulevard, Suite 200, Lanham, Maryland 20706, USA
With additional offices in Boulder, New York, Toronto (Canada), and London (UK)
www.rowman.com

British Library Cataloguing in Publication Information Available
A catalogue record for this book is available from the British Library

ISBN: HB 978-1-78348-356-3
ISBN: PB 978-1-78348-357-0

Library of Congress Cataloging-in-Publication Data Available

ISBN 978-1-78348-356-3 (cloth : alk. paper)
ISBN 978-1-78348-357-0 (pbk : alk. paper)

♾™ The paper used in this publication meets the minimum requirements of American
National Standard for Information Sciences Permanence of Paper for Printed Library
Materials, ANSI/NISO Z39.48-1992.

Printed in the United States of America

Contents

Preface

This book is the product of longstanding and recent collaborations solidified through two workshops held at the Faculty of Health Sciences, Simon Fraser University (SFU) atop Burnaby Mountain (outside Vancouver) in 2012 and 2013. We organized the first workshop as part of the Research Programme on Global Health Diplomacy, funded by the Rockefeller Foundation, and led by Richard Smith and Kelley Lee at the London School of Hygiene and Tropical Medicine. Having examined the role of governments and civil society organizations in the negotiation of global health governance (GHG) instruments, we recognized the need to better understand the role of for-profit actors, notably corporations, in global health diplomacy. The first workshop brought together a small group of established scholars who generously shared their findings to date, and ideas for developing a new research agenda on corporations and GHG. This meeting was followed by a second workshop, funded by the Canadian Institutes for Health Research (Planning Grant No. 126667), which, with the participation of additional scholars, along with graduate students and postdoctoral fellows, significantly expanded this conversation. Following each workshop, we made extensive efforts to write a paper setting out a definitive research agenda that would move thinking and practice beyond increasingly polarised debates in public health. However, given the diverse range of disciplines represented, theoretical perspectives, and business sectors studied, we found that encapsulating the full breadth of the group into a single peer-reviewed journal article proved impossible to achieve.

This book project arose from this intellectual impasse. Workshop participants agreed that there was a shared concern about the relationship between corporations and emerging forms of GHG. A loosely structured Corporations and Global Health Governance Research Network (COGH-REN) was formed. But like the parable of the blind men feeling an elephant, with each describing a different part of the same animal, the study of corporations has been approached to date from many different perspectives, generating findings within silos, and thus too often unshared across disciplines, geographies and/or sectors. Moreover, we recognized that more research is urgently needed on GHG per se, from a wider variety of disciplinary perspectives, to make sense of this rapidly shifting global governance sphere.

This book, and the accompanying *Research Guide on Corporations and Global Health Governance*, is intended to foster such research. Our aim is to encourage collaboration and dialogue in three ways. First, we want to bridge disciplinary divides and build greater understanding across discipline-focused and interdisciplinary scholars. These disciplines include anthropology, economics, history, political science, law and sociology, as well as interdisciplinary fields such as business studies, communications, development studies, international relations, public health and policy studies. Our goal is not simply to speak across disciplinary boundaries, but to build understanding of how research on corporations is undertaken by, and located within, different disciplines.

Second, we seek to broaden analytical attention beyond selected geographies and sectors. Given our understanding of global health as located within, and driven by, patterns of globalization that have impacts within and across all societies and populations, this requires a planetary approach to GHG. In doing so, we give due prominence to industrial sectors producing direct harms to human health such as tobacco, alcohol, food, pharmaceuticals and asbestos, which have been the focus of research to date on corporations and global health. Importantly, we also recognise the importance of indirect impacts generated by how corporations operate as particular forms of business organization. This extends the industries relevant to GHG to such sectors as garment making, agriculture, gambling and the extractive industries (oil and gas, lead). In reality, many industries have the potential to generate both direct and indirect impacts on health, making the challenge of creating effective GHG more complex.

Third, we seek to build intergenerational bridges, between early career and established scholars, in this subject area. The workshops actively sought participation by graduate students and early career scholars conducting research on corporations and global health, providing them with the opportunity to engage with 'battle scarred' senior researchers. We identified the important need for capacity building through training, mentoring, peer reviewing, and sharing of methodological approaches and data sources to create and support a new generation of interdisciplinary scholars. Many are currently working in relative isolation and few, if any, come from the developing world, where the health impacts of corporations can be most profound. The ensuing discussions also recognized the need to draw lessons from longer-standing bodies of knowledge, such as analysis of the tobacco industry, for research on other industries given limited attention to date. Opportunities for longitudinal and comparative analysis abound.

ACKNOWLEDGEMENTS

This book, and the accompanying volume, seeks to globalise the conversations begun at two SFU workshops. The editors would like to acknowledge the participants in these workshops who, while unable to contribute written material, substantively informed the conceptualisation and writing of these books: Doug Blanke, Dana Brown, Susan Eriksson, Ann Florini, Lee Johnston, Catherine Jones, Bruce Lanphear, Anne Roemer-Mahler, Stacey Pigg and Richard Smith.

Our appreciation to Anna Reeve, as the commissioning editor at Rowman and Littlefield International, who immediately understood and championed our vision for these books.

Finally, our warm thanks to our colleagues Ela Gohil, Natalia Botero and Linda van Vliet for all important logistical support in organizing the two workshops and their follow-up. Ela and Natalia, in particular, transcribed many hours of recorded sessions to ensure that the rich discussions were formally captured. The editors also wish to thank Jennifer Fang for so efficiently providing essential administrative support, including contractual arrangements and copyediting, underpinning the writing and delivery of this manuscript.

List of Acronyms

ABA American Beverage Association
ABB Association of British Bookmakers
ACPMA Asbestos Cement Products Manufacturers' Association
ADHD Attention-deficit hyperactivity disorder
AGOA African Growth and Opportunities Act
AI Asbestos Institute
ALAFA Apparel Lesotho Alliance to Fight AIDS
ARD Asbestos-related deaths
ART Antiretroviral therapy
ARTIST Asian Regional Tobacco Industry Science Team
ARV Antiretroviral
ASEAN Association of South-East Asian Nations
ATNI Access to Nutrition Index
BATC British American Tobacco Cambodia
BLF Beijing Liver Foundation
BMGF Bill and Melinda Gates Foundation
CLC Canadian Labour Congress
CNAPA Committee on National Alcohol Policy and Action
CNTC China National Tobacco Corporation
COP Conference of Parties
CPA Corporate political activity
CPC Communist Party of China
CPP Cambodian People's Party
CRI Chulabhorn Research Institute
CSIRO Commonwealth Scientific and Industrial Research Organisation
CSO Civil Society Organization
CSR Corporate social responsibility
CTE *Curbing the Epidemic: Governments and the Economics of Tobacco Control*
DFID Department for International Development
DG Directorates General
EAHF European Alcohol and Health Forum
ECJ European Court of Justice
EPA U.S. Environmental Protection Agency
EPASA Environment Protection Authority of South Australia
EU European Union
FAO Food and Agriculture Organization
FCTC Framework Convention on Tobacco Control
FDA Frente para la Defensa de Amazonia (Front for the Defence of Amazonia)
FENSA Framework for Engagement with Non-State Actors
FET Fair and equitable treatment
FOI Freedom of Information
FOPL Front-of-pack labelling
GAPG Global Alcohol Producers Group
GATI General Agreement of Tariffs and Trade
GAVI Global Alliance for Vaccines and Immunization
GDA Guideline Daily Allowance
GDP Gross domestic product

GFATM Global Fund to Fight AIDS, Tuberculosis and Malaria
GHG Global health governance
GM General manager
GSK GlaxoSmithKline
HIV Human immunodeficiency virus
IAVI International AIDS Vaccine Initiative
IBAS International Ban Asbestos Secretariat
IBFAN International Baby Food Action Network
ICA International Chrysotile Association
ICAP International Centre for Alcohol Policies
ICDC International Code Documentation Centre
ICIFIC International Council of Infant Food Industries
IFBA International Food and Beverage Alliance
IFPMA International Federation of Pharmaceutical Manufacturers Association
IGS International Gambling Studies
IJE *International Journal of Epidemiology*
IJOEH *International Journal of Occupational and Environmental Health*
ILO International Labour Organization
INFORMAS International Network for Food and Obesity/NCD Research, Monitoring
    and Action Support
IOCU International Organization of Consumers Unions
IRP Intellectual property rights
ISDS Investor-state dispute settlement
ITGA International Tobacco Growers' Association
JTI Japan Tobacco International
LMIC Low- and middle-income countries
LSHTM London School of Hygiene and Tropical Medicine
MDG Millennium Development Goal
MEP Global Malaria Eradication Program
MLG Multi-level governance
MNC Multinational corporation
MP Member of Parliament
MSP Member of the Scottish Parliament
MUP Minimum unit price
NAFTA North American Free Trade Agreement
NCB National coordinating body
NCD Non-communicable diseases
NCRG National Center for Responsible Gaming
NGO Non-governmental organization
NHMRC National Health and Medical Research Council
NICE National Institute for Health and Care Excellence
NRT Nicotine replacement therapy
PAC Political action committee
PATH Program for Appropriate Technology in Health
PCT Patent Cooperation Treaty
PM Philip Morris
PMA Philip Morris Asia
PPP Public-private partnership
PSI Population Services International
QFL Quebec Federation of Labour
RACGP Royal Australian College of General Physicians
RCT Randomized clinical trial
RGT Responsible Gambling Trust
SBS Sanitary and the Phytosanitary Agreement
SEATCA Southeast Asian Tobacco Control Alliance
SHS Secondhand smoke

SIRC Social Issues Research Centre
SNP Scottish National Party
SSB Sugar-sweetened beverages
STMA State Tobacco Monopoly Administration
SUTL Singapura United Trading Limited
SWA Scotch Whisky Association
TBT Agreement on Technical Barriers to Trade
TIA Trade and investment agreement
TLAP Targeted Lead Abatement Program
TNC Transnational corporation
TPP Trans-Pacific Partnership
TRIPS Trade-Related Aspects of Intellectual Property Rights
TTC Transnational tobacco company
TTM Thailand Tobacco Monopoly
UK United Kingdom
UN United Nations
U.S. United States
USTR United States Trade Representative
USWA United Steelworkers of America
VAT Value added tax
WHA World Health Assembly
WHO World Health Organization
WTO World Trade Organization

List of Figures

List of Tables

ONE

Introduction

Kelley Lee, Nora J. Kenworthy and Ross MacKenzie

The rapid rise of corporate power since the 1990s has been the defining change to the world economy brought about by globalisation. The size and scope of corporations have expanded on multiple fronts: from traditional industrial sectors to sectors hitherto deemed within the public sphere; from high- to low- and middle-income countries; and from involvement with wealth generation to increased participation in the governance of societies. As the most powerful form of business organisation, corporations hold unprecedented economic power in the early twenty-first century, and rapidly growing political legitimacy as 'citizens'. At the national level, countries such as the United States, through its *Citizens United* decision, have enshrined corporate personhood. This recognition, in turn, has become embedded in a growing number of institutional arrangements at the global level, such as multilateral trade and investment agreements. Consequently, there are profound concerns of a widening 'governance gap', between a fast-moving world economy heavily populated by transnational corporations (TNCs), and existing political institutions struggling to manage their social and environmental impacts (Urban 2014; Wiist, this volume).

This collection of case studies focuses on emerging governance gaps and growing corporate power in global health governance (GHG), a sphere where corporations have rapidly expanded their role since the 1990s. Globalisation has contributed not only to the rise of corporations, but also to the emergence of new transboundary health issues that pose acute challenges to existing forms of international health cooperation. The epidemiological transition from international to global health challenges has also prompted a governance transition, involving new institutions and a wider range of actors and resources in collective health action (Lee 2001; Brown et al. 2006). As global health has become 'firmly established on the global political agenda' (Schrecker 2012, 1), it has also emerged as a key domain of contestation and cooperation among state, market and civil society actors. The role of corporations has been seminal to debates on the appropriate structure and function of GHG. In the meantime, corporations have become major players in a wide range of global health initiatives, giving rise to concerns about fundamental conflicts between public and private interests (Richter 2001).

The existing literature on corporations and public health is already substantial, focusing on corporations' operations, goods and services, and their individual and population health outcomes. Corporate impacts on public health are increasingly diverse, ranging from the production of health-related goods and services (e.g., pharmaceuticals, medical technologies), to the marketing of goods and services that directly impact public health (e.g., food, tobacco, alcohol), to the production of goods and services that impact the social determinants of health (e.g., asbestos) (Wiist 2010; Freudenberg 2014). Although average measures of health and wellness have steadily improved around the world since the early twentieth century, recent evidence points to an unprecedented reversal in life expectancy among specific populations since the late twentieth century, largely attributed to the rise of non-communicable diseases (NCDs) such as diabetes, cancers and heart disease (Kindig and Cheng 2013). Almost all industries make decisions that have profound consequences for the social determinants of health, from choices about how much to pay workers or which occupational hazards workers will be exposed to, to decisions about whether and to what extent the industry will produce environmental harms. Thus, as the power and geographic reach of corporations has expanded over recent decades, so too have the public health harms associated with many industries.

This book is not just about '*when* corporations rule the world' (Korten 2001), but *why* and *how* they have come to do so, focusing on their rule in the domain of global health. The aims of this book are threefold. First, the case studies bring together a broader range of disciplines—including public health, political science, international relations, law, public health, social policy, anthropology—than previously assembled. Our goal is not only to share insights across disciplinary boundaries, but also to facilitate understanding of how new research can be generated and applied, to inform ongoing debates.

Second, the case studies broaden the scope of research on corporations and GHG in terms of industries and geography. Research to date has largely focused on individual industries (notably the alcohol, tobacco, food and beverage, pharmaceutical industries), resulting in specialist knowledge. We aimed to include, but not limit ourselves to, the primary 'harm industries' that have been the focus of the most extensive research on corporations and global health (Benson and Kirsch 2010). Moreover, the limited comparative analysis to date (Wiist 2010; Stuckler et al. 2012) suggests similarities across industries in terms of impacts and influence. In keeping with our understanding of corporations as operating within a world increasingly defined by economic globalisation, our geographical lens goes beyond traditional dichotomies of 'developed' and 'developing' countries, and North versus South. Undoubtedly, acute inequities persist, but in many cases the fault lines are dynamic, creating new geographies of 'haves' and 'have nots'. The case studies seek to capture this layering of old and new inequalities.

Our third aim is to build a generational bridge, across early, mid- and advanced career scholars, in the study of corporations and GHG. This book brings together established scholars with deep expertise in selected industries, and scholars emerging from a broad range of disciplines and industry interests. This cross-fertilisation of ideas, approaches, methodologies and knowledge, alongside the accompanying research guide, is intended to foster new insights and capacity.

KEY CONCEPTS: GLOBALISATION, GLOBAL HEALTH GOVERNANCE AND CORPORATIONS

This book grapples with four key concepts that have been the subject of intensely contested theorising and empirical analyses. For the purposes of this book, we focus on economic *globalisation*, by which the

> straightforward exchange between core and peripheral areas, based upon a broad division of labour, is being transformed into a highly complex, kaleidoscopic structure involving the fragmentation of many production processes and their geographical relocation on a global scale in ways which slice through national boundaries. (Dicken 1998, 2)

Since the 1990s, the restructuring of the world economy, encompassing both reterritorialisation and deterritorialisation (Scholte 2008), has intensified and extensified to embrace almost all societies and locales (Held et al. 1999).

Globalisation, *inter alia*, has led to a transformation of patterns of health and disease, and their broad determinants, on a transplanetary scale. This transition includes the territorial expansion of known health problems such as the spread of unhealthy lifestyles, as well as emergent risks that demonstrate new patterns of causation and outcome, such as antibiotic resistance and pandemic disease (Lee 2003). These *global health* dynamics suggest a certain 'levelling' of risks faced by all populations but, simultaneously, the creation of new health inequalities (Labonté and Schrecker 2007).

The advent of global health determinants and outcomes has spurred a proliferation of institutional arrangements commonly referred to as *global health governance* (GHG). Global governance per se has been the subject of intense scholarly scrutiny since the 1980s, characterised by the diffusion of authority from state-based institutions to new arrangements embracing both state and non-state actors (Rosenau and Czempiel 1992). In global health, the latter include corporations, civil society organisations (CSOs) and philanthropic organisations, which have come to play a substantial role in GHG (Biehl and Petryna 2013; Frenk and Moon 2013). Defined as a 'range of formal and informal institutional arrangements and processes operating among state and non-state actors that orient collective action on health issues which affect populations worldwide', GHG is not synonymous with formal government structures (Lee and Kamradt-Scott 2014). Nor is it singular: *governance* denotes an array of venues, institutions and processes in which power is contested and authority becomes fragmented and ephemeral.

In the context of intensified economic globalisation, and the search for effective global governance, this book focuses on the *corporation* (rather than the private sector or privatisation). Dating from the seventeenth century, the corporation has grown from 'relative obscurity to become the world's dominant economic institution' (Bakan 2004) in the early twenty-first century. In essence, a corporation is a legal entity acting for an association of individuals, created to exist and operate independently of its members. Corporations, bestowed with legal personhood, may enter into contracts, engage in transactions, exercise rights and responsibilities, and incur liabilities distinct from its members. While corporations operate in both the public and private spheres, this book is concerned with for-profit business corporations.

The unprecedented economic power of large corporations in the world economy is now widely recognised (Korten 2007). Power is also increasingly concentrated among fewer actors, with forty-three thousand transnational corporations controlling 80 percent of the world economy, and a 'super-entity' of 147 tightly knit companies controlling 40 percent of total wealth (Vitali, Glattfelder and Battiston 2011). Analyses of why and how this has occurred, however, have been 'deflected into wider debates about "globalisation" and related arguments about how the structures of global capitalism shape the capacities, resources, and even the ideologies of actors' (Bell 2012, 661). However, structural explanations have paid less attention to the precise dynamics of business power and, in particular, to corporations as actors shaping the world economy and other institutional arrangements (Fuchs and Lederer 2007). It is this dual relationship, between structure and agency, which forms a key starting point for the case studies in this book.

Another analytical contribution of this book is the dual importance given to both material and ideational power. The material power of a corporation is traditionally measured by tangible resources to pursue its business operations or further its interests, such as financial and other assets, intellectual property, goodwill and human capital. The capacity of corporations to bring together, and generate, material power on an unprecedented scale has led to present forms of economic globalisation in which they dominate. Equally important, however, is the role of ideational power. Carstensen (2015) identifies three forms of ideational power: (a) power through ideas (the capacity of actors to persuade other actors to accept and adopt their views of what they think and do); (b) power over ideas (the capacity of actors to dominate the meaning of ideas); and (c) power in ideas (the authority certain ideas enjoy in structuring thought at the expense of other ideas). As discussed in the concluding chapter of this book, corporate influence of GHG has derived from all three forms of ideational power, alongside material power.

STRUCTURE OF THE BOOK

As a collection of case studies seeking to broaden our understanding of corporations and GHG, through multidisciplinary perspectives and expanded concepts of corporate power, the structure of this book centres on three key themes. The case studies in part I examine the impacts of corporations on GHG through analyses of industries familiar to global health researchers (tobacco, pharmaceuticals and food), as well as those less familiar (garment manufacturing, lead smelting). Part II investigates the diverse ways that corporations influence GHG encompassing structural and agency power, as well as material and ideational power. Again, the case studies embrace a broad range of issue areas and institutional settings to demonstrate how corporations influence problem definition and identified solutions, which, in turn, shapes global health priority setting. Part III discusses strategies, challenges and possibilities for holding corporations to account for their impacts on global health and influence over GHG. These case studies offer important insights for ways in which to address the profound governance gaps opened up by the uncritical proliferation of institutional arrangements to strengthen collective action for global health. As readers are likely to note, however, there are significant and purposeful overlaps between these sections. For example, corporations' influence extends to the ways that public health problems and their solutions are constructed, and corporate influence itself is evident as another kind of public health harm in many of these chapters. Perhaps most importantly, as the conclusion explores in further depth, all of these cases offer lessons for how the corporate role in global health governance should be understood and contested.

REFERENCES

Bakan, Joel. 2004. *The Corporation*. New York: Penguin.

Bell, Stephen. 2012. 'The Power of Ideas: The Ideational Shaping of the Structural Power of Business'. *International Studies Quarterly* 56: 661–73. doi:10.1111/j.1468-2478.2012.00743.x.

Benson, Peter, and Stuart Kirsch. 2010. 'Capitalism and the Politics of Resignation'. *Current Anthropology* 51 (4): 459–86.

Biehl, João, and Ariana Petryna, eds. 2013. *When People Come First: Critical Studies in Global Health*. Princeton, NJ: Princeton University Press.

Brown, Theodore M., Marcos Cueto and Elizabeth Fee. 2006. 'The World Health Organization and the Transition from "International" to "Global" Public Health'. *American Journal of Public Health* 96 (1): 62–72.

Carstensen, Martin. 2015. 'Bringing Ideational Power into the Paradigm Approach: Critical Perspectives on Policy Paradigms in Theory and Practice'. In *Policy Paradigms in Theory and Practice*, edited by John Hogan and Michael Howlett, 295–314. Basingstoke, UK: Palgrave Macmillan.

Dicken, Peter. 1992. *Global Shift: The Internationalization of Economic Activity*. Berkeley, CA: University of California Press.

Frenk, Julio, and Suerie Moon. 2013. 'Governance Challenges in Global Health'. *New England Journal of Medicine* 368 (10): 936–42. doi:10.1056/NEJMra1109339.

Freudenberg N. 2014. *Lethal but Legal: Corporations, Consumption, and Protecting Public Health*. New York: Oxford University Press.

Fuchs, Doris, and Markus Lederer. 2007. 'The Power of Business'. *Business and Politics* 9 (3): 1–17. doi:10.2202/1469-3569.1214.

Held, David, Anthony McGrew, David Goldblatt and Jonathan Perraton. 1999. *Global Transformations*. London: Polity Press.

Kindig, David, and Erika Cheng. 2013. 'Even as Mortality Fell in Most U.S. Counties, Female Mortality Nonetheless Rose in 42.8 Percent of Counties from 1992 to 2006'. *Health Affairs* 32 (3): 451–58. doi: 10.1377/hlthaff.2011.0892.

Korten, David. 2001. *When Corporations Rule the World*, 2nd ed. San Francisco: Kumarian Press.

———. 2007. *The Great Turning: From Empire to Earth Community*. Bloomfield, CT: Berrett-Koehler Publishers.

Labonté, Ronald, and Ted Schrecker. 2007. 'Globalization and Social Determinants of Health: Introduction and Methodological Background (Part 1)'. *Globalization and Health* 3 (5). doi:10.1186/1744-8603-3-5.

Lee, Kelley. 2001. 'Globalisation—a New Agenda for Health?' In *International Cooperation in Health*, edited by Martin McKee, Paul Garner and Robin Stott, 14–30. London: Oxford University Press.

———. 2003. *Globalization and Health: An Introduction*. London: Palgrave Macmillan.

Lee, Kelley, and Adam Kamradt-Scott. 2014. 'The Multiple Meanings of Global Health Governance: A Call for Conceptual Clarity'. *Globalization and Health* 10 (28). doi:10.1186/1744-8603-10-28.

Richter, Judith. 2001. *Holding Corporations Accountable, Corporate Conduct, International Codes, and Citizen Action*. London: Zed Books.

Rosenau, James, and Ernst-Otto Czempiel. 1992. *Governance Without Government: Order and Change in World Politics*. Cambridge: Cambridge University Press.

Scholte, Jan Aart. 2008. 'Defining Globalisation'. *World Economy* 31 (11): 1471–502. doi:10.1111/j.1467-9701.2007.01019.x.

Schrecker, Ted, ed. 2012. *The Ashgate Research Companion to the Globalization of Health*. Burlington, VT: Ashgate.

Stuckler David, Martin McKee, Shah Ebrahim and Sanjay Basu. 2012. 'Manufacturing Epidemics: The Role of Global Producers in Increased Consumption of Unhealthy Commodities Including Processed Foods, Alcohol, and Tobacco'. *PLoS Medicine* 9 (6): e1001235. doi: 10.1371/journal.pmed.1001235.

Urban, Greg, ed. 2014. *Democracy, Citizenship, and Constitutionalism: Corporations and Citizenship*. Philadelphia: University of Pennsylvania Press.

Vitali, Stefania, James Glattfelder and Stefano Battiston. 2011. 'The Network of Global Corporate Control'. *PLoS One* 6 (10): e25995. doi: 10.1371/journal.pone.0025995.

Wiist, William H. 2010. *The Bottom Line or Public Health*. Oxford: Oxford University Press.

I

Impacts of Corporations on Global Health

TWO

Governing through Production

A Public-Private Partnership's Impacts and Dissolution in Lesotho's Garment Industry

Nora J. Kenworthy

A common critique of global health programs is that they are short-lived and vertically implemented, due to budget timelines and shifting global priorities (Pfeiffer and Nichter 2008; Biesma et al. 2009). This situation was exacerbated when donor funding plateaued following the 2008 financial crisis, and programs faced further threats to their longevity (IHME 2012). Against this backdrop, public-private partnerships (PPPs) in global health continue to gain popularity (Richter 2004) based on perceptions of greater sustainability, in part due to their private financing models (Buse and Harmer 2007). Yet few studies have examined the sustainability of PPPs, or the conditions under which corporate-led partnerships come to an end, and empirical research on the impacts of global health program closures is rare (Abramowitz 2015; Prince 2014; Qureshi 2015).

This chapter examines the closure of a successful PPP providing HIV services in Lesotho's garment industry, the Apparel Lesotho Alliance to Fight AIDS (ALAFA).[1] Rather than interrogate the internal micropolitics that may have contributed to its dissolution, this chapter asks what ALAFA's closure reveals about the political and moral governance of HIV programmes in Lesotho. The moment of program closure provides unique insight into PPPs' impacts on the governance of struggling health systems and the health of populations, beyond the direct provision of services. To fully understand PPPs' political impacts, we must examine the broader health and social systems in which they are embedded. This chapter argues that, rather than simply offering technical solutions or convenient collaborations, PPPs produce specific and varying health outcomes in populations, and manufacture certain notions of responsibility for population health.

Drawing on ethnographic data gathered intermittently over six years, this chapter describes the conditions under which ALAFA provided care to the garment industry's heavily HIV-affected workforce. It then discusses ALAFA's closure, drawing on garment factory workers' perspectives. Findings suggest that PPPs are directly involved in the consumerisation of health and disease, producing specific kinds of health in a transnational industry reliant on the marketing of clothing produced by HIV-affected workers. The chapter concludes by discussing how PPPs have altered the moral and practical politics that underlie Lesotho's urban health system.

BACKGROUND

The debate on PPPs is highly polarised. A prominent form of corporate involvement in global health governance (GHG), PPPs vary greatly, and empirical research on their forms, purposes and impacts remains limited (Brada 2011; Ramiah and Reich 2005). Context-specific and data-rich ethnographic research can provide insight into the complicated and productive 'frictions' (Tsing 2004) of partnerships. Following the work of Rajak (2011a), this chapter focuses on PPPs as a driving force behind moral and ethical shifts within local and transnational governance systems. As Rajak (2011a, 13) argues with regard to Corporate Social Responsibility (CSR), the power of corporations' ethical engagements exists in the way these efforts provide 'them with a moral mechanism through which their authority is extended over the social order'.

PPPs are a popular institutional arrangement for the management of CSR activities, though CSR can also encompass charitable donations and more ad-hoc contributions by corporations to specific causes. PPPs offer corporations an institutional structure for CSR activities that privileges the roles and voices of private stakeholders and, like CSR, creates a moral governance regarding whether, how and to whom entitlements will be granted. This form of GHG is enacted at transnational and national levels, but also individually, changing citizens' expectations of the health system and their rights. It intersects with Foucault's theories of governmentality, wherein the modern state (and, in this case, its partners) wields a power that extends into social and personal realms, influencing individual dispositions and behaviours (Foucault 2008). This chapter is less concerned with how PPPs impact the 'conduct of conduct' (Foucault

1994, 237), and instead asks how they influence a country's collective understanding of the health system and the rights of citizens.

Anthropologists studying HIV and global health initiatives have noted the ways that systems of care in low-income settings are increasingly 'projectified', composed of 'archipelagos' of services (Whyte et al. 2013; Geissler 2014). Care 'landscapes' shift constantly as projects arrive and depart; patients must expertly navigate temporal and spatial geographies where care is partial and insecure. While scholarship primarily focuses on NGOs as producing 'projectified' care, PPPs are increasingly common within global health landscapes (Whyte et al. 2013). Proponents argue that they can efficiently fill gaps in existing health systems, yet claims of longevity and sustainability are rarely interrogated (Swidler and Watkins 2009). PPPs can also partition care, implementing parallel systems (Brada 2011; Buse and Harmer 2007). A single case study cannot provide a definitive verdict regarding PPP impacts, but this analysis demonstrates the temporal fragilities and political impacts of one such arrangement.

This chapter combines the two framing concepts of projectified landscapes and PPPs as a form of moral governance to study ALAFA as embedded within, and altering, a 'moral landscape' of care in Lesotho (Fassin 2012; Livingston 2005). This conceptual framework embraces the 'local moral worlds' (Kleinman and Kleinman 1997, 7) of patients seeking treatment, and the normative power of PPPs at local, national and transnational levels. Notably, even when services are no longer provided, a program's normative residues remain, influencing social mores about who should be responsible for care, and which entitlements are deserved. These are an important, though frequently overlooked, form of GHG.

METHODS

Drawing on theories and methods from medical anthropology, this chapter presents data from a larger research project on the political impacts of HIV programming in Lesotho. This project has involved ethnographic research in Lesotho since 2008, including: analysis of primary and secondary sources regarding the industry and ALAFA (from 2008 to the present); in-depth, semi-structured interviews with more than seventy-five factory workers, union leaders, factory managers, clinic and program staff, factory inspectors and HIV peer educators (from 2010 to 2011); participant observation at a factory, referred to here as New Century to protect workers' identities (2010–2011); and three focus group discussions with approximately thirty workers from other factories (2011). In 2014, follow-up research was conducted to understand how ALAFA's closing impacted workers' access to care and treatment services. All primary data was transcribed and analysed using open-ended coding.

FINDINGS

PPPs and the Moral Landscapes of Care in Lesotho

Lesotho is a landlocked country of 1.8 million people, bordered on all sides by South Africa. Colonialism, labour migration and relations with South Africa have heavily impacted Lesotho's economy and health (Ferguson 2006; Murray 1981). Its unremittingly high HIV prevalence—Lesotho recently surpassed Botswana to claim the world's second-highest adult HIV prevalence—reflects persistent social inequities (National AIDS Commission 2011). HIV is largely responsible for dramatic declines in adult life expectancy, from sixty-one years in 1990 to forty-nine years in 2015 (WHO 2015), but a range of other diseases also contribute heavily to mortality figures (IHME 2013).

Lesotho's health system is composed of a network of hospitals, health centres and rural health posts. The Christian Health Association of Lesotho (CHAL), under the auspices of the Ministry of Health and Social Welfare (MOHSW), runs 38 percent of facilities. Most of the remainder are run directly by the MOHSW (Government of Lesotho [GoL] 2013). The abolition of user fees for basic services in 2008 increased uptake of primary health care (GoL 2013). By 2009, Lesotho transitioned its HIV care and treatment programs to a nurse-led, clinic-based model, enabling antiretroviral therapy (ART) to be offered in all clinics. Nevertheless, persistently high and at times increasing rates of maternal, child, and infant mortality have underscored problems of access and service delivery in the primary health system during the past decade (GoL 2013; MOHSW 2015).

Two PPPs distinguish Lesotho's urban health system. ALAFA, established in 2006, provides HIV care, treatment, and prevention services to workers in Lesotho's garment industry, the country's largest private-sector employer. The garment sector employs between thirty-five thousand and fifty thousand workers, nearly 50 percent of the formally employed workforce in the country (International Labour Office 2009). More than 80 percent of workers are women. As will be described below, ALAFA is uniquely embedded in this industry, and central to new efforts to make the garment sector production 'ethical'.

In 2011, Queen 'Mamohato Memorial Hospital, a new PPP and Lesotho's only tertiary care facility, was opened.[2] The International Finance Corporation helped establish 'Mamohato Hospital to replace the aging and under-resourced Queen Elizabeth II Hospital; it is the first public hospital in a low-income country to be financed and run through a PPP. Since opening, 'Mamohato has been plagued by inefficiencies, costing nearly three times a year more than the hospital it replaced, yet failing to provide essential services to many patients (Oxfam 2014; Webster 2015). Even with minimal service delivery, 'Mamohato Hospital now monopolises more than half of Lesotho's health budget (Oxfam 2014). It promises enormous dividends to initial investors, some of whom are reportedly the ministerial staff responsible for approving the project contract. While this chapter focuses primarily on ALAFA, and the two PPPs are very different, both partnerships shape the landscape of care in urban Lesotho.

As a PPP, ALAFA's services, and its very existence, are shaped by the history and contemporary politics of the industry in which it is embedded. Taiwanese, Chinese and South African factory owners began moving garment manufacturing to Lesotho in the 1980s, drawn by preferential trade conditions and a cheap but flexible workforce. The U.S. African Growth and Opportunities Act (AGOA), introduced in 2000, gave preferential trade deals to manufacturers on the continent and, as Seidman (2009, 583) notes, 'reimagined [trade] as a form of development aid', allowing U.S. companies to 'help' Africa, while sourcing cheap goods from the continent with minimal oversight.

Lesotho's industry remained vulnerable to competition from other countries despite AGOA (Bennet 2006) and factory owners argued that extraordinarily high HIV prevalence (40 percent), among the largely female factory workforce, undermined productivity. Turnover due to illness and death was continual, and workers frequently missed work to visit public clinics (ALAFA 2010). In 2006, a feasibility study to assess the practicality of HIV prevention and treatment services within the factories returned promising results (Colvin et al. 2006). With this evidence, trade partners, the World Bank and the International Labour Organisation (ILO) proposed that Lesotho begin to market itself as a new 'ethical' production site for western, and mostly U.S., clothing labels (Seidman 2009). This marketing strategy was particularly appealing to U.S. brands like Gap that were investing heavily in CSR projects in the hopes of resuscitating brands tarnished by labour scandals.

With this shift towards ethical marketing, Lesotho signed additional ILO conventions,[3] and factories pledged to adhere to U.S. buyer 'codes of conduct', with oversight largely reliant on voluntary standards and internal auditing (Seidman 2009). In many cases, factories still cut corners and violated safety regulations, resulting in significant and widespread health hazards. As experts predicted (Seidman 2009), and as previous research for this project documented (Kenworthy 2014), the new 'ethical' standards created an environment in which workplace violations were routine but silenced. Factories, and the industry as a whole, enacted a 'theatre of virtue' (Rajak 2011b) in which workers, labour unions and factory management colluded in maintaining an image of factory compliance and ethical practice to protect jobs.

This ethical theatre was rooted in an almost-myopic focus on addressing HIV within the factories. In 2006, the first pilot program for providing HIV prevention and treatment services to factory workers was launched at New Century Factory, under the aegis of ALAFA. Gap announced that its Product(RED) line, created in partnership with Bono's (RED) initiative (with 50 percent of proceeds donated to the Global Fund to Fight AIDS, Tuberculosis and Malaria [GFATM]), would be produced at New Century. Bono helped launch ALAFA, along with the CEO of the GFATM and other dignitaries. Gap provided initial funding for the pilot program, and ALAFA quickly became a centrepiece of its global CSR efforts.

ALAFA itself was emblematic of a new kind of PPP. Formed as a cooperative initiative between U.S. clothing brands, garment factory owners, government ministries and labour representatives, ALAFA maintained its own staff and board, but managed programs in the factories through a diverse set of partnerships and contributions. ARVs were sourced from the MOHSW and provided on-site in factories by private doctors, hired to avoid depleting human resources from the public system. Factories provided space for a clinic and salaries for some support staff. ALAFA paid doctors, peer educators and program staff out of grants received from U.S. corporations and donor agencies. Partnerships with other organisations like Population Services International (PSI), supported the provision of condoms and prevention awareness activities in the factories. As ALAFA expanded, it was able to leverage partnerships to encourage factories to participate in care and treatment services, and promoted workplace policies preventing discrimination against workers living with HIV. Consequently, ALAFA gained international recognition as a successful CSR initiative (ALAFA 2015). Among workers, ALAFA was remarkably popular, offering a high level of care that allowed them to maintain their jobs and miss less work when seeking care. Ultimately, treatment was provided to around 5,800 workers, and prevention to thousands more, each year (ALAFA 2015).

ALAFA linked provision of HIV treatment with the marketing of an 'ethical' country brand, the survival of a fragile transnational market, and the provision of care through a complex web of partnerships. This meant that workers navigated a complex moral, economic and therapeutic geography as they sought out HIV services. The provision of those services was possible because it satisfied two economic, rather than moral, principles: first, factories embraced treatment because it promised to improve worker productivity; second, treatment enabled factories to market products made by a heavily HIV-affected workforce at a premium. These conditions enabled a uniquely attractive form of humanitarian marketing and capitalism. In this way, ALAFA represented an unprecedented consumerisation of disease, linking humanitarian consumers in U.S. markets to diseased workforces in Lesotho. Many would argue that ALAFA was an innovative and, for workers, fortunate intervention that harnessed divergent interests among consumers, manufacturers, and workers toward a common goal. Yet, as argued elsewhere, it also equated industry ethics and labour rights with the provision of a limited program of treatment (Kenworthy 2014). By providing a circumscribed, commodified form of care that relied on workers maintaining jobs in an unsafe industry, the program relieved factories and clothing corporations of a broader responsibility to protect workers' welfare.

Sustainability and Program Closures

ALAFA's reliance on external funding made it vulnerable to shifts in global health aid after 2008. When a key grant from Department for International Development (DFID) ended in 2011, the European Union offered an eleventh-hour grant to continue services, with the explicit intention of building 'local funding sustainability' (ALAFA 2015). ALAFA considered diverse fiscal arrangements for continuing services, including contributions from worker salaries and support from other donors. In subsequent years, however, *sustainability* came to mean that the Lesotho government, specifically the MOHSW, would take on the program. In some ways, this made sense: the MOHSW already provided ARVs to ALAFA and managed HIV care in the public sector. But many local onlookers, including some ALAFA staff, insisted that *sustainability* meant that partnerships and donor commitments, once forged, should be upheld, rather than cut short by budget shortfalls and shifting priorities. Despite lengthy negotiations between ALAFA and the government, a new agreement never materialised. Political instabilities and funding shortfalls at the time likely contributed to government resistance to extending ALAFA's services, but no clear explanation was offered.

By October 2014, ALAFA had officially terminated programs, and workers had spent several months struggling to access care and avoid disruptions in their treatment. The moral impacts of ALAFA's closure are best understood through the perspectives of workers trying to maintain access to care. The remainder of this section focuses on those perspectives before turning to a discussion of how they relate to larger shifts in the moral landscape of care and the corporate governance of health in Lesotho.

As it ceased operations, ALAFA crafted painstaking plans for the transition of services, and posted detailed letters on clinic walls describing where workers could access services after closure. Nevertheless, access to care was uneven and unpredictable. One former employee reported that ALAFA's departure 'left management [in the factories] to negotiate with doctors and figure [things] out' on their own. Some factories opted to pay doctors to continue providing services; however most factories (including New Century) simply passed costs on to workers, deducting doctors' fees from their pay. Workers were encouraged to continue coming to factory clinics rather than travel to public clinics, which could result in absences and decreased productivity.

Nonetheless, most workers wanted to be transferred to local public clinics, because they could not afford doctors' fees. Those seeking transfers had to secure letters from their former doctors, and present them at local clinics. Because the vast majority of factories in Lesotho are located in two urban areas, local clinics were quickly overrun. 'Patients were sent out to other clinics, transferred, and some were accepted, but some were not', a factory nurse told me. 'It gave us such a headache', a worker commented. While it is difficult to accurately gauge the numbers of workers turned away from public clinics, New Century and other factories were rife with rumours of workers unable to get into clinics and falling ill. Though some of these stories likely reflected anticipatory fears, many clinics in the area were genuinely struggling under patient loads. Some of the increased pressure on clinics was due to difficulties accessing services at 'Mamohato Hospital. Service delivery problems became so acute in 2014 that the abandoned hospital that 'Mamohato replaced, Queen Elizabeth II Hospital, reopened as an HIV and maternal health facility to fill gaps in care for urban residents. Yet even these measures could not adequately meet the needs of an unexpected influx of thousands of patients.

Facing health system barriers, workers travelled further to find services. 'Some of us asked for transfers but were rejected, including myself. . . . We were told that the clinics were full', Lebohang reported. 'I even tried to go to Ramabanta [nearly 70 kilometres away], but the transport was too heavy [expensive]'. Going to public clinics meant lost wages and the additional cost of transport. Though workers were entitled to sick leave with a signed letter from a health care provider, managers frequently denied sick leave requests. 'The firm [factory] just gives us time to go and take our pills from this [factory] clinic. If we go outside [to another clinic], we are not paid. The doctors have to come here', one worker noted. Another reported that New Century was pulling out 'much more from my pay cheque than I earn in a day' when she missed work to go to the clinic: 'When the ALAFA services stopped, I had to go out to get services from the clinic. But the factories were deducting too much from our pay cheques for going out, so I stopped my treatment for a month. . . . We were just told to go to [the factory doctor], but they didn't tell us why'. Factories carefully policed workers' therapeutic itineraries in the wake of ALAFA's closing, punitively incentivising workers to continue seeking treatment from the factory clinics, in order to ensure productivity remained high.

While continuity of care might be considered the best possible outcome in the wake of ALAFA's closing, workers' wages were so low that doctors' fees presented significant barriers. 'It was terrible, it was not good at all. It was so hard for the patients to pay the doctors, because they are earning nothing as it is', one factory nurse reported. Many workers relied on self-rationing. 'I'm not able to pay', a worker stated. 'I went there [to the doctor] but I didn't even let him draw blood [for routine tests]. . . . People with HIV are probably going to die'. Many interviewees noted that they had no choice but to pay for visits, though they did not know how long they could continue incurring loans and cutting out basic necessities.

ALAFA's closure revealed tensions over duties and responsibilities for worker welfare. At a clinical level, the shift from a PPP to privatised services altered the quality of care, even when the very same clinicians provided it. At an industry level, closures revealed fissures in the existing fabric of care, as HIV treatment remained primary, and occupational health services were neglected. Nationally, as the fragile balance ALAFA had struck between partners evaporated, it became clear that the industry would bear no lasting responsibility for HIV programs, though it had benefitted from them the most. While the closure made many workers nostalgic for the care they had once received, ALAFA had altered the governance of care in ways that worsened the crisis. Patients struggled to access the public system because they were no longer considered the 'responsibility' of the public sector; through the PPP, they lost some of the recognition as rights-bearing citizens they had once merited from Lesotho's health system. Because it was arranged as a PPP, ALAFA shifted responsibility for worker welfare out of the direct realm of garment industry representatives; thus, when it closed, these same industry actors felt a limited responsibility to continue supporting care. These changes revealed the broader impacts of the PPP on the governance of worker health and the moral landscapes of care. The narrative of one worker at New Century elaborates some of these tensions.

Puleng

Puleng, a woman in her mid-thirties, received HIV treatment through ALAFA for three years while working at New Century. She was deeply concerned about ALAFA's closure, stating that 'some' workers had already 'passed away . . . [because] they couldn't afford to pay for services. When they went to the government clinics, they were not received very nicely'. She explained that patients coming from ALAFA frequently faced discrimination from clinic nurses. Nurses resented not only the influx of patients, but also their former access to private physicians, whose higher salaries and capitalist approaches to care engendered suspicion. 'The nurses told us that the private doctors didn't teach us how to take our medicines, so they don't like people coming from [them]. They wanted us to go through the patient training [before getting ARVs] and they said that people [like us] don't know how to take ARVs'. Training and education sessions are frequently used as an informal means of sorting and triaging patients, selecting those most likely to be successful with adherence, given treatment scarcity (Nguyen 2010). But Puleng admitted that the training for factory workers was more limited, especially once ALAFA closed. 'The private doctors don't care about educating patients because it costs [them] money. They really could have done better with that . . . and once ALAFA left, the doctors just stopped caring about the patients entirely'.

Puleng decided to continue paying her private doctor after being turned away from a few public clinics. But she felt that the care was rushed, and poorly overseen. She experienced two months of 'high blood [pressure]' recorded by the nurse at the factory clinic, but her doctor did nothing to treat it. Turned away from the public clinic for her presumed lack of knowledge, Puleng confidently monitored her own hypertension, identified it as a serious but common co-morbidity, and sought out treatment. 'I knew it was dangerous, and I was feeling very sick. So I tried to go elsewhere'. She eventually paid to see another doctor in Maseru in order to obtain high blood pressure medications, thus continuing two separate but interrelated fee-for-service treatment regimens.

Puleng's account reveals the increasing distrust with which ALAFA's former doctors were held. An HIV counsellor within the factories corroborated this impression, stating that doctors were now unregulated, and the care uneven. Two doctors served patients at New Century: one charged for routine tests like CD4 counts in addition to monthly visits; the other did not. They capitalised on a significant gap in governance: 'Now that ALAFA is gone, the doctors are just doing what they like. There is no oversight. We need standards to say who should pay what', she insisted. Without funding from ALAFA, supplemental services and goods that helped to support workers in adhering to treatment—including formula for the infants of workers living with HIV—were disappearing. Even under ALAFA, primary care services for conditions like diabetes and hypertension did not receive the same support that HIV services did. Though many workers attributed their hypertension to stressful work conditions, Puleng knew her blood pressure would merit more attention as a side effect of treatment, not working conditions. Thus, the services that remained after ALAFA's closure retained an air of unevenness, untrustworthiness, and partiality. Reduced to the most rudimentary, biomedical routines of HIV treatment, ALAFA's doctors came to be seen as crudely capitalistic in their care. Puleng's story reflects the broader consumerisation of care in urban Lesotho, which required patients to be more independent and educated, even as the public sector continued to view them with distrust due to the suboptimal care they were receiving.

Privatisation and the Production of Health

Puleng's experience underscores the ways that PPPs are producing health for garment workers in Lesotho, and also altering broader health systems. Much of this production involves what has been called, in other contexts, 'boundary-work', institutional labours to define, police and reinforce boundaries of legitimacy and belonging (Gieryn 1983). Here, boundary work is most evident in the (mis-)recognition of health problems and hazards. Despite the provision of services for HIV, tuberculosis and reproductive health, ALAFA never succeeded in convincing the industry to tackle other health issues, let alone occupational health and safety concerns. Its fragile and negotiated position as a PPP made it difficult to finance the expansion of services, or to acknowledge the full extent of occupational harms (Kenworthy, 2014). Many factories directly opposed such efforts, worried that screening for health issues might inadvertently document the extent and impact of occupational hazards. Under ALAFA, HIV therapeutics produced workers' productivity, but also produced ideas about worker health in which HIV was primary and occupational hazards became invisible.

Lesotho's garment workers, like many Africans, routinely move among multiple private, public and traditional health care providers in attempting to get health problems recognised and treated. But PPPs have the power to considerably alter those therapeutic itineraries. The influx of patients into the public sector following ALAFA's closure intersected with 'Mamohato Hospital's failures, such that both PPPs created additional gaps in workers' health care. Given workers' claims that they were skipping routine tests, hoarding pills, and simply being turned away from care, it is likely that the increasingly privatised and fractured system of care provided fertile conditions for the emergence of treatment resistance, and the resurgence of viral loads in patient bodies.[4] Thus, it seems possible, if not likely, that the closure of HIV treatment programs will impact population health beyond those populations directly served by such programs, even when extensive plans are made for patients' care transitions.

In late 2014, a partial solution to the gaps in HIV care emerged from an unlikely source. The private doctors formerly employed by ALAFA approached the MOHSW, and successfully convinced ministry officials to fund rudimentary free HIV treatment for workers. Where ALAFA's nearly two-year-long efforts to negotiate with the government had failed, a small number of private doctors, seeking to redress a significant source of revenue that was lost when ALAFA closed, prevailed. The responsiveness of Lesotho's government officials to the requests of private actors thus enabled not only the launch of 'Mamohato Hospital, but also the successful resuscitation of HIV treatment within the factories.[5] On the one hand, this compromise offered welcome support for programs, and indicated that the government was willing to consider factory workers as at least partially within its purview of responsibility; on the other hand, services remained circumscribed, limited to HIV treatment provision. In addition, the 'private' partners of the initial partnership—factories, clothing brands, and even private physicians—could be said to have gained the upper hand, benefitting from treatment availability and remaining immune from financial or moral responsibility, while Lesotho's cash-strapped government shouldered the bulk of the expense of treatment, funnelling fees to private physicians instead of the public health system. Ironically, this turn of events also accomplished the kind of 'sustainability' the PPP had hoped for in the first place, but not the kind garment workers imagined to be fairest. While workers also wanted fair access to health care beyond HIV treatment and broader protections from workplace hazards, the PPP had changed the moral landscape for these aspects of care by prioritising HIV treatment above all else, and marketing the workforce as HIV-infected and ART-treated. Consequently, other health concerns became less visible.

CONCLUSION

PPPs can pose a direct challenge to health system strengthening through public-sector institutions as envisioned in the 1978 Declaration of Alma Ata, which called for governments and the world community to protect and promote the health of all people through rights-based, equitable primary health care (WHO 1978). Substantial evidence demonstrates that PPPs and other privatisation efforts transform citizens into consumers within increasingly fractured systems of care (Birn 2013; Pfeiffer 2004; Richter 2004). Despite abundant critiques of PPPs, detailed ethnographic accounts of how specific partnerships operate at the local level and impact care are relatively scarce (Brada 2011). As this chapter describes, studies of PPPs in context offer insight into the socio-political legacies of global health privatisation and consumerisation. PPPs can fill gaps in health care in under-resourced health systems, albeit with varying success (Oxfam 2014). They can also alter perceptions of obligations and entitlements in global health, even when they cease to provide care.

This analysis suggests that rather than regard corporations simply as entities that threaten or undermine the welfare of populations, it may be more useful to examine them as institutions that are deeply engaged in the production of certain ideas about health, responsibility and belonging. Their discursive and pragmatic efforts constitute 'boundary work' that polices the borders of what constitutes health and illness. Their engagement in health provision is also producing new biological realities (productive bodies, or emergent drug resistance) within complicated global health systems. In these new institutional arrangements, corporations must be recognised as manufacturers of new biological, political and moral worlds.

FUNDING

This material is based on work supported by the National Science Foundation under Grant No. 1024097, the American Association of University Women, and the U.S. Fulbright/IIE program. Sabina Monts'i, Ponts'o Tseounyane and Thabo Liphoto assisted with translation. Findings, opinions and errors are solely my own.

NOTES

1. It is worth noting that ALAFA's services had more longevity than other global health initiatives.
2. 'Mamohato Hospital is frequently referred to as 'Tsepong' hospital in Maseru, after the name of private entity set up to run the hospital, a consortium led by South African private health care giant Netcare.
3. See Seidman (2009) for additional details. As Seidman notes (2009, 587), 'Far too many member states have ratified ILO conventions without ensuring that labour laws are implemented'.
4. Nguyen (2010) notes how the 'triage' politics HIV treatment prior to widespread access to ART in the public health system in West Africa likely encouraged rampant treatment resistance. Few studies, however, have examined whether and to what extent treatment resistance emerges as ART programs are shuttered or transitioned to other institutions.
5. The familiarity between ALAFA's private physicians and government officials likely helped in both cases. One of ALAFA's former doctors was named the new minister of health just months after this negotiation.

REFERENCES

Abramowitz, Sharon. 2015. 'What Happens When Médecins Sans Frontières Leaves? Humanitarian Departure and Medical Sovereignty in Postconflict Liberia'. In *Medical Humanitarianism: Ethnographies of Practice,* edited by Sharon Abramowitz and Catherine Panter-Brick, 137–54. Philadelphia: University of Pennsylvania Press.
ALAFA. 2010. *ALAFA: An Industry Model for Fighting HIV/AIDS and TB.* Maseru.
———. 2015. *ALAFA: End of Project Report 2006-2014.* Maseru.
Bennet, Mark. 2006. 'Lesotho's Export Textiles & Garment Industry'. In *The Future of the Textile and Clothing Industry in Sub-Saharan Africa,* edited by Herbert Jauch and Rudolf Traub-Merz, 165–77. Bonn: Friedrich-Ebert-Stiftung.
Biesma, Regien G., Ruairí Brugha, Andrew Harmer, Aisling Walsh, Neil Spicer and Gill Walt. 2009. 'The Effects of Global Health Initiatives on Country Health Systems: A Review of the Evidence from HIV/AIDS Control'. *Health Policy and Planning* 24 (4): 239–52.
Birn, Anne-Emanuelle. 2013. 'Philanthrocapitalism, Past and Present: The Rockefeller Foundation, the Gates Foundation, and the Setting(s) of the International/Global Health Agenda'. *Hypothesis* 10 (1).
Brada, Betsey. 2011. '"Not Here": Making the Spaces and Subjects of "Global Health" in Botswana'. *Culture, Medicine and Psychiatry* 35 (2): 285–312.
Buse, Kent, and Andrew M. Harmer. 2007. 'Seven Habits of Highly Effective Global Public-Private Health Partnerships: Practice and Potential'. *Social Science & Medicine* 64 (2): 259–71.
Colvin, Mark, Genieve Lemmon and Julian Naidoo. 2006. 'The Private Sector Response to HIV and AIDS in Lesotho'. London: ALAFA/ComMark Trust.

Fassin, Didier. 2012. *Humanitarian Reason: A Moral History of the Present.* Berkeley: University of California Press.

Ferguson, James. 2006. *Global Shadows: Africa in the Neoliberal World Order.* Durham, NC: Duke University Press.

Foucault, Michel. 1994. *Dits et écrits IV.* Paris: Gallimard.

———. 2008. *The Birth of Biopolitics: Lectures at the College De France, 1978-79.* New York: Picador.

Geissler, Wenzel P. 2014. 'The Archipelago of Public Health: Comments on the Landscape of Medical Research in Twenty-First-Century Africa'. In *Making and Unmaking Public Health in Africa: Ethnographic and Historical Perspectives,* edited by Ruth Prince and Rebevva Marsland, 231–56. Athens: Ohio University Press.

Gieryn, Thomas F. 1983. 'Boundary-Work and the Demarcation of Science from Non-Science: Strains and Interests in Professional Ideologies of Scientists'. *American Sociological Review* 48 (6): 781–95.

Government of Lesotho. 2013. *Health Sector Strategic Plan 2012/13-2016/17.* Maseru.

Institute for Health Metrics and Evaluation (IHME). 2012. *Financing Global Health 2012: The End of the Golden Age?* Seattle.

———. 2013. *GBD Profile: Lesotho.* Seattle.

International Labour Office. 2009. *Decent Work Country Programme: Lesotho.* Geneva.

Kenworthy, Nora J. 2014. 'A Manufactu(RED) Ethics: Labor, HIV, and the Body in Lesotho's "Sweat-Free" Garment Industry'. *Medical Anthropology Quarterly* 28 (4): 459–79.

Kleinman, Arthur, and Joan Kleinman. 1997. 'The Appeal of Experience; the Dismay of Images: Cultural Appropriations of Suffering in Our Times'. In *Social Suffering,* edited by Arthur Kleinman, Veena Das and Margaret Lock. Berkeley: University of California Press.

Livingston, Julie. 2005. *Debility and the Moral Imagination in Botswana.* Bloomington: Indiana University Press.

Ministry of Health and Social Welfare (MOHSW). 2015. *Demographic and Health Survey 2014: Key Indicators Report.* Maseru.

Murray, Colin. 1981. *Families Divided: The Impact of Migrant Labour in Lesotho.* Cambridge: Cambridge University Press.

National AIDS Commission. 2011. National HIV and AIDS strategic plan 2011/12-2015/16. Maseru.

Nguyen, Vinh-Kim. 2010. *The Republic of Therapy: Triage and Sovereignty in West Africa's Time of AIDS.* Durham, NC: Duke University Press.

Oxfam. 2014, April 7. 'A Dangerous Diversion: Will the IFC's Flagship Health PPP Bankrupt Lesotho's Ministry of Health?' *Oxfam Briefing Note.* Accessed April 21, 2014. http://oxf.am/Zf6P.

Pfeiffer, James. 2004. 'Condom Social Marketing, Pentecostalism, and Structural Adjustment in Mozambique: A Clash of AIDS Prevention Messages'. *Medical Anthropology Quarterly* 18 (1): 77–103.

Pfeiffer, James, and Mark Nichter. 2008. 'What Can Critical Medical Anthropology Contribute to Global Health?' *Medical Anthropology Quarterly* 22 (4): 410–15.

Prince, Ruth. 2014. 'Navigating "Global Health" in an East African City'. In *Making and Unmaking Public Health in Africa: Ethnographic and Historical Perspectives,* edited by Ruth Prince and Rebevva Marsland, 208–30. Athens: Ohio University Press.

Qureshi, Ayaz. 2015. 'AIDS Activism in Pakistan: Diminishing Funds, Evasive State'. *Development and Change* 46 (2): 320–38.

Rajak, Dinah. 2011a. *In Good Company: An Anatomy of Corporate Social Responsibility.* Redwood City, CA: Stanford University Press.

———. 2011b. 'Theatres of Virtue: Collaboration, Consensus, and the Social Life of Corporate Social Responsibility'. *Focaal* 2011 (60): 9–20.

Ramiah, Ilavenil, and Michael R. Reich. 2005. 'Public-Private Partnerships and Antiretroviral Drugs for HIV/AIDS: Lessons from Botswana'. *Health Affairs* 24 (2): 545–51.

Richter, Judith. 2004. 'Public–Private Partnerships for Health: A Trend with No Alternatives?' *Development* 47 (2): 43–48.

Seidman, Gay W. 2009. 'Labouring under an Illusion? Lesotho's "Sweat-Free" Label'. *Third World Quarterly* 30 (3): 581–98.

Swidler, Ann, and Susan Cotts Watkins. 2009. '"Teach a Man to Fish": The Doctrine of Sustainability and Its Effects on Three Strata of Malawian Society'. *World Development* 37 (7): 1182–96.

Tsing, Anna Lowenhaupt. 2004. *Friction: An Ethnography of Global Connection*. Princeton, NJ: Princeton University Press.

Webster, Paul C. 2015. 'Lesotho's Controversial Public-Private Partnership Project'. *The Lancet* 386: 1929–31.

Whyte, Susan Reynolds, Michael Whyte, Lotte Meinert and Jenipher Twebaze. 2013. 'Belonging in Uganda's Projectified Landscape of AIDS Care'. In *When People Come First: Critical Studies in Global Health*, edited by João Biehl and Adriana Petryna, 140–65. Princeton, NJ: Princeton University Press.

World Health Organization. 1978, September 6–12. Declaration of Alma-Ata: International Conference on Primary Health Care, Alma-Ata, USSR. www.who.int/hpr/NPH/docs/declaration_almaata.pdf.

World Health Organization. 2015. *World Health Statistics 2015*. Geneva.

THREE

Medicalisation and Commodification of Smoking Cessation

The Role of Industry Actors in Shaping Health Policy

Ross MacKenzie and Benjamin Hawkins

Smoking remains the leading preventable cause of death worldwide, and is predicted to claim an estimated 1 billion lives during this century (World Health Organization [WHO] 2013). With almost 1 billion existing smokers in 2015, and 30 million new smokers annually (Giovino et al. 2012), cessation remains a critical public health priority. Almost 70 percent of smokers wish to quit (WHO 2013) and significant funding has been invested in cessation research and promotion. However, long-term success rates remain modest, with 80–95 percent of those who give up relapsing within twelve months of quitting (Hendershot et al. 2011; Lee and Kahende 2007). It is important to note, however, that while success *rates* of quit attempts remain unremarkable, the *aggregate number* of ex-smokers nonetheless continues to rise so that in some countries, including the United States (U.S. Department of Health 2014), United Kingdom (Office for National Statistics 2013) and Australia (Scollo and Winstanley 2015), former smokers now outnumber current smokers.

Cessation methods are categorised as either assisted or unassisted. *Assisted* cessation includes use of prescribed or non-prescribed pharmaceutical interventions, such as nicotine replacement therapy (NRT) in the form of patches, gum or sprays; medication such as varenicline and bupropion; individual or group counselling; calling a quitline; use of self-help materials; or natural or alternative therapies (Smith, Chapman and Dunlop 2013). *Unassisted* refers to quit attempts made without recourse to

27

these devices and services.[1] Historically, most ex-smokers have quit without assistance, yet policy and practice are dominated by an emphasis on pharmaceutical intervention, primarily NRT. The recent emergence of electronic cigarettes (e-cigarettes) and their promotion as an alternative to smoking has added a new dimension to cessation debates, particularly in countries where they now occupy dominant market positions (Milenkovic 2014). While some users and advocates consider e-cigarettes not as a method of medicalised cessation, but as consumer products, policy debates have largely been framed in terms of their role as substitutes for conventional cigarettes, and as a means of 'harm reduction' for smokers who cannot (or will not) quit (Rodu and Godshall 2006). The limited, albeit rapidly expanding, literature on e-cigarettes has sought to address questions about the effects and potential harms of e-cigarette use (McNeill et al. 2015; Grana et al. 2014).

In this chapter, we argue that pharmaceutical corporations that manufacture NRT and other cessation aids have, in recent decades, successfully shaped the discourse around how smokers quit. As a result, smoking cessation has become both medicalised and commodified. That is, it has become defined as a treatable medical condition for which manufactured remedies are available for purchase. The framing of e-cigarettes as harm-reduction products for current smokers is a further example of commodification. This is particularly relevant to transnational tobacco corporations (TTCs), which now own many of the leading e-cigarette brands, which serves to offset declines in consumption of traditional tobacco products.

Based on their respective products, pharmaceutical and tobacco corporations are seeking to shape the changing cessation landscape in ways that further their particular commercial interests, and this is likely to pit them against each other in efforts to influence policy. There is also the potential for conflicts of interest through the involvement of these industries in the policy-making process, which could serve to undermine public health. This is especially true if governments engage with tobacco corporations, even in their capacity as e-cigarette producers, and potentially significant implications exist for compliance with Article 5.3 of the Framework Convention on Tobacco Control (FCTC), which states that public health bodies and policy must be protected from the vested interests and influence of the tobacco industry.

METHODS

This chapter undertakes a narrative review (Green et al. 2006) of peer-reviewed articles, systematic reviews, market analyses, reports on smoking cessation published by government agencies and non-governmental organisations, and grey literature. We identified relevant material by searching MEDLINE and Google Scholar using search terms and phrases including *smoking cessation, quitting smoking, nicotine replacement therapy, NRT, electronic (e)-cigarettes* and *vaping*. This analysis was conducted with the aim of synthesising exiting research on smoking cessation in order to critically assess the dominant 'medicalised' model of smoking cessations and the increasing commodification of quitting both via NRT and, more recently, e-cigarettes. The majority of the material available relates to high-income countries but this analysis has global implications, particularly as corporations that manufacture cessation aids and e-cigarettes look to expand into the markets of low- and middle-income countries (LMICs)

FINDINGS

Research Production and the Medicalisation of Smoking Cessation

Disagreements between proponents of assisted versus unassisted cessation reflect differences in how research and data on quitting are produced. For many researchers and practitioners, data from randomised clinical trials (RCTs) are considered the only reliable indicator of quit rates. Clinical trials typically report that pharmacotherapy-assisted cessation increases success rates, compared to placebo or no assistance, by as much as 50–70 percent (Stead et al. 2012). However, concerns exist regarding the dependability of RCT results because trial settings can be far removed from the real-world environments in which smokers seek to quit. RCT participants are, generally, unrepresentative of the broader population (Rothwell 2005) and are, for instance, more likely to complete a prescribed drug schedule than in a real-world setting (Smith and Chapman 2014; Walsh 2011). Participants also receive free medication, travel and other expenses, and have regular contact with supportive researchers, which can create 'Hawthorne effects', namely 'the additional clinical response that results from increased attention provided by participation in the clinical trial' (Wolfe and Michaud 2010). Reported limitations specific to NRT trials include (1) poor blindness integrity, that is, participants are often aware when they receive placebo (Mooney, White and Hatsukami 2004), and (2) that potential participants with mental health problems are routinely screened out (Lembke and Humphreys 2015) despite their over-representation among smokers.

Impressive quit rates obtained in trial conditions are not replicated in population-level surveys of pharmacotherapy-assisted cessation, and most of those attempting to give up cigarettes report continued smoking six to twelve months after using pharmaceutical assistance (Smith and Chapman 2014). Population-level studies also show that unassisted cessation is the most successful means of quitting, with between two-thirds and three-quarters of former smokers having stopped smoking without recourse to medication or counselling (Edwards et al. 2014). U.S. studies report unassisted quit attempts to be 2.8 times more successful than those using NRT (Shiffman et al. 2008) and that NRT had no effect on successful cessation (Alpert, Connolly and Biener 2013), while a 2013 Gallup poll found that 48 percent of ex-smokers had quit without pharmacotherapy, compared to 6 percent who used NRT patches or gum, and another 3 percent who used prescription drugs (Newport 2013). Analysis of U.S. census data by Pierce et al. (2012) found that, three months after quitting, light smokers (fewer than fifteen cigarettes per day) who quit unassisted were 37 percent more likely to be successful than those who used some form of assistance; heavier smokers who quit unassisted were 50 percent more successful than those who used assistance.

Despite the historical reality that most ex-smokers quit without assistance, and relapse at a lower rate, the pharmaceutical industry enthusiastically cites RCT results in the extensive promotion of their products. Pierce et al. (2012) note that pharmaceutical corporations were the largest purchasers of advertising related to smoking cessation in the United States between 1992 and 2005, far outspending tobacco-control organisations. The message actively conveyed to consumers that pharmacotherapy dramatically improves the chances of quitting successfully has gained broad acceptance, and has made cessation a lucrative business for a small number of manufacturers. NRT sales of US$2.369 billion in 2014 are expected to rise by more than US$100 million by 2019 (Strobel 2015), and more than two-thirds (70.6 percent) of cessation products are manufactured by Johnson & Johnson (33.9 percent of market share), GlaxoSmithKline (GSK) (22.8 percent) and Novartis (13.9 percent) (Euromonitor 2015a).

A key related concern is that much of the evidence used to support the industry's message derives from research funded by pharmaceutical corporations. Previous studies (Silverman et al. 2010; Stamatakis, Weller and Ionnadis 2013) have demonstrated that corporate-funded research is several times more likely to report findings favourable to the sponsoring company than studies supported by government or not-for-profit organisations. Reasons cited include publication bias, that is, releasing positive results while withholding unfavourable outcomes (Lexchin et al. 2003); use of methodological approaches more likely to return favourable results; utilisation of inappropriate comparators, for example, non-equivalent doses; selection of outcomes that favour the trial drug; or use of statistical methods that conceal or downplay adverse results (DeVries and Lemmens 2006). Finally, researchers gravitate to well-supported fields of enquiry (Russo 2005), raising concerns about potential conflicts of interest (Norris et al. 2011; Cosgrove et al. 2013). These issues are relevant to NRT research, as suggested by a 2007 review of selected trials that found that 51 percent of industry-funded trials reported significant cessation effects, compared to 22 percent of trials not funded by pharmaceutical corporations (Etter, Burri and Stapleton 2007).

Industry funding has also resulted in a significant imbalance in evidence available on assisted versus unassisted quit attempts. A review by Chapman and MacKenzie (2010) of 511 original articles, meta-analyses and reviews on smoking cessation published during 2007–2008 found 91.4 percent focused on assisted cessation, while 8.6 percent investigated the impact of unassisted quit attempts. Of these, almost one-half (48 percent) of pharmacotherapy intervention studies, compared to 10.3 percent of non-pharmacotherapy intervention studies, involved at least one author who declared funding or support from a pharmacotherapy cessation manufacturer. None of the research into unassisted cessation reported industry funding. This focus on assisted cessation has contributed to a lack of understanding of *why* most smokers quit unassisted, and research into related habits, attitudes and social environments that contributed to the success of unassisted quitting may reveal important information that could help current smokers (Chapman and MacKenzie 2010). Results of a small-scale study of ex-smokers published in 2015 provide some indication. Unassisted quitters reported that they had not been convinced by professional advice on cessation; that they took into account the cost of unassisted versus assisted strategies; and that they believed that they had a personal responsibility to take charge of quitting (Smith et al. 2015).

The Commodification of Smoking Cessation

Pharmacotherapy-assisted cessation is a relatively recent innovation and millions of smokers had quit prior to its availability. In the United States, some 30 million people had given up smoking before NRT was launched in the 1980s (Smith and Chapman 2014), and the American Cancer Society (2003) noted that 91.4 percent of the estimated 40 million ex-smokers in the country by 2003 had quit 'unaided' after the U.S. Surgeon-General's 1964 report on smoking and lung cancer. Yet the 'historical amnesia' (Chapman and Wakefield 2013) that obscures the reality that the overwhelming majority of ex-smokers have quit unassisted has allowed the 'no success without assistance' message to dominate the cessation debate with real implications for national and global health policy.

At the national level, U.S. guidelines in 2015 for medical advice and hospital-based quit programs recommend that *every* smoker be treated or offered pharmacotherapy other than pregnant women, smokeless tobacco users, light smokers and adolescents (Pierce et al. 2012). In the United Kingdom, the National Institute for Health and Care Excellence (NICE) advises general practitioners (GPs) to offer NRT, varenicline or bupropion to smokers seeking to quit, and to refer them to a national stop-smoking program (NICE 2013). Smokers consulting the National Health Service website (NHS 2015a) are directed to either contact an NHS Stop

Smoking Service, which will make it 'easy and affordable' to obtain pharmaceutical products (NHS 2015b), or consult a GP who 'can prescribe several different stop smoking treatments' (NHS 2015c). Nowhere on the NHS website was unassisted cessation mentioned at the time of this writing.

A similar situation exists in Australia. The Royal Australian College of General Physicians (2014) advises GPs that pharmacotherapy be recommended as first-line therapy for smokers expressing an interest in quitting. The National Tobacco Campaign (2012) maintains that smokers can double the chances of quitting by using medication, and even questions the authenticity of ex-smokers' claims about having quit without assistance. Varenicline has been subsidised under the national Pharmaceutical Benefits Scheme (PBS) since 2007, while NRT was added to the PBS list of subsidised medicines in 2010 following lobbying by Cancer Council Australia, the Heart Foundation and Quit Victoria (MacKenzie and Rogers 2015). Yet widespread availability of subsidised cessation medication in Australia has not been statistically associated with smoking prevalence (Wakefield et al. 2014).

NRT remains predominantly sold in high-income countries, with North America (38 percent, US$906 million) and Western Europe (44 percent, US$1 billion) accounting for the bulk of global sales in 2014 (Euromonitor 2015a). However, pharmacotherapy is increasingly being recommended for use across all countries, representing a significant shift in global health policy. WHO (2013) recommends that 'at least three clinical interventions should be included in any tobacco control programme', including pharmacological therapy, and recommends that the essential medicine list of each country include NRT. Similarly, Article 14 of the FCTC requires parties to take action to promote smoking cessation and to 'facilitate accessibility and affordability for treatment of tobacco dependence including pharmaceutical products' (WHO 2003).

Many LMICs, some with the highest smoking rates in the world, have remained indifferent to pharmacotherapy for reasons of cost, poor access to health care and lack of awareness (Wang et al. 2015). In China and Indonesia, the entrenched popularity of smoking has limited efforts to promote cessation generally, while the uptake of e-cigarettes in the Philippines (Euromonitor 2015b) represents a major obstacle to sales of NRT. Relatively strong uptake in South Korea has been attributed to consumer response to an 80 percent rise in cigarette taxes announced in 2014 (Euromonitor 2015c); uptake in Taiwan appears to be due to government subsidisation of cessation products (Euromonitor 2015d). Mixed results notwithstanding, NRT manufacturers are aware of the opportunities represented by LMIC markets to compensate for slowing growth in traditional markets (Strobel 2014), effectively echoing the tobacco industry's shift from traditional to emerging LMIC markets since the mid-twentieth century.

The Marketing of Electronic Cigarettes as Harm Reduction

Debates around smoking cessation have been both invigorated and complicated by the emergence of e-cigarettes and their increasing popularity. E-cigarettes are hand-held, battery-operated devices, in which liquid nicotine is vaporised and inhaled by the user (or 'vapers') (Brown and Cheng 2014). Research suggests that toxicity levels of e-cigarette vapour are significantly lower than tobacco smoke (Orr 2014; Callahan-Lyon 2014), which has led some public health advocates to suggest that they offer a less harmful alternative for smokers unable or unwilling to quit.

Models vary greatly in form and appearance, with some products (known as 'cigalikes') closely resembling conventional cigarettes in shape and appearance, while larger, modifiable, refillable devices bear little visual similarity (Zhu et al. 2014; Grana et al. 2014). Regardless of the model, replication of the smoking experience offered by e-cigarettes (Bell and Keane 2012) marks a significant departure from nicotine substitution derived from patches, gum and sprays. Their emergence as an alternative form of nicotine delivery has been hailed by advocates as a 'disruptive technology' that marks a potentially decisive shift in smoking behaviour (Abrams 2014), and widening appeal is reflected by the reported doubling of e-cigarette use in Europe and North America between 2008 and 2012 (Grana, Benowitz and Glantz 2014).

In contrast, many public health actors have expressed reservations about their population health effects (Aktan 2014). Concerns centre on the extent to which using e-cigarettes will supplement, rather than replace, traditional cigarettes among smokers or encourage them to reduce consumption, rather than quit. There is also the potential for the maintenance of nicotine addiction via e-cigarettes, and the ability to use them as 'bridge products' in smoke-free environments may also remove an important incentive to quitting. Moreover, it is argued that e-cigarettes may appeal to non-smokers including youth, effectively acting as a gateway to nicotine addiction and eventually to cigarette smoking as a more effective form of nicotine delivery (Fairchild, Bayer and Colgrove 2014; Dutra and Glantz 2014). Concerns have also been raised regarding the extent to which marketing and public use of such products that are, in many cases, visually similar to conventional cigarettes, may undermine tobacco marketing bans and clean-air legislation (i.e., indoor smoking bans), resulting in the 'renormalisation' of smoking (Fairchild, Bayer and Colgrove 2014). As the popularity and promotion of e-cigarettes has grown, government approaches to regulating their sale, use and marketing have differed radically and include outright prohibition such as in Australia and Brazil. In countries where the sale and use of e-cigarettes is legal, they may be treated as consumer products, tobacco products or medical devices, with each potential categorisation having implications for production standards, availability for purchase, product labelling and the marketing claims that can be made. In the United States, there has been considerable debate about the classification of e-cigarettes and confusion among regulators about how to proceed in developing a regulatory framework, while the European Union tobacco products directive (2014) allows for the regulation of e-cigarettes as either tobacco products or medical devices depending on product characteristics. Strategies by manufacturers to bring e-cigarettes to market as either medical devices or tobacco products have significant implications for policy because of the different standards and regulations that apply to advertising of consumer versus medical goods. That it is only possible to market medically licensed products as cessation aids and to make claims about their efficacy, makes clear the commercial advantages of having e-cigarettes registered as medical devices.

Development of effective e-cigarette policies is complicated by two further factors. First, because of the novelty of these devices, there remains a dearth of clear, robust evidence about their long-term health effects and their patterns of use. Further studies are needed to establish the relative toxicity of vapour emitted by e-cigarettes compared with smoked cigarettes, the health impacts of their use over time in real-world situations, and their potential effect on population-level health and smoking rates. Ideally, this would include multi-disciplinary research aimed at understanding the usage patterns of vapers; the extent to which e-cigarettes are used as substitutes, rather than supplements, for continued (or dual) tobacco use; the longevity of tobacco abstinence by e-cigarette users; and the impacts of e-cigarette advertising.

Second, significant investment by the tobacco industry in the e-cigarette industry has received insufficient attention from policy makers and researchers. British American Tobacco (BAT) became the first tobacco company to launch an e-cigarette in the UK in 2013 (Manning 2013), and was soon followed by Philip Morris International, Japan Tobacco International and Imperial Tobacco. This development reflects wider moves by TTCs to enter the e-cigarette market globally, primarily through promotion of 'cigalikes' that closely resemble traditional cigarettes (Tobacco Tactics 2015), which would potentially allow for brand synergies and marketing overlaps between conventional and electronic products. Strategic investment in e-cigarettes is in keeping with past attempts by tobacco producers to use the development of allegedly reduced-harm products (e.g., 'light' and 'low tar' cigarettes) to shift policy debate away from effective tobacco-control measures, and deflect attention from the harmful nature of their core products (Savell, Gilmore and Fooks 2014; Smith, Chapman and Dunlop 2013). TTC ownership has raised concerns that e-cigarettes may be marketed not as substitute products to help smokers quit, but as ancillary products designed to keep them smoking (i.e., to maintain addiction and be used as bridge products in smoke-restricted environments). In other words, e-cigarettes may become a vital tool for the tobacco industry in sustaining their core tobacco businesses in highly regulated markets.

Tobacco industry investment also has implications for the medicalisation of harm reduction. The process of gaining medical approval is beyond the resources of many smaller, independent e-cigarette producers who lack the financial resources to undertake trials of their products and fulfil licensing requirements. TTCs face no such restrictions, and regulating e-cigarettes may prove to be beneficial to their attempts to control the market. The decision by BAT subsidiary Nicoventures to seek medical licensing for its Voke brand of e-cigarette in the UK, for example, demonstrates TTC intentions to take this route to market. The licencing of Voke as a medical device, if approved, could mean that they are made available on the NHS and provided to smokers via doctors' prescriptions (McNeill et al. 2015).

Investment in e-cigarettes and their promotion as harm-reduction products allows TTCs to reposition themselves as part of the solution to the smoking epidemic, and to use this as a means through which to re-establish contact with policy makers. Whilst meetings with the tobacco industry are precluded by Article 5.3 of the FCTC, TTCs may argue such restrictions do not extend to their e-cigarette subsidiaries. Their potential status as producers of medical devices endorsed by the NHS will provide another powerful argument for TTCs to use in their attempts to regain their seat at the decision-making table.

The existing evidence is unclear as to whether e-cigarettes, when used in real-world conditions over the long term, offer smokers a safe alternative to tobacco use, or whether they can lead to long-term reductions in smoking prevalence. What is apparent is that proponents of e-cigarettes share the assumptions promoted by the pharmaceutical industry that nicotine substitution is essential to quitting smoking. Proponents also identify the pharmaceutical industry as a key vested interest that opposes the promotion of e-cigarettes on the grounds that they represent a more effective form of nicotine substitution than the patches, gum and other products sold by leading corporations. Evolving debates about smoking-cessation policy thus pit two powerful industries against one another, each attempting to commodify the process of smoking cessation and to place their product at the heart of government policy.

CONCLUSION

Smoking cessation is an important case study of how the strategies, actions and economic imperatives of transnational corporations can undermine effective and cost-effective global health governance. This chapter argues that the widely held misperception that successfully quitting smoking depends on pharmacotherapy can be traced to longstanding

efforts by pharmaceutical corporations to frame the discourse on cessation through research funding and marketing. In practice, the use of medication to stop smoking is a relatively recent innovation, and millions of
smokers were able to quit prior to tobacco use becoming pathologised,
and cessation medicalised. The definition of smoking as a condition that
requires medical intervention reflects the increasingly broad influence of
biomedical approaches to health care that are characterised by reduction-
ism, individualism and bias towards technological solutions that coincide
with, and indeed overlap with, the economic interests of the pharmaceutical industry and other commercial interests (Clark 2014).

In the case of e-cigarettes, medicalisation has been more contentious.
Some user groups have resisted what they perceive to be attempts to
regulate e-cigarettes as medical devices and to pathologise their use, rejecting the idea that they should be treated as sick people trying to get
well. Instead, they consider themselves to be consumers choosing to use
nicotine via what they consider a safer form of delivery. This message has
been embraced by producers who see growing commercial opportunities
in the consumer and lifestyle market. As with smoking cessation, the
logic of consumption underlies the marketing of e-cigarettes as less harmful alternatives to combustible tobacco. Increasingly, routes away from
smoking are being commodified, packaged and sold by transnational
pharmaceutical and tobacco corporations whose past strategies to influence the regulatory environment for their products, and the scientific
content of policy debates, are now well documented (Sell 2003). In the
case of the tobacco industry this includes myriad attempts to develop
ostensibly less harmful products (Peeters and Gilmore 2014) with limited,
if any, evidence of reductions in harm for smokers. While the commodification of smoking cessation has clear commercial benefits for corporate
actors, the extent to which it serves the interests of public health remains
unclear.

The involvement of powerful economic actors, capable of funding research and lobbying policy makers as described above, poses fundamental conflicts in which the interests of public health are shaped by the
pursuit of corporate profits. In the case of the tobacco industry in particular, a history of past mendacity and the strictures of Article 5.3 of the
FCTC mean that governments must proceed with extreme caution when
developing regulations for electronic and non-combustible product categories. This includes clear limitations on the extent to which corporations
in these sectors should be able to engage, as stakeholders, in the policy-
making process. At the same time, those responsible for policy formulation will need robust independent studies of the relative efficacy of these
products as cessation aids, compared to unassisted methods, to facilitate
evidence-informed decision making. In the case of e-cigarettes, this must
be matched with emerging evidence about the effects of long-term vap-

ing and its impact, not just on current smokers, but on the wider public health.

NOTE

1. Quitting 'cold turkey' is frequently used in the literature to refer to quitting abruptly both with and without pharmacological assistance, and is therefore not used in this analysis.

REFERENCES

Abrams, David. 2014. *Statement from Specialists in Nicotine Science and Public Health Policy*. http://nicotinepolicy.net/documents/letters/MargaretChan.pdf.

Aktan, Özdemir . 2014. *129 Public Health and Medical Authorities from 31 Countries Write WHO DG Chan Urging Evidence-Based Approach to Ecigs*. https://tobacco.ucsf.edu/129-public-health-and-medical-authorities-31-countries-write-who-dg-chan-urging-evidence-based-appro.

Alpert, Hillel, Gregory Connolly and Lois Biener. 2013. 'A Prospective Cohort Study Challenging the Effectiveness of Population-Based Medical Intervention for Smoking Cessation'. *Tobacco Control* 22 (1): 32–37. doi: 10.1136/tobaccocontrol-2011-050129.

American Cancer Society. 2003. Cancer Facts and Figures. Atlanta: American Cancer Society. http://whyquit.com/studies/2003_ACS_Cancer_Facts.pdf.

Bell, Kirsten, and Helen Keane. 2012. 'Nicotine Control: E-cigarettes, Smoking and Addiction'. *International Journal of Drug Policy* 23: 242–47. doi: 10.1016/j.drugpo.2012.01.006.

Brown, Christopher, and James Cheng. 2014. 'Electronic Cigarettes: Product Characterisation and Design Considerations'. *Tobacco Control* 23: ii4–ii10. doi:10.1136/tobaccocontrol-2013-051476.

Callahan-Lyon, Priscilla. 2014. 'Electronic Cigarettes: Human Health Effects'. *Tobacco Control* 23: ii36–ii40. doi:10.1136/tobaccocontrol-2013-051470.

Chapman, Simon, and Melanie Wakefield. 2013. ' Large-Scale Unassisted Smoking Cessation over 50 Years: Lessons from History for Endgame Planning in Tobacco Control'. Tobacco Control 22 : i33–i35. doi:10.1136/tobaccocontrol-2012-050767.

Chapman, Simon, and Ross MacKenzie. 2010. 'The Global Research Neglect of Unassisted Smoking Cessation: Causes and Consequences'. *PLoS Medicine* 7: e1000216. doi:10.1371/journal.pmed.1000216.

Clark, Jocelyn. 2014. 'Medicalization of Global Health 1: Has the Global Health Agenda Become Too Medicalized?' *Global Health Action* 7: 23998. doi: 10.3402/gha.v7.23998.

Cosgrove, Lisa, Harold Bursztajn, Deborah Erlich, Emily Wheeler and Allen Shaughnessy. 2013. 'Conflicts of Interest and the Quality of Recommendations in Clinical Guidelines'. *Journal of Evaluation in Clinical Practice* 19 (4): 674–81. doi: 10.1111/jep.12016.

DeVries, Raymon, and Trudo Lemmens. 2006. 'The Social and Cultural Shaping of Medical Evidence: Case Studies from Pharmaceutical Research and Obstetric Science'. *Social Sciences & Medicine* 62: 2694–706. doi:10.1016/j.socscimed.2005.11.026.

Dutra, Lauren, and Stanton Glantz. 2014. 'Electronic Cigarettes and Conventional Cigarette Use among US Adolescents: A Cross-Sectional Study'. *JAMA Pediatrics* 168 (7): 610–17. doi: 10.1001/jamapediatrics.2013.5488.

Edwards, Sarah, Susan Bondy, Russell Callaghan and Robert Mann. 2014. 'Prevalence of Unassisted Quit Attempts in Population-Based Studies: A Systematic Review of the Literature'. *Addictive Behaviors* 9: 512–19. doi: 10.1016/j.addbeh.2013.10.036.

Etter, Jean-François, Mafaldi Burri and John Stapleton. 2007. 'The Impact of Pharmaceutical Company Funding on Results of Randomized Trials of Nicotine Replacement Therapy for Smoking Cessation: A Meta-Analysis'. *Addiction* 102: 815–22. doi:10.1111/j.1360-0443.2007.01822.x.

Euromonitor. 2015a. *NRT Smoking Cessation Aids. Company shares. Global, 2014*. London: Euromonitor International.

———. 2015b. *NRT Smoking Cessation Aids in the Philippines*. London: Euromonitor International.

———. 2015c. *NRT Smoking Cessation Aids in South Korea*. London: Euromonitor International.

———. 2015d. *NRT Smoking Cessation Aids in Taiwan*. London: Euromonitor International.

European Union. 2014. *Directive 2014/40/EU of the European Parliament of 3 April 2014 on the Approximation of the Laws, Regulations and Administrative Provisions of the Member States Concerning the Manufacture, Presentation and Sale of Tobacco and Related Products and Repealing Directive 2001/37/EC*.

Fairchild, Amy, Ronald Bayer and James Colgrove. 2014. 'The Renormalization of Smoking? E-cigarettes and the Tobacco "Endgame"'. *New England Journal of Medicine* 370: 293–95 .

Giovino, Gary, Sara Mirza, Jonathan Samet and Prakash Gupta, for the GATS Collaborative Group. 2012. 'Tobacco Use in 3 Billion Individuals from 16 Countries: An Analysis of Nationally Representative Cross-Sectional Household Surveys'. *The Lancet* 380: 668–79. doi:http://dx.doi.org/10.1016/S0140-6736(12)61085-X.

Grana, Rachel, Neal Benowitz and Stanton Glantz. 2014. 'Electronic Cigarettes'. *Circulation* 129: e490–e492. doi:10.1161/CIRCULATIONAHA.114.007667.

Green, Bart, Claire Johnson and Alan Adams. 2006. 'Writing Narrative Literature Reviews for Peer-Reviewed Journals: Secrets of the Trade'. *Journal of Chiropractic Medicine* 5 (3): 101–17. doi: 10.1016/S0899-3467(07)60142-6.

Hendershot, Christian , Katie Witkiewitz, William George and G. Alan Marlatt. 2011. 'Relapse Prevention for Addictive Behaviors'. Substance Abuse Treatment, Prevention, and Policy 6 (17). doi:10.1186/1747-597X-6-17.

Lee, Chung-won, and Jennifer Kahende. 2007. 'Factors Associated with Successful Smoking Cessation in the United States'. *American Journal of Public Health* 97: 1503–9. doi: 10.2105/AJPH.2005.083527.

Lembke, Anna, and Keith Humphreys. 2015. 'A Call to Include People with Mental Illness and Substance Use Disorders alongside 'Regular' Smokers in Smoking Cessation Research'. *Tobacco Control*. doi:10.1136/tobaccocontrol-2014-052215.

Lexchin, Joel, Lisa Bero, Benjamin Djulbegovic and Otavio Clark. 2003. 'Pharmaceutical Industry Sponsorship and Research Outcome and Quality: Systematic Review'. *British Medical Journal* 326. doi:http://dx.doi.org/10.1136/bmj.326.7400.1167.

MacKenzie, Ross, and Wendy Rogers. 2015. 'Potential Conflict of Interest and Bias in the RACGP's Smoking Cessation Guidelines: Are GPs Provided with the Best Advice on Smoking Cessation for Their Patients?' *Public Health Ethics* 8 (3): 319–31. doi:10.1093/phe/phv010.

Manning, Sanchez. 2013. 'British American Tobacco Enters Electronic Cigarette Market in Britain with the "Vype"'. *The Independent*, 30 July. http://tinyurl.com/nsrovbo.

McNeill, Anne, Leonie Brose, Robert Calder, Sara Hitchman, Peter Hajek and Hayden McRobbie. 2015. *E-cigarettes: An Evidence Update. A Report Commissioned by Public Health England*. London: Public Health England.

Milenkovic, Zora. 2014. *Imperial Propelled to Top of E-cigarettes Tree with Surprise Acquisition of Blu in Reynolds/Lorillard Divesture*. London: Euromonitor International.

Mooney, Marc, Thom White and Dorothy Hatsukami. 2004. 'The Blind Spot in the Nicotine Replacement Therapy Literature: Assessment of the Double-Blind in Clinical Trials'. *Addictive Behaviors* 29: 673–84. doi:10.1016/j.addbeh.2004.02.010.

National Health Service. 2015a. *Stop Smoking Treatments*.www.nhs.uk/conditions/Smoking-%28quitting%29/Pages/Treatment.aspx.

———. 2015b. *NHS Stop Smoking Services Help You Quit*. www.nhs.uk/Livewell/smoking/Pages/NHS-stop-smoking-adviser.aspx.
National Institute for Health and Care Excellence. 2013. *Smoking: Harm-Reduction*. Nice public health guidance 45. Manchester, UK: NICE. www.nice.org.uk/guidance/ph45.
National Tobacco Campaign Australia. 2012. *National Tobacco Strategy: 2012–2018*. http://tinyurl.com/az6rqyj.
Newport, Frank. 2013. *Most US Smokers Want to Quit, Have Tried Multiple Times*. Gallup Well-Being. www.gallup.com/poll/163763/smokers-quittried-multiple-times.aspx.
Norris, Susan, Haley Holmer, Lauren Ogden and Brittany Burda. 2011. 'Conflict of Interest in Clinical Practice Guideline Development: A Systematic Review'. *PLoS One* 6 (10). doi:10.1371/journal.pone.0075284.
Office for National Statistics. 2013. *Adult Smoking Habits in Great Britain*. http://tinyurl.com/pol5fuy.
Orr, Michael. 2014. 'Electronic Cigarettes in the USA: A Summary of Available Toxicology Data and Suggestions for the Future'. *Tobacco Control* 23: ii18–ii22. doi:10.1136/tobaccocontrol-2013-051474.
Peeters, Sylvie, and Anna Gilmore. 2014. 'Understanding the Emergence of the Tobacco Industry's Use of the Term Tobacco Harm Reduction in Order to Inform Public Health Policy'. *Tobacco Control*. doi:10.1136/tobaccocontrol-2013-051502.
Pharmaceutical Benefits Scheme. *Varenicline*. Australia Department of Health.www.pbs.gov.au/medicine/item/5469W-9128K-9129L.
Pierce, John, Sharon Cummins, Martha White, Aimee Humphrey and Karen Messer. 2012. 'Quitlines and Nicotine Replacement for Smoking Cessation: Do We Need to Change Policy?' *Annual Review of Public Health* 33: 341–56. doi:10.1146/annurev-publhealth-031811-124624.
Rodu, Brad, and William Godshall. 2006. 'Tobacco Harm Reduction: An Alternative Cessation Strategy for Inveterate Smokers'. *Harm Reduction Journal* 3 (37). doi:10.1186/1477-7517-3-37.
Rothwell, Peter. 2005. 'External Validity of Randomised Controlled Trials: "To Whom Do the Results of This Trial Apply?"' *The Lancet* 365: 82–93. doi:10.1016/S0140-6736(04)17670-8.
Russo, Eugene. 2005. 'Follow the Money—the Politics of Embryonic Stem Cell Research'. *PLoS Biology* 3: e234. doi:10.1371/journal.pbio.0030234.
Savell, Emily, Anna Gilmore and Gary Fooks. 2014. 'How Does the Tobacco Industry Attempt to Influence Marketing Regulations? A Systematic Review'. *PloS ONE* 9: e87389. doi:10.1371/journal.pone.0087389.
Scollo, Michelle, and Margaret Winstanley. 2015. *Tobacco in Australia: Facts and issues*. Melbourne: Cancer Council Victoria. www.TobaccoInAustralia.org.au.
Sell, Susan. 2003. *Private Power, Public Law: The Globalization of Intellectual Property*. Cambridge: Cambridge University Press.
Shiffman Saul, Sarah Brockwell, Janine Pillitteri and Joseph Gitchell. 2008. 'Use of Smoking-Cessation Treatments in the United States'. *American Journal of Preventative Medicine* 34: 102–11. doi:10.1016/j.amepre.2007.09.033.
Silverman, Gabriel, George Loewenstein, Britta Anderson, Peter Ubel and Stanley Zinberg. 2010. 'Failure to Discount for Conflict of Interest When Evaluating Medical Literature: A Randomised Trial of Physicians'. *Journal of Medical Ethics* 36: 265–70. doi:10.1136/jme.2009.034496.
Smith, Andrea, and Simon Chapman. 2014. 'Quitting Smoking Unassisted: The 50-Year Research Neglect of a Major Public Health Phenomenon'. *Journal of the American Medical Association* 32 :1137 – 38. doi: 10.1001/jama.2013.28261.
Smith, Andrea, Simon Chapman and Sally Dunlop. 2013. ' What Do We Know about Unassisted Smoking Cessation in Australia? A Systematic Review, 2005–2012'. *Tobacco Control*. doi:10.1136/tobaccocontrol-2013-051019.
Smith, Andrea, Stacey Carter, Simon Chapman, Sally Dunlop and Becky Freeman. 2015. 'Why Do Smokers Try to Quit Without Medication or Counselling? A Qualita-

tive Study with Ex-Smokers'. *BMJ Open* 5: e007301 doi:10.1136/bmjopen-2014-007301.

Stamatakis, Emmanuel, Richard Weller and John Ionnadis. 2013. 'Undue Industry Influences That Distort Healthcare Research, Strategy, Expenditure and Practice: A Review'. *European Journal of Clinical Investigation* 43: 460–74. doi:10.1111/eci.1207.

Stead, Lindsay, Rafael Perera, Christopher Bullen, David Mant, Jamie Hartmann-Boyce, Kate Cahill and Tim Lancaster. 2012. 'Nicotine Replacement Therapy for Smoking Cessation'. *Cochrane Database of System Reviews* 11: CD000146. doi:10.1002/14651858.CD000146.pub4.

Strobel, Mark. 2014. *Nicotine Replacement Therapy Smoking Cessation Aids: Challenges and Opportunities*. 16 January. Euromonitor.

———. 2015. *Overhyping the Impact of E-Cigarettes on NRT Smoking Cessation Aids*. 23 January. Euromonitor.

Tobacco Tactics. 2015. *E-cigarettes*. www.tobaccotactics.org/index.php/E-cigarettes.

U.S. Department of Health and Human Services. 2014. *The Health Consequences of Smoking—50 Years of Progress: A Report of the Surgeon General* . Atlanta: U.S. Department of Health and Human Services, Centers for Disease Control and Prevention, National Center for Chronic Disease Prevention and Health Promotion.

Wakefield, Melanie, Kerri Coomber, Sarah Durkin, Michelle Scollo, Megan Bayly, Matthew Spittal, Julie Simpson and David Hill. 2014. 'Time Series Analysis of the Impact of Tobacco Control Policies on Smoking Prevalence among Australian Adults, 2001–2011'. *Bulletin of the World Health Organization* 92: 413–22. http://dx.doi.org/10.2471/BLT.13.118448.

Walsh, Raoul. 2011. 'Australia's Experience with Varenicline: Usage, Costs and Adverse Reactions'. *Addiction* 106: 451–52. doi:10.1111/j.1360-0443.2010.03282.x.

Wang, Ling, Yue Jin, Bo Lu and Amy Ferketich. 2015. 'A Cross-Country Study of Smoking Cessation Assistance Utilization in 16 Low and Middle Income Countries: Data from the Global Adult Tobacco Survey (2008–2012)'. *Nicotine & Tobacco Research*. doi: 10.1093/ntr/ntv139.

Wolfe, Frederick, and Kaleb Michaud. 2010. 'The Hawthorne Effect, Sponsored Trials, and the Overestimation of Treatment Effectiveness'. *Journal of Rheumatology* 37: 2216–20. doi: 10.3899/jrheum.100497.

WHO. 2003. *Framework Convention on Tobacco Control*. Geneva: WHO.

———. 2013. *Report on the Global Tobacco Epidemic, 2013*. Geneva: WHO.

Zhu, Shu-Hong, Jessica Sun, Erika Bonnevie, Sharon Cummins, Anthony Gamst, Lu Yin and Madeleine Lee. 2014. 'Four Hundred and Sixty Brands of E-cigarettes and Counting: Implications for Product Regulation'. *Tobacco Control* 23: iii3–iii9. doi:10.1136/tobac cocontrol-2014-051670.

FOUR

The Influence of the Food Industry on Public Health Governance

Insights from Mexico and the United States

Courtney Scott, Angela Carriedo and Cécile Knai

Unhealthy diets play a major role in the current global non-communicable diseases pandemic (Swinburn et al. 2011). The rapidly expanding multinational food and non-alcoholic beverage industry (hereafter referred to as the processed food industry) has been referred to as a global vector of diseases such as diabetes, obesity and certain types of cancer (Mialon, Swinburn and Sacks 2015), due to its increasing sales of inexpensive, nutrient-poor ultra-processed foods (Stuckler and Nestle 2012) and political activities to shape relevant policies in its favour (Mialon, Swinburn and Sacks 2015). This chapter analyses some of the common political tactics used by the food industry through case studies from Mexico and California, USA.

METHODS

This chapter uses a qualitative policy analysis and literature review to explore corporate political strategies in the processed food industry and their impact on global health governance. In order to illustrate a range of corporate political tactics used by the processed food industry, the chapter presents two case studies. Case study 1 assesses the process around nutrition labelling regulation in Mexico based on documentary analysis and twelve interviews conducted in 2014, as part of a larger study conducted by the National Institute of Public Health in Mexico. Ethical approval for this research was obtained from their research ethics committee. The case study explores the role of the food industry in influencing the regulation and the contextual factors that enabled their influence. Case study 2 analyses efforts to enact soda tax legislation in California using a literature and media review conducted in 2015. It illustrates how the beverage industry used well-funded campaigns and strategic messaging to prevent soda taxes from being adopted.

BACKGROUND

How the Processed Food Industry Influences Public Health Governance

Governance of public health, food and nutrition policies is a political process subject to constraints and competing priorities, both from external stakeholders and within the political system. Corporate political strategies commonly employed by the processed food industry include: participating in drafting agricultural and nutrition policies and constructing favourable trade agreements (Clark et al. 2012); lobbying; funding and/or partnering with health organizations or academics (Knai et al. 2010); and creating or discrediting scientific evidence (Wiist 2010). Food and beverage industry use of lobbyists and sponsored academics to challenge the evidence underpinning Chile's 2014 front-of-package nutrition labelling criteria, and Mexico's 2010 School Food Guidelines to restrict sales of ultra-processed foods at schools (Castillo 2014; Ministry of Education of Mexico 2010) are two examples in which eventual guidelines were less rigorous than intended. These strategies are analysed in case study 1.

Furthermore, as case study 2 illustrates, the processed food industry portrays attempts to control the availability and affordability of ultra-processed foods as a form of government paternalism or 'nanny statism', using terms that infer unwarranted government intrusion into everyday life (Hoek 2015). The industry instead promotes self-regulation and public-private partnerships with government on public health issues (Kraak et al. 2012). Such arrangements, however, often involve inherent conflicts of interest. Nor are they always effective approaches (Jensen and Ronit 2015; Knai et al. 2015).

DISCUSSION

Case Study 1: Regulation for a Front-of-Pack Nutrition Labelling System in Mexico

Front-of-pack nutrition labelling (FOPL) is widely supported internationally as a strategy for helping consumers make healthier food purchases. Though there is mixed evidence on its effectiveness at doing so, it may contribute to product reformulations that reduce nutrients such as sugar, salt and fat in processed foods (Mozaffarian et al. 2012). In an effort to reduce the high burden of obesity in Mexico, where nearly three-quarters of adults are either overweight or obese (Rivera Dommarco et al. 2012), the newly elected government launched a national strategy to address this problem in October 2013 (SSA México 2014). The strategy includes a regulation on food advertising and promotion of foods to children, fiscal measures (including soda and snack taxes) and the implementation of a mandatory FOPL system. The latter includes: (a) indication of content as a percentage of a 'standard diet' of four nutrients, and (b) a voluntary logo that can be used on the front of packaged foods to signal to consumers it complies with the criteria defined by the government. Food companies were given one year starting from February 2014 to implement the regulation.

In 2009, prior to these regulatory measures being developed, the largest consortium of food industries in Mexico, and other local and transnational food producers and retailers, had voluntarily implemented an alternative FOPL based on the Guideline Daily Allowance (GDA) system, an industry-designed labelling scheme that has now been adopted by food corporations internationally (El Poder del Consumidor 2012; Stern, Tolentino and Barquera 2011). GDAs define the proportion of a 'standard diet' for each nutrient, but present a number of problems primarily because they are not aligned with WHO dietary recommendations (WHO 2003), and, because they are based on the daily recommended amounts for women with moderate physical activity, they are inappropriate for use by all adults or by children (Stern, Tolentino and Barquera 2011). Moreover, consumers cannot easily understand GDAs because they may lack understanding of what the percentages refer to, and if they are by package or by portion (Cruz-Gongora et al. 2012; Stern, Tolentino and Barquera 2011). Nutrition experts and civil society organisations recommended that the Mexican government not use the GDA system, as explained by a civil society organisation representative: 'First we made a public demand [against the voluntary GDA FOPL scheme] to the Ministry of Health; we were concerned that the GDA FOPL labelling used by the industries was misleading and that it represented a health risk for consumers because they underestimated the amount of sugar in products'. Despite these concerns, the food industry continued to use and promote the voluntary strategy for two years and in 2013 argued strongly for the GDA to be adopted as the national regulatory FOPL during negotiations on the new labelling regulation (Carriedo and Barquera 2013; Barquera, Campos and Rivera 2013).

FOPL Strategy, Implementation and Reactions

When President Enrique Peña Nieto presented the 2013 national obesity strategy, the Ministry of Health appointed its food and drug regulatory agency (COFEPRIS) to coordinate its implementation. This regulatory agency opened a consultation process whereby any person or organisation, including civil society groups, academics and food industry members, could submit their views and recommendations (Barragán 2015). A range of arguments, at times contradictory, were presented, with several stakeholders giving and supporting evidence-based recommendations for various FOPL systems, including warning logos and the traffic light system (Rivera Dommarco et al. 2012; WHO 2004).

Though the head of COFEPRIS publicly stated that they met with all key actors including civil society organisations and food industry leaders (Barragán 2015), several civil society groups stated that they were excluded from the policy design phase, as were academics. For example, as one civil society representative explained, many did not have the opportunity to attend private or public meetings with COFEPRIS: 'COFEPRIS went through a process which was not crystal clear; civil society [organisations] were never consulted, academia was not consulted . . . and now we see that the labelling [regulation] favours the industry. . . . COFEPRIS chose their [food industry] nutrient criteria'. Another civil society representative reported that the food and beverage industry had participated in the process: 'Some legislators that were in the meetings, and that have had a close relationship with industry people, confirmed that they [the food industry] participated in the design of these criteria'.

The final FOPL regulation was published in February 2014. It included a numeric system that reported total energy, saturated fats, sugar and sodium, and the percentage of these nutrients as a proportion of the 'standardized diet' using the GDA criteria, as well as a voluntary health logo. It used a mix of the GDA-based criteria, used previously by the food industry for the voluntary FOPLs, as well as the criteria of the European Union (EU) pledge (www.eu-pledge.edu), a voluntary pledge made by food industries to limit food marketing to children in the European Union, which has since been found to be unlikely to be effective as a public health measure (Jensen and Ronit 2015).

Following the launch of the FOPL strategy, public health experts and civil society groups publicly denounced the final regulation for lacking the rigour required to address the Mexican obesity epidemic. Their main concerns were that stricter criteria were needed in light of the extreme prevalence of obesity in Mexico; that the FOPL did not include added sugars or trans fats, two nutrients known to have adverse health effects; and that the system lacked a colour-coded format, despite evidence that consumers find it easier to understand. To date, these concerns, although publicly disclosed, have not had an impact on changing the regulation.

This case study illustrates the ways in which the processed food industry in Mexico was involved in the design and formulation of food and nutrition regulations. As a result, regulations may not be based on expert recommendations, and therefore are not as effective in modifying food consumption or the prevalence of obesity in Mexico (Rivera Dommarco et al. 2012). This case study also highlights a lack of transparency in the policy process, such as the reported exclusion of key actors from the process of setting the labelling regulation, despite claims of a consultation process open to civil society actors. This underscores the importance of having open public debates during the policy process that include civil society observers as a means of improving transparency, particularly given the inherent competing interests underlying nutrition policy.

Case Study 2: Soda Tax in California

Excessive consumption of sugar-sweetened beverages (SSB) is associated with numerous adverse health outcomes including diabetes and strokes (Wang et al. 2012). There is growing evidence that a soda tax, like those implemented in Barbados, Egypt, France, Hungary and Mexico, represents an effective public health response (Popkin 2015). A comprehensive evidence synthesis concluded, for instance, that a well-designed tax is likely to increase the price of an unhealthy food, and in turn reduce its consumption (Cornelsen and Carriedo 2015).

In California, policy makers and advocates have proposed a statewide soda tax on four occasions since 2010, as well as numerous tax proposals at the local municipality level (Rudd Policy Center 2015). Soda tax propositions were on the ballot in San Francisco and Berkeley in November 2014, both large, politically liberal cities. The proposals garnered immense interest from beverage corporations and the media, as well as public health policy makers and advocates in other states and countries. The bill in Berkeley proposed a one-cent tax per ounce on all SSBs sold with revenues to go into the city's general fund, and towards creating a board of nutrition and health experts tasked with addressing child health (YesOnD 2015). The San Francisco bill proposed a tax of two-cents per ounce, with revenues earmarked for nutrition and health programmes in the city (San Francisco Board of Supervisors 2014).

In response to these initiatives, the American Beverage Association (ABA) contributed $9.24 million to fight the soda tax in San Francisco, and an additional $2.43 million in Berkeley. These funds supported financial contributions to and direct lobbying of legislators (Duan 2015), mass media campaigns, billboards, leaflets and door-to-door organising, and targeting of local businesses in an attempt to have them speak out against the tax (Harrington 2014). Much of this work in influencing the public debate was carried out by front groups paid for by the ABA, such as the Coalition for an Affordable City in San Francisco (NoOnE 2015), and the

No Berkeley Beverage Tax (NoOnD 2015) whose billboards and advertising campaigns were reportedly 'plastered on the walls across from the trains, pinned to spaces near the ticket machine, and laid out on the floor of the station' (Aubrey 2014).

Despite the beverage industry's sustained efforts, the soda tax bill in Berkeley passed with support from 75 percent of voters. This was an unprecedented victory for soda tax initiatives, which many credited to the grassroots community organizing done by the 'Yes on Measure D' campaign (YesOnD 2015). Success was the result of a combination of factors. At a practical level, the Yes campaign received funding from donors such as Bloomberg Philanthropies, which enabled them to counter the beverage industry's messaging on TV (Aubrey 2014). The stated intention to use associated tax revenues to support health campaigns was significant as such allocation has been shown to increase public support for soda taxes (Jou et al. 2014). Finally, the Berkeley campaign was successful because its key message—'Berkeley v. Big Soda'—positioned the soda tax as a local social justice issue (Dinkelspiel 2014). Campaigns reminded voters, 'This tax is charged to the industry that profits off of drinks that promote diabetes and obesity, diseases that disproportionately affect people with limited incomes and communities of colour' (YesOnD 2015). Unlike other campaigns that have focused on health messaging, the social justice framing of the Berkeley soda tax was unique in addressing the impacts of beverage corporations' actions on local community members. Many credit the success of the initiative to this social justice approach (Nestle 2015).

Richmond and El Monte Tax Initiatives

In nearby Richmond and El Monte, socioeconomically diverse cities in California, each with just over one hundred thousand people, local governments and advocates also attempted to pass soda taxes in 2012. In these relatively small cities, the beverage industry spent $4 million over a period of approximately six months to defeat the proposed taxes (Zingale 2012). As in San Francisco and Berkeley, beverage industry strategies to fight the initiatives were largely conducted through two front groups: the Community Coalition Against Beverage Taxes in Richmond, and the El Monte Citizens Against Beverage Taxes (Mejia et al. 2014). After a high-profile and strongly contested campaign, only 23 percent of voters in El Monte and 33 percent in Richmond supported the soda tax (Jou et al. 2014).

Analyses of these initiatives (Jou et al. 2014; Mejia et al. 2014) highlighted the industry's appropriation of terms like *community* or *citizen* to portray the campaign of front groups as grassroots-driven. The industry also challenged the legitimacy of the tax on multiple fronts through messages that the tax would not only be ineffective but also result in economic harm and job loss, was racist and regressive in that it would dispropor-tionately affect lower socioeconomic groups, and would limit personal choice and freedom. There were also accusations of dishonesty, claiming that the money raised by the tax would not be spent on obesity preven-tion programs but were instead a 'blank check' for the government.

Advocates in Richmond and El Monte attempted to counter such mes-sages by emphasising that the tax could fund health programs, and chal-lenging the regressivity arguments made by the industry. One advocate argued, for example, 'A sugar-sweetened beverage tax may be regressive, but . . . what's really regressive is the health disparities that we document in Richmond and throughout the country that are caused to a consider-able extent by sugar-sweetened beverages. That's the real regressive tax: a tax on our health' (Jou et al. 2014).

The anti-tax messages in Richmond and El Monte were found to 'ap-peal to ideological or political beliefs', for instance, by focusing on the importance of personal choice (Jou et al. 2014). In this way, the anti-tax messages invoked broader individualistic values prominent in the Unit-ed States and implied questions about the role that government should or could play in dietary choices. These value-based messages resonate deep-ly with individuals, more so than the predominant pro-tax messages on the health consequences of SSBs (Dorfman, Wallack and Woodruff 2005). In addition, significant funding from the beverage industry allowed anti-tax messages to be targeted to particular groups and to play upon exist-ing socioeconomic concerns and tensions in the community. For example, an advocate, as cited by Jou et al. (2014), described how anti-tax bill-boards in Richmond featured African American men with messaging about the tax 'unfairly targeting . . . low income communities', while messages about how the tax would be 'an empty check' to the govern-ment featured a middle-age white woman. Furthermore, the beverage companies had been sponsoring local sports teams and community events in Richmond for a number of years, and advocates suggest that the goodwill generated by these sponsorships improved the reception of the industry's anti-tax messages among community members (Jou et al. 2014).

Lessons Learned

These case studies present only a small sample of the many examples of the beverage industry's response to soda tax initiatives in California. Strikingly similar tactics have been shown in other states and countries (Nixon, Mejia and Dorfman 2014; Donaldson 2015). Although the process around each initiative has unique aspects that reflect the context and circumstances specific to each jurisdiction, the industry has employed common approaches such as intense pushback, campaigning and lobby-ing. An 'emerging "playbook" for opposing soda tax' includes creating 'industry-funded coalitions of local residents and leaders' (Nixon, Mejia and Dorfman 2014), arguing that beverage consumption is an issue of personal responsibility (Koplan and Brownell 2010), and that a tax would have a disproportionate impact on lower socioeconomic groups (Jou et al. 2014). The industry also adapts their messages to the local social and economic context by 'reframing the soda tax to capitalize on existing issues or tensions in the community' (Nixon, Mejia and Dorfman 2014). In Richmond, a working-class city, the industry was able to exploit 'a history of racial and ethnic divisions [and] fuelled allegations that the tax was paternalistic and discriminatory to low income residents of color' (Nixon, Mejia and Dorfman 2014). In contrast, in El Monte, a city that at the time was facing bankruptcy, 'tax opponents framed the tax as a money grab from a city government mired in financial mistrust' (Nixon, Mejia and Dorfman 2014).

Understanding these strategies can help to frame future soda tax initiatives, or other equally crucial nutrition policies, by highlighting the need to prepare effective counter-messaging strategies. Advocates will have an advantage if they can set value-based campaign messages, rather than responding to messaging crafted by the beverage industry (Dorfman, Wallack and Woodruff 2005). The successful 2014 Berkeley soda tax campaign, which focused on social justice issues and the culpability of the beverage industry, highlights the importance of connecting pro-tax messages to issues broader than personal health. These points may be particularly important for low- and middle-income countries, which are target markets for beverage company expansion and will need to consider effective regulatory responses (Studdert, Flanders and Mello 2015).

CONCLUSION

This chapter discusses political strategies used by the processed food industry to influence public health governance. The industry employs multiple strategies to influence nutrition and public health evidence, and to shape policy negotiations in order to ensure that they do not infringe upon their ability to sell, market and promote their products. The Mexican case study illustrates how the industry uses voluntary, self-created measures and concerted lobbying to influence the design and implementation of mandatory regulations. Analysis of the tax initiatives in California underlines the importance of two additional strategies, namely creating front groups and using targeted messaging to weaken calls for legislation.

Findings from this chapter underscore the need for improved public health efforts to monitor and analyse corporate political activity in the processed food industry (Mialon, Swinburn and Sacks 2015), and to adopt strategies to understand coalition and network building in public health policy (Weishaar, Amos and Collin 2015). The chapter also illustrates the importance of openly acknowledging any inherently competing goals among sectors and mitigating the processed food industry's ability to undermine public health policies. This requires drafting clear rules of engagement (Adams 2007; Oshaug 2009), strengthening regulatory capacity, monitoring compliance with existing voluntary agreements, and ensuring evidence-based, well-defined and measurable policy targets (Bryden et al. 2013).

REFERENCES

Adams, Peter. 2007. 'Assessing Whether to Receive Funding Support from Tobacco, Alcohol, Gambling and Other Dangerous Consumption Industries'. *Addiction* 102 (7): 1027–33. doi: 10.1111/j.1360-0443.2007.01829.x.

Aubrey, Allison. 2014. 'How Did Berkeley Pass a Soda Tax? Bloomberg's Cash Didn't Hurt'. Washington: National Public Radio.

Barquera, Simon, Ismael Campos and Juan A. Rivera. 2013. 'Mexico Attempts to Tackle Obesity: The Process, Results, Push Backs and Future Challenges'. *Obesity Reviews* 14: 69–78. doi:10.1111/obr.12096.

Barragán, Daniela. 2015. 'Entrevista a Comsionado de Coferpis rechaza estar al servicio de la industria, como dice ONGs'. *Animal Polítio.* www.sinembargo.mx/09-03-2015/1273606.

Bryden, Anna, Mark Petticrew, Nicholas Mays, Elizabeth Eastmure and Cecile Knai. 2013. 'Voluntary Agreements between Government and Business—a Scoping Review of the Literature with Specific Reference to the Public Health Responsibility Deal'. *Health Policy* 110 (2–3): 186–97. doi:10.1016/j.healthpol.2013.02.009.

Carriedo, Ana, and Simon Barquera. 2013. 'Sistema voluntario de etiquetado frontal de alimentos en méxico: antecedentes, bases técnicas y propuesta de implementación'. Mexico: Instituto Nacional de Salud Pública.

Castillo, Cecilia L. 2014. 'Para la historia: La ley de alimentos y su reglamento pasará a la historia de Chile y sus nombres, los de ustedes, quedarán inmortalizados'. Comité De Abogacía Por La Medicina Familiar Y Las Políticas Públicas.

Clark, Sarah E., Corinna Hawkes, Sophia M. E. Murphy, Karen A. Hansen-Kuhn and David Wallinga. 2012. 'Exporting Obesity: U.S. Farm and Trade Policy and the Transformation of the Mexican Consumer Food Environment'. *Int J Occup Environ Health* 18: 53–65. doi: http://dx.doi.org/10.1179/1077352512Z.0000000007.

Cornelsen, Laura, and Ana Carreido. 2015. 'Health-Related Taxes on Food and Beverages'. 5 May. Food Research Collaboration Policy Brief. http://foodresearch.org.uk/wp-content/uploads/2015/06/Food-and-beverages-taxes-final-amended.pdf.

Cruz-Gongora, Vanessa de la, Salvado Villalpando, Guadalupe Rodriguez-Oliveros, Marcia Castillo-Garcia, Veronica Mundo-Rosas and Sergio Meneses-Navarro. 2012. 'Use and Understanding of the Nutrition Information Panel of Pre-packaged Foods in a Sample of Mexican Consumers'. *Salud Publica de Mexico* 54 (2): 158–66.

Dinkelspiel, Frances. 2014. 'Why Berkeley Passed a Soda Tax While Other Cities Failed'. *Berkeley Side,* 5 November. www.berkeleyside.com/2014/11/05/why-berkeley-passed-a-soda-tax-where-others-failed.

Donaldson E. 2015. *Advocating for Sugar-Sweetened Beverage Taxation: A Case Study of Mexico.* John Hopkins Bloomberg School of Public Health. www.jhsph.edu/departments/health-behavior-and-society/_pdf/Advocating_For_Sugar_Sweetened_Beverage_Taxation.pdf.

Dorfman, Lori, Lawrence Wallack and Katie Woodruff. 2005. 'More Than a Message: Framing Public Health Advocacy to Change Corporate Practices'. *Health Education and Behavior* 32 (3): 320–36. doi:0.1177/1090198105275046.

Duan, Mary. 2015. 'How the Soda Industry Spends Millions to Crush Laws That Warn Us about the Dangers of Sugar. Lawmakers Try to Put Warning Labels on Soda and Sweetened Drinks, but So Far Have Been Unsuccessful against the Soda Lobby'. Sacramento: News & Review.

El Poder del Consumidor. 2012. 'Atenta contra la salud, nuevo etiquetado de Conméxico'. El Poder del Consumidor. http://elpoderdelconsumidor.org/saludnutricional/atenta-contra-la-salud-nuevo-etiquetado-de-conmexico.

Harrington, Elissa. 2014. 'Billboards Feature Small Business Owners to Fight Sf Soda Tax'. *ABC 7 News*, 9 September. http://abc7news.com/politics/billboards-feature-small-business-owners-to-fight-sf-soda-tax/302056.

Hoek, Janet. 2015. 'Informed Choice and the Nanny State: Learning from the Tobacco Industry'. *Public Health* 129 (8): 1038–45. doi: 10.1016/j.puhe.2015.03.009.

Jensen, Jørgen D., and Karsten Ronit. 2015. 'The EU Pledge for Responsible Marketing of Food and Beverages to Children: Implementation in Food Companies'. *Eur J Clin Nutr*. 69: 896–901. doi:10.1038/ejcn.2015.52.

Jou, Judy, Jeff Niederdeppe, Colleen L. Barry and Sarah E. Gollust. 2014. 'Strategic Messaging to Promote Taxation of Sugar-Sweetened Beverages: Lessons from Recent Political Campaigns'. *Am J Public Health* 104: 847–53. doi: 10.2105/AJPH.2013.301679.

Knai, Cecile, Anna Gilmore, Karen Lock and Martin McKee. 2010. 'Public Health Research Funding: Independence Is Important'. *Lancet* 376: 75–77. http://dx.doi.org/10.1016/S0140-6736(09)62063-8.

Knai, Cecile, Mark Petticrew, Mary Alison Durand et al. 2015. 'Has a Public–Private Partnership Resulted in Action on Healthier Diets in England? An Analysis of the Public Health Responsibility Deal Food Pledges'. *Food Policy* 54. doi:10.1016/j.foodpol.2015.04.002.

Koplan Jeffrey P., and Kelley Brownell. 2010. 'Response of the Food and Beverage Industry to the Obesity Threat'. *JAMA* 304: 1487–88. doi:10.1001/jama.2010.1436.

Kraak, Vivika I., Paige B. Harrigan, Mark Lawrence, Paul J. Harrison, Michaela A. Jackson and Boyd Swinburn. 2012. 'Balancing the Benefits and Risks of Public-Private Partnerships to Address the Global Double Burden of Malnutrition'. *Public Health Nutr* 15: 503–17. doi: 10.1017/S1368980011002060.

Mejia, Pamela, Laura Nixon, Andrew Cheyne, Lori Dorfman and Fernando Quintero. 2014. 'Issue 21: Two Communities, Two Debates: News Coverage of Soda Tax Proposals in Richmond and El Monte'. Berkeley, CA: Berkeley Media Studies Group.

Mialon, Melissa, Boyd A. Swinburn and Gary Sacks. 2015. 'A Proposed Approach to Systematically Identify and Monitor the Corporate Political Activity of the Food Industry with Respect to Public Health Using Publicly Available Information'. *Obesity Review* 16 (7): 519–30. doi:10.1111/obr.12289.

Ministry of Education of Mexico. 2010. 'Comunicado 130—lineamientos generales para el expendio o distribuciòn de alimentos y bebidas en los establecimientos de consumo escolar de los planetes de eduacaciòn bàsica'. 13 August. www.sep.gob.mx/es/sep1/C1300810#.VhabchN_Okp.

Mozaffarian, Dariuz, Ashkan Afshin, Neal L. Benowitz et al. 2012. 'Population Approaches to Improve Diet, Physical Activity, and Smoking Habits: A Scientific Statement from the American Heart Association'. *Circulation* 126: 1514–63. doi:10.1161/CIR.0b013e318260a20b.

Nestle, Marion. 2015. 'Interview with Columbia University Public Health Students'. www.Foodpolitics.Com/2015/04/Interview-with-Columbias-Mailman-School-of-Public-Health.

Nixon, Laura, Pamela Mejia and Lori Dorfman. 2014. 'Soda Tax Debates: An Analysis of News Coverage of the 2-13 Soda Tax Proposal in Telluride, Colorado'. Berkeley, CA: Berkeley Media Studies Group.

NoOnD. 2015. 'Vote No on D'. http://noberkeleybeveragetax.com.

NoOnE. 2015. 'At a Time When Many San Franciscans Confront a Growing Affordability Gap—the Last Thing We Need Is a New Beverage Tax'.

Oshaug, Arne. 2009. 'What Is the Food and Drink Industry Doing in Nutrition Conferences?' *Public Health Nutr* 12 (7): 1019–20. doi:10.1017/S136898000900593X.

Popkin, Barry. 2015. 'Global Consumption Patterns, Policies, Taxes and Other Issues'. Presentation at World Obesity Hot Topic Conference on Dietary Sugars, Obesity and Metabolic Disease, 29 June, Berlin.

Rivera Dommarco, Juan A., Anabel Velasco Bernal, Mauricio Hernández Ávila, Carlos Alberto Aguilar Salinas, Felipe Vadillo Ortega and Ciro Murayama Rendón. 2012. 'Obesidad en México: Recomendaciones para una política de estado'. Mexico: Universidad Nacional Autónoma de México.

Rudd Policy Center. 2015. 'Rudd Policy Center Legislation Database'. www.uconnruddcenter.org/legislation-database.

San Francisco Board of Supervisors. 2014. 'Initiative Ordinance—Business and Tax Regulations Code—Tax on Sugar-Sweetened Beverages to Fund Food and Health Programs. File No. 140098. Amended in Committee 9 July 2014'.

SSA, Secretaría de Salud, México. 2014. 'Estrategia nacional para la prevención y el control del sobrepeso, la obesidad y la diabetes México 2013 [4 February 2014]'. Gobierno Fedeera, Secrteraría de Salud.

Stern, Dalia, Lizbeth Tolentino and Simón Barquera. 2011. 'Revisión del etiquetado frontal: Análisis de las Guias Diarias de Alimentación (GDA) y su comprensión por estudiantes de nutrición'. Mexico: National Institute of Public Health.

Stuckler, David, and Marion Nestle. 2012. 'Big Food, Food Systems, and Global Health'. *PLoS Med* 9: e1001242. doi:10.1371/journal.pmed.1001242.

Studdert, David M., Jordan Flanders and Michelle M. Mello. 2015. 'Searching for Public Health Law's Sweet Spot: The Regulation of Sugar-Sweetened Beverages'. *PLoS Medicine* 12 (7): e1001848. doi:10.1371/journal.pmed.1001848.

Swinburn, Boyd A., Gary Sacks, Kevin D. Hall, Klim McPherson, Diane T. Finegood, Marjory L. Moodie and Steven L. Gortmaker. 2011. 'The Global Obesity Pandemic: Shaped by Global Drivers and Local Environments'. *Lancet* 378 (9793): 804–14. doi: http://dx.doi.org/10.1016/S0140-6736(11)60813-1.

Wang, Y. Clare, Pamela Coxson, Yu-Ming Shen, Lee Goldman and Kirsten Bibbins-Domingo. 2012. 'A Penny-Per-Ounce Tax on Sugar-Sweetened Beverages Would Cut Health and Cost Burdens of Diabetes'. *Health Aff (Millwood)* 31: 199–207. doi: 10.1377/hlthaff.2011.0410.

Weishaar, Heide, Amanda Amos and Jeff Collin. 2015. 'Best of Enemies: Using Social Network Analysis to Explore a Policy Network in European Smoke-Free Policy'. *Soc Sci Med* 133: 85–92. doi:10.1016/j.socscimed.2015.03.045.

WHO. 2003. 'Diet, Nutrition and the Prevention of Chronic Diseases'. Technical Report Series 916. Geneva: World Health Organization.

———. 2004. 'Global Strategy on Diet, Physical Activity and Health'. Report by the Secretariat. 57th World Health Assembly (A57/9). Geneva: World Health Organization.

Wiist, William H. 2010. *The Bottom Line or Public Health: Tactics Corporations Use to Influence Health and Health Policy, and What We Can Do to Counter Them*. Oxford: Oxford University Press.

YesOnD. 2015. 'Berkeley vs. Big Soda'. www.berkeleyvsbigsoda.com.

Zingale, Daniel. 2012. 'Gulp! The High Cost of Big Soda's Victory'. *Los Angeles Times*, 9 December. http://articles.latimes.com/2012/dec/09/opinion/la-oe-zingale-soda-tax-campaign-funding-20121209.

FIVE

Examples of Failures to Regulate Mining and Smelting Emissions and Their Consequent Effects on Human Health Outcomes

Mark Patrick Taylor and Steven George

Australia has been a world leader in lead mining, smelting and processing for over a century. The industry, government agencies and officials, and regulators have historically downplayed the adverse health impacts associated with production (Taylor 2012; Taylor et al. 2014a). This is despite longstanding and well-documented evidence of the adverse health effects of lead exposure, especially in children. Today, there are ongoing concerns for three Australian communities that are severely lead contaminated—Broken Hill, Port Pirie and Mount Isa (Taylor et al. 2011; Taylor et al. 2014a; Taylor et al. 2014b; Earl et al. 2015). Port Pirie in South Australia particularly illustrates the conflicting objectives faced by regulators. Lead smelting in Port Pirie has been ongoing since 1889, producing over a century of environmental emissions that continue to blanket the community with lead and other toxic metal dust. This has earned Port Pirie the dubious title of Australia's most lead contaminated town (Taylor 2012).

This chapter sets out the lengthy histories of toxic pollution, conflicts over evidence, and ultimately regulatory failures in Port Pirie. It begins by describing the recognized methods for measuring lead exposure, and the results for this specific community. Data show that emissions of lead and smelting-related toxic substances, including sulphur dioxide, continue to regularly exceed acceptable levels (Taylor et al. 2014a). The chapter then argues that, despite decades of clear evidence of harmful health effects (Landrigan 1983; Fowler and Grabosky 1989; Taylor 2012), there has been a history of ineffective government action. Until recently, the government has remained relatively passive to these risks or, at worst, complicit in ignoring them (Taylor 2012). It shows that at the heart of Port Pirie's ongoing contamination lies powerful corporate interests that have been given precedence over effective environmental and health protections. This chapter offers lessons regarding the challenges of holding corporations to account, even in well-resourced settings of high-income countries where public health evidence abounds (cf. Sullivan 2014).

BACKGROUND

Port Pirie is a seaport approximately 220 kilometres north of Adelaide. The city hosts one of the world's largest lead smelters, currently owned and operated by Nyrstar Port Pirie. As a result, it has experienced a long history of industrial emissions and associated lead exposure. As early as 1925, the South Australian Royal Commission on Plumbism (lead poisoning) identified fine lead dust as the principal cause of poisoning (South Australia Royal Commission on Plumbism 1925). In 1976 and 1981, the Commonwealth Scientific and Industrial Research Organisation (CSIRO) demonstrated that the smelter was the source of lead contamination in soils, crops and vegetables around the Port Pirie area (ECOS 1976, 1981), thus requiring locally produced grains to be blended to meet international food export standards (Crikey 2004). Throughout the 1980s and 1990s, government officials argued that historic lead smelter dust emissions, held in the city's soils and home environments, were the primary cause of elevated blood lead in children (Body et al. 1991). However, the Environment Protection Authority of South Australia's (EPASA) published lead-in-air data, and SA Health blood lead measures in children aged zero to four years, show that contemporary and historical lead-in-air emissions are the primary causes of elevated blood-lead levels in Port Pirie children (Taylor 2011; Taylor et al. 2013; Taylor et al. 2014a).

EPASA data indicate that atmospheric emissions of lead have been rising in Port Pirie since 2013 (Taylor and Isley 2014; EPASA 2014). According to EPASA monitoring, lead-in-air values have exceeded the annual National Environmental Protection Measures (NEPM) guidelines every year since monitoring was implemented in 2007 (Mitchell 2014). Consequently, more than three thousand children in Port Pirie during the previous decade have been lead poisoned (Taylor 2012). The data shows at least 47.5 percent of the city's children between zero to four years have blood lead (PbB) levels of >5 µg/dL (micrograms per decilitre), the new intervention value (above which intervention is recommended) for Aus-

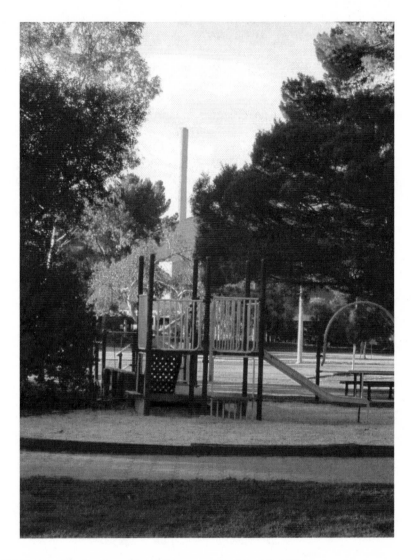

Figure 5.1. The lead smelter chimney overlooking Port Pirie

tralians (National Health and Medical Research Council 2015; Simon, Lewis and Pumpa 2015).

Moreover, although children are born with relatively low PbB levels (well below 5 µg/dL), blood lead rises rapidly after two to three months of age, demonstrating that environmental lead emissions are difficult to avoid (Simon et al. 2007). At this age, children are not mobile and thus primarily exposed in their cots to lead dust deposits on their own and their parent's clothing and skin. By the time children are twenty-four months old, the geometric mean PbB level is 6.6 μg/dL (above the new NHMRC guidelines) and are at risk of neurocognitive damage (National Toxicology Program [NTP] 2012a).

Childhood exposure to lead has been linked to lower intelligence measures and academic achievement, and to a range of socio-behavioural problems such as attention deficit hyperactivity disorder (ADHD), learning difficulties, oppositional/conduct disorders and delinquency (Baghurst et al. 1992; Lanphear et al. 2002; Lanphear et al. 2005; Jusko et al. 2003; Zahran et al. 2009; Lucchini et al. 2012; NTP 2012b; Zhang et al. 2012). Disabling mental health issues from lead exposure often persist into adolescence and adulthood. The economic costs arising from childhood lead exposure are also significant. Lead toxicity is estimated to cost US$50 billion per annum in the United States and up to €22.7 billion in France (Pichery et al. 2011; Trasande and Liu 2011). Fortunately, lead exposures are entirely preventable and cost-effective. Each dollar spent on lead exposure reductions in housing has been found to return estimated societal benefits of between US$17 and US$220 (Gould 2009).

In 2012, the U.S. Centers for Disease Control and Prevention (CDC) lowered its designated action threshold for blood-lead (PbB) to 5.0 μg/dL after reviewing accepting research evidence that there is no safe threshold. The CDC also acknowledged the need for earlier interventions to limit damage to children. In May 2015, the Australian National Health and Medical Research Council (NHMRC) followed suit, lowering the level for intervention to 5.0 μg/dL, but took a slightly different policy approach. Internationally, most agree that there is 'no safe level' of exposure (Taylor, Winder and Lanpear 2014). While this phrase was present in previous NHMRC-led advisories, it was absent in the 2015 report (NHMRC 2015). The NHMRC contends that evidence of health effects at exposures < 10 μg/dL is less clear than for exposures above this level, a position in conflict with a range of respected bodies including the CDC, U.S. Environmental Protection Agency (EPA), Health Canada and WHO.

Methods

To analyse the role of corporate interests in the regulation of lead exposure in Australia, we draw together works published by the first author since 2010, with new and updated perspectives based on additional information gathered since 2014. We use a 'multiple methods' approach to understand the health risks associated with environmental smelter emissions and subsequent exposure. The chapter draws on published data from dust and soil sampling, ambient air monitoring and childhood blood lead testing and reporting. This data is triangulated with Australian and international standards drawn from numerous sources including peer-reviewed articles and South Australian government reports. The source data in this chapter has typically been tested in accredited laboratories using certified reference materials and quality assurance approaches. Details of the methods used can be found in the referenced articles by the first author.

Importantly, we set out how recognized methods for, and results from, the measurement of lead exposure have been influenced by industry interests. We describe the role of the industry in collecting, analysing and using the above data to influence regulatory measures. These practices are compared with those in other countries and internationally by recognized authorities.

PROBLEMS WITH METHODS USED TO MONITOR ENVIRONMENTAL EMISSIONS

Appropriate methods and data sources for monitoring environmental emissions are essential for effective regulation. The EPASA's lead-in-air monitoring has been undertaken at four sites in Port Pirie—Ellen Street (2001), Frank Green Park (1999), Oliver Street (1998) and Pirie West Primary (1995) (figure 5.2). At Oliver Street, emissions of sulphur dioxide (SO_2), another environmental contaminant emitted to the atmosphere from smelting operations, is also measured. Exposure to SO_2 is known to adversely affect respiratory and lung system function, and cause irritation of the eyes (Williams et al. 2012). Although Australia has set national standards for SO_2 emissions, these are not enforceable unless reflected in state or territory legislation, or in individual facility licence arrangements. Relevantly, air quality standards pertaining to SO_2 are absent from the Nyrstar licence (EPASA 2012). At the Oliver Street SO_2 monitoring station, the NEPM 0.2 ppm SO_2 one-hour standard was exceeded forty-three and sixty-eight times in 2013 and 2014, respectively (figure 5.3). Other neurotoxic metals such as arsenic and cadmium are not routinely measured although are known to exceed acceptable international air quality concentrations (Taylor et al. 2014a). Lead-in-air data is collected every sixth day according to methods detailed in Standards Australia (Australian Government 2005) and reported in the annual NEPM statements. The EPASA also collects lead-in-air data from West Pirie Primary School and Ellen Street as part of its routine monitoring but these are not part of the national reporting for the NEPMs.

It is notable that lead-in-air monitoring for the purpose of assessment against Nyrstar's licence requirements is based on industry, rather than EPA, data. Nyrstar maintains a monitoring network of thirteen sites across Port Pirie, with four co-located next to EPASA sites (figure 5.2). Industry data reported to EPAs are typically not made publicly available. An exception is New South Wales, where monitoring data, collected as part of a facility's licence, is required to be published since 2012 (New South Wales EPA 2012). To remain licensed, Nyrstar must provide data

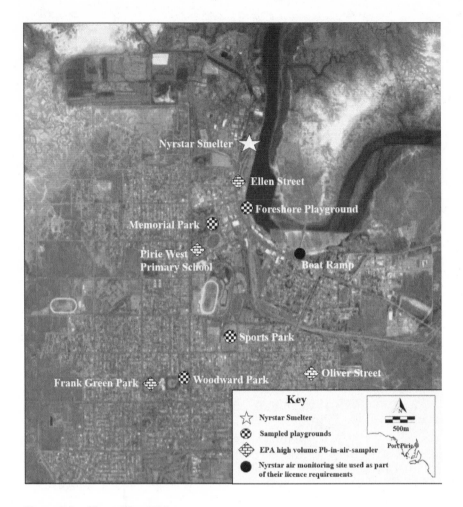

Figure 5.2. Map of Port Pirie

from its air monitoring sites located at the Boat Ramp, Pirie West Primary School, Oliver Street and Ellen Street (EPASA 2012). For regulatory purposes, only data from the Frank Green Park and Oliver Street sites are used for national air quality monitoring and reporting (NEPM) purposes. This is problematic for two reasons.

First, these NEPM sites are located more than three kilometres from the smelter, in areas considered medium risk for lead exposures (Maynard, Franks and Malcolm 2006). The use of these more distant sites, for NEPM reporting, underestimates the industry's total impact on local air quality. As a result, although the whole city is impacted by emissions, this is not properly captured in the annual NEPM reporting using the data only from Frank Green Park and Oliver Street. Recent assessments

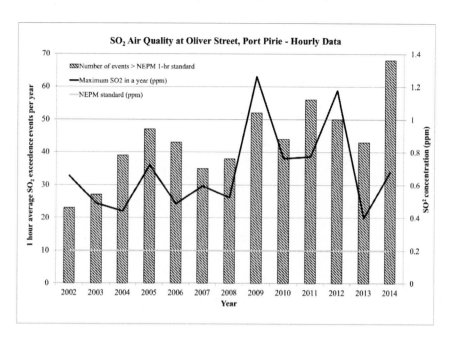

Figure 5.3.   Port Pirie air quality, hourly data

of aerosol and dust data from playgrounds (Taylor et al. 2013; Taylor et al. 2014a; Taylor et al. 2015) confirm that although these locations have lower levels of contamination, they frequently remain above acceptable values. Assessment of hand lead levels following fixed play routines at public playgrounds show that they decline with distance from the smelter. However, values remain at levels that pose a clear risk to human health, even after playgrounds have been subject to washing routines executed by the local council and Nyrstar (Taylor et al. 2015).

Second, as part of Nyrstar's licensing, the South Australian EPA uses a rolling annual average to determine acceptable lead-in-air results (set at 0.5 µg/m³). This does not properly capture the impact from significantly elevated short-term pollution spikes. Admittedly, this approach is better than the existing national standard, which is set at 0.5 µg/m³ and calculated as an average concentration over a calendar year. Nevertheless, air quality data from 2011 (Taylor et al. 2014a, see figure 10 therein) shows that the whole of the city of Port Pirie experienced multiple short-term lead-in-air concentration spikes exceeding the 0.5 µg/m³ annual standard. The site closest to the smelter, Ellen Street, recorded a twenty-four-hour lead-in-air spike of > 22 µg/m³. An Australian review of health data for air quality standards acknowledged that ambient levels should not exceed 0.5 µg/m³ 'at any time' (Streeton 2000). Nevertheless, spikes in emis-

sions are still not considered as part of existing environmental licences in
Port Pirie or anywhere elsewhere in Australia.

UNDERREPORTING AS A RESULT OF MISLEADING STATISTICS

The aforementioned shortcomings, with respect to field sampling problems, are also reflected in the underreporting of blood lead exposures in
Port Pirie children by government and media. Typically, reports cite the
percentage of children with a blood lead > 10 µg/dL, inclusive of maternal surrogate values (in May 2015 the reporting value was changed to 5
µg/dL in light of the NHMRC lowering the intervention value). Surrogate
values include a mother's blood lead level, in place of a child's (Simon,
Lewis and Pumpa 2015), for children less than nine months old whose
blood has not yet been tested (David Simon, personal communication).
Figure 5.4 clearly shows the effect of using surrogate blood lead levels for
reporting purposes, in that it clearly reduces the number of children who
present with 'elevated blood lead levels'. This approach also does not
take into account the fact that childhood blood lead levels rise markedly
after the first thirty-five days of a child's life (Simon et al. 2007).

Additionally, for SA Health's end-of-year (annual) blood lead reporting, only the last test for a child that year is reported. Again, this results
in a lower reporting of the percentage of children impacted by elevated
blood lead values. Typically, when a child presents with an elevated
blood lead level, SA Health will intervene and provide advice and awareness training for parents. Under such circumstances, a child would be

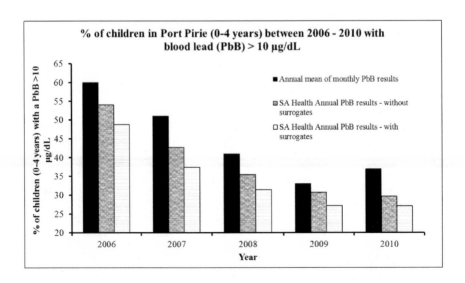

Figure 5.4.   Blood lead levels in children of Port Pirie

followed up and retested multiple times to ensure exposure levels are reduced. However, for the purposes of periodic blood lead reports, only the most recent blood lead result is used to calculate the percentage of children above or below > 10 µg/dL, even where a child has been tested multiple times in a year (Simon et al. 2015). By contrast, the data in figure 5.4 reflect the annual mean monthly percentages of all children who returned a blood lead test > 10 µg/dL, and include repeat measures on the same child in any one year. This selective use of data is misleading, deflating the blood lead levels reported from 2006 to 2010. SA Health has perpetuated this method of health assessment despite clear evidence of its problematic nature (Taylor et al. 2014a).

FAILURE OF REGULATORY APPROACHES TO REDUCE EXPOSURE

It is argued that the flaws in the above-described methods and data sources, resulting in the underreporting of environmental emissions in Port Pirie, reflect failures in the regulatory approaches taken by the Australian government over many decades. Historically, inadequate actions to limit or eliminate Port Pirie's significant smelter emissions, totalling forty-seven tonnes of lead into the air in 2013–2014, have allowed lead-rich particulates to contaminate indoor and outdoor surfaces, soils and the atmosphere over a long period of time (National Pollutant Inventory 2015; Taylor et al. 2013; Taylor et al. 2015). In 1983, paediatrician Phillip Landrigan (1983) called for urgent action in a report commissioned by the Australian Minister of Health. Landrigan identified airborne lead, and its accidental ingestion from atmospherically contaminated dust and soil, as the main sources of exposure. While the report acknowledged that some useful work was undertaken by a task force set up in 1983 to deal with the problem, the goal of reducing blood lead levels in 95 percent of children <5 years old, to below 10 µg/dL by 2010, was never reached. Although blood lead levels had fallen by 2010, more than 25 percent of children were still presenting each year with blood lead levels above 10 µg/dL, placing them at serious risk of neurological damage.

Taylor et al. (2013; 2015) identified highly elevated dust deposits containing arsenic, cadmium and lead on playgrounds across Port Pirie. As a result, the local council and the Nyrstar smelter company have undertaken regular washing of playgrounds. Subsequent checks found, however, that the benefits of washing was time-limited and did little to reduce pervasive and persistent contaminations that blanket the city (Taylor et al. 2014a; Taylor et al. 2015). Residents are currently advised to protect themselves by washing hands, surfaces and food, and limiting the transport of dust and soil from outside (Targeted Lead Abatement Program 2015). This approach has proven problematic for two reasons. First, a recent review of household interventions for preventing domestic lead exposure in children found that household interventions showed that educational advice and related practices are not effective at reducing exposures over time (Yeoh et al. 2012). Second, this approach inappropriately pushes primary responsibility onto local residents to protect themselves from a seriously polluting industry, rather than implementing effective emission capture. Indeed, such an approach runs contrary to the principles of primary prevention, the gold standard of public health policy, which is to address a known problem at its source and before consequences become apparent in the population.

THE PORT PIRIE SMELTER TRANSFORMATION PROJECT: A CHANGE FOR A HEALTHIER FUTURE OR BUSINESS AS USUAL?

The methods of data collection, analysis and reporting described above, much of which has been influenced by industry interests, continue to downplay the true nature and extent of Port Pirie's environmental problems. Substantial research now available, however, challenges official data and provides clear evidence of the urgent need for more effective regulatory action by government (e.g., van Alphen 1999; Maynard, Franks and Malcolm 2006; Simon et al. 2007). As Simon et al. (2007) write, residing in Port Pirie is akin to 'living in a sea of lead' from which there is no escape. Nevertheless, some continue to deny the scale of the problem. For example, member of the South Australian Parliament for Frome Geoff Brock maintained that Port Pirie does not deserve its negative image: 'I think it is unwarranted, quite frankly. We have got that stigma of . . . a polluted city, and we are not a polluted city. It is an inherited issue through the lead smelter over many, many years' (Sara 2012). Such dismissals of the pollution problem, as simply a legacy of the past, reflect why effective action has been difficult to implement for over three decades.

Following a 2011 report to the EPASA on lead-in-air exposure (Taylor et al. 2011) and the publication of independent evidence of the problem and associated extensive media coverage, a number of government-industry collaborations to clean up Port Pirie have been initiated. Notably, this includes an upgrade of the smelter at an estimated cost of AU$514 million, which was approved in 2015 (Government of South Australia 2015). Nyrstar has also committed AU$3 million annually over ten years to a Targeted Lead Abatement Program (TLAP), with additional start-up funds of AU$5 million to accelerate the TLAP objectives (Targeted Lead Abatement Program 2015). The South Australia government has also committed AU$1.5 million per year for ten years towards the TLAP.

While these commitments mark a clear shift by the government and industry, in recognising and responding to the persistent environmental and human health issues in Port Pirie, there remain a number of concerns. Notably, existing and new statutory instruments used to frame the smelter upgrade remain problematic. Although the smelter upgrade and proposed clean-ups in the city are positive outcomes, state government capture appears to remain evident.

At the federal level, the government stipulated that air quality standards were legally binding at each level of government, and set a goal that states and territories would meet all standards by 2008 (Australian Government 2005). While these standards are legally binding, there is no mechanism for enforcement unless the relevant values have been stipulated in a facilities environmental protection licence, such as those for the Nyrstar operations (e.g., Environment Protection Authority South Australia [EPASA] 2012). Therefore, in practical terms, it is clear that the individual states of the Australian Commonwealth retain significant discretion in terms of enforcement of the NEPM (1998) air quality standards.

At the state level, as part of the Port Pirie smelter transformation project, the South Australian government introduced new legislation and adopted new obligations regarding smelter management. The state government announced that it would to provide a guarantee/indemnity of up to AUS$115 million for potential environmental, health and property liabilities, to help attract external financing for the proposed Port Pirie smelter upgrade (Weatherill 2013). This amount also includes protection for the minister and related staff from any future litigation regarding the *Port Pirie Smelting Facility (Lead-in-Air Concentrations) Act 2013* (South Australia) (box 5.1). The legislation was designed to provide environmental certainty (e.g., guarantees in regard to air quality standards) for the operation of the new smelter. Of particular concern, in light of the long history of South Australia not addressing environmental and human health concerns appropriately or adequately, are sections 4 and 5 of the act. These sections reveal that the South Australia government curtailed the independent power of South Australia's EPA to alter Nyrstar's conditions in regard to the maximum allowable lead-in-air concentrations.

Box 5.1. Extracts from the *Port Pirie Smelting Facility (Lead-in-Air Concentrations) Act 2013* (SA).

4 – Provisions relating to reduction of maximum lead-in-air condition by Environment Protection Authority

1. The Environment Authority may not, during the period commencing on the project completion date and ending on the commencement day, vary a maximum lead-in-air condition in a way that would have the effect of reducing the maximum specific in the condition unless the Environment Protection Authority has consulted with –

---

a. the Manufacturing Minister; and
b. the Company

2. The Environment Protection Authority may not, during the prescribed period, vary a maximum lead-in-air condition in a way that would have the effect of reducing the maximum specified in the condition.
3. Subsection (2) does not apply if –

a. the Manufacturing Minister approves the variation; or
b. the Company consents to the variation

5 – Maximum lead-in-air condition not affected by other laws of State

1. The law of the State is modified so that any requirements applying (whether directly or indirectly) to the Company under –

a. a law of the State; or
b. a relevant authorisation,

that would have the effect of reducing the maximum permissible air concentration of lead at a location or locations in Port Pirie specific in a condition of a relevant environmental authorisation (a *relevant requirement*), is taken not to apply (but only to the extent that the relevant requirement has that effect and except as provided in sub-section (3) to the Company during the prescribed period).

These administrative and legal decisions appear to place the opera-tions of a smelter company ahead of the rights and interests of the com-munity and public health outcomes. In particular, the limitations applied to the functions of South Australia's Environment Protection Authority under the *Port Pirie Smelting Facility Act* would appear to contradict the *Environment Protection Act 1993* (South Australia) that was enacted to define the Environment Protection Authority's functions and powers (box 5.2). The *Environment Protection Act 1993* (South Australia) states that the act's objective is to 'to facilitate the adoption and implementation of environment protection measures agreed on by the State under inter-governmental arrangements for greater uniformity and effectiveness in environment protection'. This statement appears to relate to schedule 4 of the Intergovernmental Agreement on the Environment (1992) (Austra-lian Government 2010). The Intergovernmental Agreement, ratified by all Australian states and territories, explicitly states that there should be harmonization of legislation across the Commonwealth of Australia, and that all Australians should have equal protection from environmental pollution. Thus, it would appear that the construction of the *Port Pirie*

Smelting Facility (Lead-in-Air Concentrations) Act 2013 (South Australia) is specifically designed to erode these established rights. Further, the legislation provides an environmental emissions gift by offering Nyrstar a competitive advantage compared to other industries or locations in the state of South Australia.

Box 5.2. Extracts from the Objects from the *Environment Protection Act 1993* (SA).

10 – Objects of Act

1. The object of this Act are –

    a. to promote the following principles (***principles of ecologically sustainable development***):

        a. that the use, development and protection of the environment should be managed in a way, and at a rate, that will enable people and communities to provide for their economic, social and physical wellbeing and for their health and safety while –

            a. sustaining the potential of natural and physical resources to meet the reasonably foreseeable needs of the future generations; and

            b. safeguarding the life-supporting capacity of air, water, land and ecosystems; and

            c. avoiding, remedying or mitigating any adverse effects of ativities on the environment;

        b. that proper weight should be given to both long and short term economic, environmental, social and equity considerations in deciding all matters relating to environmental protection, restoration and enhancement; and

    b. to ensure that all reasonable and practicable measures are taken to protect, restore and enhance the quality of the environment having regard to the principles of ecologically sustainable development, and - ...

1. to coordinate activities, policies and programmes necessary to prevent, reduce and minimise or eliminate environmental harm and ensure effective environmental protection, restoration and enhancement; and

---

> 2. to facilitate the adoption and implementation of environmen-
> tal protection measures agreed on by the State under inter-
> governmental arrangements for greater uniformity and effec-
> tiveness in environment protection; and ...

There are clear analogies between this piece of South Australian legislation and the *Mount Isa Mines Limited Agreement Act 1985, 1997* in Queensland. Mount Isa's Transitional Environmental Program permits smelter
emissions to exceed Queensland state-wide standards (Taylor et al.
2014a). In both of these environmental licence arrangement examples, the
needs of a specific industry and their economic requirements are placed
ahead of known environmental and health concerns. The special arrangements, in effect, provide a business advantage by virtue of not requiring
more stringent and immediate environmental management controls on
pollution, which of course increase operating costs.

CONCLUSION

Exposure to preventable emissions that result in elevated blood lead values is unacceptable for anyone, notably children. The longstanding
source and extent of Port Pirie's lead pollution problem is well-documented, and the well-known solutions available to government and industry are supported by clear evidence. The smelter is located too close to
the community, a situation unlikely to be permitted under contemporary
environmental and human health standards. To eliminate exposures, either the smelter must be closed or the most vulnerable populations
moved several kilometres away from operations. While both solutions
may appear to be radical options to government and industry, they are
consistent with the long-established opinions of Landrigan (1983) and
also those of Turner (1909), who asserted more than a century ago: 'The
curative treatment consists essentially in removing the child from the
source of the poison. We adopt also other measures calculated to encourage the elimination of lead from the system, but to what extent these are
efficacious must be a matter of doubt. By themselves they are useless'.

This chapter argues that at the heart of this issue lies a conflict between the private interests of industry and individuals and the public
health concerns of communities. For more than a century, the failures of
governance and regulation of Port Pirie's lead smelting operations can be
seen to reflect the government's decision to give greater value to the
economic gains from the lead mining, smelting, and processing industry
than to the environmental and public health costs to local communities.
From the recurrent experiences of mining and smelter communities, it is
argued that economic objectives have taken precedence over human
health needs, resulting in clear examples of environmental injustice (cf.

Sicotte 2009). This is particularly evident in small, isolated communities such as Port Pirie where economic alternatives to dominant industries are virtually non-existent.

Importantly, Port Pirie's history exemplifies a systemic failure of government to effectively tackle pollution and well-known human health risks (e.g., Fowler and Grabosky 1989; Sullivan 2014; Taylor, Winder and Lanpear, 2014; Taylor et al. 2014a; Taylor et al. 2014b; Spear, Thomas and Shrader-Frechette 2015). This chapter highlights the subtle, but real impact corporations have in influencing the methods for collecting, analysing and reporting data on the problem. The government, in turn, has long accepted such approaches despite evidence suggesting substantial under-reporting of the public health impacts of lead-in-air exposures.

This chapter contends that, despite the continued accumulation of evidence and profound public health impacts, this situation persists, despite recent improvements. The South Australian government's approval of a smelter transformation project in 2015, which includes a refit with modern, clean technology, coupled with remediation across the city, is intended to reduce lead exposures from air, dust and soil significantly. Reconciling the persistent gap between evidence and practice will require fundamental changes to the production of knowledge about environmental contamination problems, in this case lead, and how it is reported and used by government. This chapter concludes that these changes are urgently needed before appropriate improvements can be achieved in regulatory action. Further, better data transparency (collection and reporting methods) is required to facilitate better public understanding of the problem, which will help drive long-term reductions in environmental lead exposures.

REFERENCES

Australian Government. 2005. 'National Standards for Criteria Air Pollutants in Australia'. Department of Sustainability, Environment, Water, Population and Communities. www.environment.gov.au/atmosphere/airquality/publications/standards.html.

Australian Government. 2010. 'Intergovernmental Agreement on the Environment 1992'. Department of Sustainability, Environment, Water, Population and Communities. Canberra, Australia. www.environment.gov.au/node/13008.

Baghurst, Peter, Shilu Tong, Andrew J. McMichael, Evalyn F. Robertson, Neil R. Wigg and Graham Vimpani. 1992. 'Determinants of Blood Lead Concentrations to, Age 5 Years in a Birth Cohort Study of Children Living in the Lead Smelting City of Port Pirie and Surrounding Areas'. *Archives of Environmental Health* 47: 203–10. doi:10.1080/00039896.1992.9938350.

Body, Peter. E., Geoffrey Inglis, Peter R. Dolan and Denis E. Mulcahy. 1991. 'Environmental Lead: A Review'. *Critical Reviews in Environmental Control* 5: 299–310. doi:10.1080/10643389109388403.

Crikey. 2004. 'Port Pirie and SA Grains Blending'. www.crikey.com.au/2004/11/09/port-pirie-and-sa-grains-blending.

Earl, Rachel, Nicholas Burns, Ted Nettelbeck and Peter Baghurst. 2015. 'Low-Level Environmental Lead Exposure Still Negatively Associated with Children's Cognitive Abilities'. *Australian Journal of Psychology*. doi: 10.1111/ajpy.12096.

ECOS. 1976. 'Toxic Metals around Port Pirie'. *ECOS* 7: 27–31. www.ecosmagazine. com/?act=view_file&file_id=EC07p27.pdf.

———. 1981. 'Pollution of Crops and Pasture by a Smelter'. *ECOS* 28: 27–28. www. ecosmagazine.com/?act=view_file&file_id=EC28p27.pdf.

Environment Protection Authority South Australia (EPASA). 2012. 'Licence EPA 775— Nyrstar Port Pirie Pty Ltd. Environment Protection Act 1993'. www.epa.sa.gov.au/ licence_docs/EPA775%20-%20Nyrstar%20Port%20Pirie%20Pty%20Ltd%20- %20Port%20Pirie.pdf.

Fowler, Rob, and Peter Grabosky. 1989. 'Lead Pollution and the Children of Port Pirie'. In *Stains on a White Collar: Fourteen Studies in Corporate Crime or Corporate Harm*, edited by Peter Grabosky and Adam Sutton, 143–59. Sydney: Federation Press.

Gould, Elise. 2009. 'Childhood Lead Poisoning: Conservative Estimates of the Social and Economic Benefits of Lead Hazard Control'. *Environmental Health Perspectives* 117: 1162–67. doi:10.1289/ehp.0800408.

Government of South Australia. 1993. 'Environment Protection Act (South Australia)'. www.austlii.edu.au/au/legis/sa/consol_act/epa1993284.

———. 2013. 'Port Pirie Smelting Facility (Lead-In-Air Concentrations) Act'. www.austlii.edu.au/au/legis/sa/consol_act/ppsfca2013526.

———. 2015. 'SA Strategic Plan'. http://saplan.org.au/targets/42-minerals-production-and-processing.

Jusko, Todd A., Charles R. Henderson Jr., Bruce P. Lanphear, Deborah A. Cory-Slechta, Patrick J. Parsons and Richard L. Canfield. 2008. 'Blood Lead Concentrations < 10 µg/dL and Child Intelligence at 6 Years of Age'. *Environmental Health Perspectives* 116: 243–48.

Landrigan, Philip J. 1983. *Lead Exposure, Lead Absorption and Lead Toxicity in the Children of Port Pirie: A Second Opinion*. Adelaide: South Australian Health Commission.

Lanphear, Bruce P., Richard Hornung, Jane Khoury et al. 2005. 'Low-Level Environmental Lead Exposure and Children's Intellectual Function: An International Pooled Analysis'. *Environmental Health Perspectives* 113: 894–99. doi:10.1289/ ehp.7688.

Lanphear, Bruce P., Richard Hornung, Mona Ho, Cynthia R. Howard, Shirley Eberly and Karen Knauf. 2002. 'Environmental Lead Exposure during Early Childhood'. *The Journal of Pediatrics* 140: 40–47. doi:10.1067/mpd.2002.120513.

Lucchini, Roberto G., Silvia Zoni, Stefano Guazzetti et al. 2012. 'Inverse Association of Intellectual Function with Very Low Blood Lead but Not with Manganese Exposure in Italian Adolescents'. *Environmental Research* 118: 65–71. doi:10.1016/ j.envres.2012.08.003.

Maynard, Edward, Lynda J. Franks and Mark S. Malcolm. 2006. 'The Port Pirie Lead Implementation Program: Future Focus and Directions.' South Australian Department of Health. www.sahealth.sa.gov.au/wps/wcm/connect/651e880048 f416a3a672e70e3d7ae4ad/ptpirie-future-focus-06.pdf?MOD=AJPERES&CACHEID= 651e880048f416a3a672e70e3d7ae4ad.

Mitchell, R. 2014. *Air Monitoring Report for South Australia 2013: Compliance with the National Environment Protection (Ambient Air Quality) Measure, June 2014*. Adelaide, South Australia: South Australia Environmental Protection Authority. www.scew.gov.au/system/files/resources/7c4e85af-5d11-9074-d171-0184e06fc243/ files/sa-aaq-nepm-sir-monitoring-report-2013.pdf.

National Environment Protection Measure (NEPM). 1998. 'Ambient Air Quality Standards'. Department of Sustainability, Environment, Water, Population and Communities. www.environment.gov.au/protection/air-quality/air-quality-standards.

National Health and Medical Research Council (NHMRC). 2015. 'NHMRC Statement: Evidence on the Effects of Lead on Human Health'. www.nhmrc.gov.au/_files_

nhmrc/publications/attachments/eh58_nhmrc_statement_lead_effects_human_
health_a.pdf.
National Pollutant Inventory. 2015. '2013/2014 Report for Nyrstar Port Pirie Pty Ltd,
Nyrstar Port Pirie—Port Pirie, SA'. www.npi.gov.au/npidata/action/load/individu-
alfacilitydetail/criteria/state/SA/year/2014/jurisdiction-facility/SA0018.
National Toxicology Program (NTP). 2012a. 'NTP Monograph: Health Effects of Low-
Level Lead'. U.S. Department of Health and Human Services. http://
ntp.niehs.nih.gov/ntp/ohat/lead/final/monographhealtheffectslowlevel-
lead_newissn_508.pdf#search=health%20effects%20of%20lowlevel%20lead.
———. 2012b. 'National Toxicology Program Monograph on Health Effects of Low-
Level Lead'. http://ntp.niehs.nih.gov/NTP/ohat/Lead/Final/MonographHealthEf-
fectsLowLevelLead_prepublication_508.pdf.
New South Wales Environment Protection Authority. 2012. 'Requirements for Publishing Pollution Monitoring Data'. www.environment.nsw.gov.au/resources/legis-
lation/20120263reqpubpmdata.pdf.
Pichery, Celine, Martine Bellanger, Denis Zmirou-Navier, Philippe Glorennec, Philippe Hartemann and Philippe Grandjean. 2011. 'Childhood Lead Exposure in
France: Benefit Estimation and Partial Cost-Benefit Analysis of Lead Hazard Control'. *Environmental Health* 10: 1–12. doi:10.1186/1476-069X-10-44.
Sara, Sally. 2012. 'Towns' Fate Tied to Struggling Smelter'. *ABC News*, 10 July.
www.abc.net.au/news/2012-07-10/pirie-smelter-pm/4122114.
Sicotte, Diane. 2009. 'Power, Profit and Pollution: The Persistence of Environmental
Injustice in a Company Town'. *Human Ecology Review* 16 (2):141–50.
Simon, David L., Edward J. Maynard and Katherine D. Thomas. 2007. 'Living in a Sea
of Lead—Changes in Blood- and Hand-Lead of Infants Living Near a Smelter'.
Journal of Exposure Science and Environmental Epidemiology 17: 248–59. doi:10.1038/
sj.jes.7500512.
Simon, David, Carolyn Lewis and Lucy Pumpa. 2015. *Port Pirie Blood Lead Levels—
Analysis of Blood Lead Levels for the First Half of 2015 (1 January–30 June 2015)*. Government of South Australia: SA Health. www.sahealth.sa.gov.au/wps/wcm/connect/
fba2f5004987061fa943a94564a15cee/Port+Pirie+Blood+Lead+Levels+Analysis+of+
blood+lead+levels+for+the+first....pdf?MOD=AJPERES&CACHEID=
fba2f5004987061fa943a94564a15cee.
South Australia Royal Commission on Plumbism. 1925. 'Report of the Royal Commission on Plumbism, together with Minutes of Evidence and Appendices'. Adelaide:
Government Printer.
Spear, Michael, Rebecca Thomas and Kristin Shrader-Frechette. 2015. 'Commentary:
Flawed Science Delays Smelter Cleanup and Worsens Health'. *Accountability in Re-
search: Policies and Quality Assurance* 22 (1): 41–60. doi:10.1080/08989621.2014.939746.
Streeton, Jonathan A. 2000. 'A Review on Existing Health Data on Six Pollutants'.
www.scew.gov.au/system/files/resources/9947318f-af8c-0b24-d928-04e4d3a4b25c/
files/aaq-rpt-review-existing-health-data-6-pollutants-report-streeton-199705-re-
print-200006.pdf.
Sullivan, Marianne. 2014. *Tainted Earth: Smelters, Public Health and the Environment*.
New Brunswick: Rutgers University Press.
Targeted Lead Abatement Program. 2015. www.tlap.com.au.
Taylor, Mark P. 2011. 'Report for the Environment Protection Authority, South Austra-
lia: Examination of the Relationship between Nyrstar Port Pirie Pty Ltd Smelter,
Airborne Lead Emissions and Environmental Health Impacts'.
———. 2012. 'Lead Poisoning of Port Pirie Children: A Long History of Looking the
Other Way'. *The Conversation*, 19 July. http://theconversation.edu.au/lead-poison-
ing-of-port-pirie-children-a-long-history-of-looking-the-other-way-8296.
Taylor, Mark P., Carolyn A. Schniering, Bruce P. Lanphear and Alison Jones. 2011.
'Lessons Learned on Lead Poisoning in Children: One-Hundred Years on from
Turner's Declaration'. *Journal of Paediatrics and Child Health* 47 (12): 849–56.
doi:10.1111/j.1440-1754.2010.01777.x.

Taylor, Mark P., Chris Winder and Bruce Lanphear. 2014. 'Australia's Leading Public Health Body Delays Action on the Revision of the Public Health Goal for Blood Lead Exposures'. *Environment International* 70: 113–17. doi:10.1016/j.envint.2014.04.023.

Taylor, Mark P., and Cynthia Isley. 2014. 'Measuring, Monitoring and Reporting but Not intervening: Air Quality in Australian Mining and Smelting Areas'. *Air Quality and Climate Change Journal* 48 (2): 35–42.

Taylor, Mark P., Danielle Camenzuli, Louise J. Kristensen, Miriam Forbes and Sammy Zahran. 2013. 'Environmental Lead Exposure Risks Associated with Children's Outdoor Playgrounds'. *Environmental Pollution* 178: 447–54. doi:10.1016/j.envpol.2013.03.054.

Taylor, Mark P., Peter J. Davies, Louise J. Kristensen and Janae L. Csavina. 2014a. 'Licenced to Pollute but Not to Poison: The Ineffectiveness of Regulatory Authorities at Protecting Public Health from Atmospheric Arsenic, Lead and Other Contaminants Resulting from Mining and Smelting Operations'. *Aeolian Research* 14: 35–52. doi:10.1016/j.aeolia.2014.03.003.

Taylor, Mark P., Sammy Zahran, Louise J. Kristensen and Marek Rouillon. 2015. 'Evaluating the Efficacy of Playground Washing to Reduce Environmental Metal Exposures'. *Environmental Pollution* 202: 112–19. doi:0.1016/j.envpol.2015.02.029.

Taylor, Mark P., Simon A. Mould, Louise J. Kristensen and Marek Rouillon. 2014b. 'Environmental Arsenic, Cadmium and Lead Dust Emissions from Metal Mine Operations: Implications for Environmental Management, Monitoring and Human Health'. *Environmental Research* 135: 296–303. doi:10.1016/j.envres.2014.08.036.

Trasande, Leonardo, and Yinghua Liu. 2011. 'Reducing the Staggering Costs of Environmental Disease in Children, Estimated at $76.6 billion in 2008'. *Health Affairs* 30: 863–70. doi:10.1377/hlthaff.2010.1239.

Turner, Alfred J. 1909. 'On Lead Poisoning in Childhood'. *BMJ* 1: 895–97.

van Alphen, Mike. 1999. 'Atmospheric Heavy Metal Deposition Plumes Adjacent to a Primary Lead-Zinc Smelter'. *Science of the Total Environment* 236: 119–34. doi:10.1016/S0048-9697(99)00272-7.

Weatherill, Jay. 2013. '2013–14 Budget Statement: Budget Paper 3'. Department of Treasury and Finance, South Australian Government. www.treasury.sa.gov.au/__data/assets/pdf_file/0020/2873/Budgetp3_201314.pdf.

Williams, Gail, Guy B. Marks, Lyn Denison and Bin Jalaludin. 2012. 'Australian Child Health and Air Pollution Study (ACHAPS)'. www.scew.gov.au/resource/australian-child-health-and-air-pollution-study-achaps-final-report.

Yeoh, Berlinda, Susan Woolfenden, Bruce Lanphear, Greta F. Ridley, Nuala Livingstone and Emile Jorgensen. 2014. 'Household Interventions for Preventing Domestic Lead Exposure in Children'. *Cochrane Database of Systematic Reviews 2014* 12 (CD006047). doi:10.1002/14651858.CD006047.pub4.

Zahran, Sammy, H. W. Mielke, Stefan Weiler, K. J. Berry and C. Gonzales. 2009. 'Children's Blood Lead and Standardized Test Performance Response as Indicators of Neurotoxicity in Metropolitan New Orleans Elementary Schools'. *NeuroToxicology* 30: 888–97. doi:10.1016/j.neuro.2009.07.017.

Zhang, Xiuwu, Linsheng Yang, Yonghua Li, Hairong Li, Wuyi Wang and Bixiong Ye. 2012. 'Impacts of Lead/Zinc Mining and Smelting on the Environment and Human Health in China'. *Environmental Monitoring and Assessment* 184 (4): 2261–73. doi:10.1007/s10661-011-2115-6.

II

Corporate Influence of Global Health Governance

SIX

Informal Channels of Corporate Influence on Global Health Policymaking

A Mapping of Strategies across Four Industries

Elina Suzuki and Suerie Moon

It is not just Big Tobacco anymore. Public health must also contend with Big Food, Big Soda, and Big Alcohol. All of these industries fear regulation, and protect themselves by using the same tactics. Research has documented these tactics well. They include front groups, lobbies, promises of self-regulation, lawsuits, and industry-funded research that confuses the evidence and keeps the public in doubt. —Margaret Chan, director-general of the World Health Organization, 2013

Traditionally, governments have been almost solely responsible for establishing rules (e.g., laws, policies, and regulations) to govern society at the national level. Classic international relations theory further considers governments to be the primary actors for creating rules at the international level. Since the start of the twenty-first century, however, new arrangements in global health[1] have signalled a shift, from purely public-based, to hybrid (public-private) or even wholly private forms of governance. Prominent examples of hybrid governance include the Global Fund to Fight AIDS, Tuberculosis and Malaria and Gavi, the Vaccine Alliance (Gavi), multibillion-dollar initiatives governed by representatives of state and non-state actors (e.g., corporations, civil society organizations and foundations). Public-private partnerships, also known as multi-stakeholder governance models, are now relatively common in global health (Buse and Tanaka 2011).

This trend has raised concerns about the risks of giving for-profit corporations a formal role in global governance processes (Buse and Tanaka 2011). While such partnerships can bring substantial new resources to health challenges, they have raised concerns about potential conflicts of interest, protection of the public interest and undue influence on policymaking (Buse and Walt 2000). Such concerns have come to the fore in debates over engagement by the World Health Organization (WHO) with the private for-profit sector. Since 2013, among the most contentious issues at the annual World Health Assembly (WHA) has been the draft 'Framework for Engagement with Non-State Actors' (FENSA), proposed rules for regulating how WHO works with industry, not-for-profit nongovernmental organizations (NGOs), foundations and academia (Ngo 2013; Saez 2014; Saez and New 2015; WHO 2015a). The most controversial point of debate regarding FENSA at the 2015 WHA pertained to the relationship between for-profit companies and WHO (Gopakumar and Alas 2015). WHO's policy for engaging with industry is particularly important because of the organization's influential normative work. WHO technical committees issue guidelines that can profoundly impact the business interests of corporations. For example, HIV treatment guidelines or the Model List of Essential Medicines influence which company's drugs will be purchased with billions of dollars in donor and government funds. WHO's non-binding codes of conduct can also wield significant normative force at the national level, as illustrated by the 1981 International Code of Marketing of Breastmilk Substitutes. One hundred and thirty countries adopted national legislation or policies restricting baby formula advertising within the three-year period after adoption of the code (Brady 2012). Finally, WHO has the constitutional authority to make binding international law through treaty negotiations, such as the 2003 Framework Convention on Tobacco Control (FCTC).

WHO is the lead organization for international rulemaking on public health, but rules adopted by organizations in the trade, agriculture and environment sectors also have health impacts (Lee, Sridhar and Patel 2009; Ottersen et al. 2014). It is therefore also important to consider the ways private for-profit interests shape rulemaking in trade and investment agreements, climate change negotiations, and other relevant forums.

In this chapter we define 'formal' channels as visible, sanctioned modes of participation such as voting seats on governing bodies, public participation in policy debates, or membership on technical advisory committees. We define 'informal' channels as less visible, not formally sanctioned, but nevertheless legal means of influencing rulemaking processes. We exclude illegal channels, such as bribery of government officials, from our analysis. Significant scholarly and policy attention has been paid to the rise of formal participation by private for-profit entities in global health governance (GHG). For example, FENSA largely focuses on regulating the formal ways in which corporations may influence WHO's normative work, such as restrictions on their participation in norm-setting or advisory bodies, or financing of such work. Critics have also raised concerns about industry participation, and absence of health representatives, in trade advisory committees to the U.S. government. Shaffer and Brenner (2004) argue that corporations use this channel to wield enormous influence over the positions that the U.S. government pursues in international trade talks. While attention to formal participation is merited, this chapter argues that insufficient attention is paid to *informal* channels used to shape global rulemaking processes. Indeed, neither the FENSA debate nor the literature on public-private partnerships in health adequately wrestles with the many informal channels of influence that have been raised as concerns. Through an analysis of four industries, this chapter seeks to better understand the strategies used to exert such influence. It concludes that protecting the integrity of policymaking processes from informal channels of influence can be more difficult precisely because they are less visible.

METHODS

We selected four health-related industries (tobacco, alcohol, food and non-alcoholic beverages, and pharmaceuticals) based on their transnational nature and direct relevance to health.[2] We then searched Google Scholar, JSTOR, and Web of Science, as well as industry- and health-specific literatures, using relevant search terms (e.g., 'alcohol/beverage/food/tobacco industry' AND 'global governance', 'regulation' and 'influence') to identify strategies used by these industries to influence global rulemaking processes. A snowball-sampling approach identified additional sources through a review of bibliographies.

Using an inductive approach, we identified four categories of strategies that emerged from this literature, and illustrate these strategies using specific examples. We highlight specific cases to underscore the similarities of tactics used across different sectors, despite the varied purposes, structures and histories of these industries. While the focus of this chapter is transnational, we highlight examples from both the national and global levels, given the cross-border impacts domestic policies and strategies can have. Evidence of informal channels of influence is best documented for the tobacco industry due to the public availability of internal documents, a result of litigation, whistle-blower disclosures and the Master Settlement Agreement in the United States (Hurt et al. 2009). For other industries there is far less public information available, but existing evidence is nonetheless informative. Commonalities across the four indus-

tries suggest that use of informal channels of influence is neither idiosyn-
cratic nor exceptional. It also suggests that policies to govern the influence of corporations in global health rulemaking should span multiple
industries rather than targeting individual sectors.

INFORMAL CHANNELS OF POLICY INFLUENCE

Lobbying

The scale of corporate spending on lobbying at the national level
underscores their enormous financial power and potential to influence
policy. More than US$170 million was spent in the United States on to-
bacco lobbying efforts between 1999 and 2007 (Holden and Lee 2009). The
pharmaceutical and health industry spent more money lobbying the U.S.
government in 2011, over US$200 million, than the governments of sixty-
four countries each spent on health expenditures (Center for Responsive
Politics n.d.; WHO 2015b). Importantly, other strategies for influencing
policy makers—such as donating to politicians' favoured charitable
causes (Fooks et al. 2011)—are not disclosed in lobbying documents, suggesting that lobbying budgets likely extend beyond publicly declared
efforts (Corporate Europe Observatory 2009).

National-level lobbying of influential governments such as the United
States is a commonly used route to influence global policy making. The
Global Alcohol Producers Group (GAPG), for example, spent at least
US$1.16 million on lobbyists from 2005 to 2015 for 'alcohol related issues
at the World Health Organization', including alcohol harm reduction policies in 2014 and 2015.[3] During the 1980s and 1990s, the pharmaceutical
industry successfully lobbied the United States, European, and Japanese
governments to push for stringent intellectual property provisions during the Uruguay round of trade negotiations. These negotiations resulted
in the 1994 creation of the WTO and Agreement on Trade-Related Aspects of Intellectual Property Rights (TRIPS), requiring many low- and
middle-income countries (LMICs) to grant patent monopolies on medicines for the first time (Sell 2003). The pharmaceutical industry has since
succeeded in lobbying the U.S. trade representative to demand—and
usually secure—intellectual property protections extending beyond
TRIPS (TRIPS-plus provisions) in bilateral and regional trade negotiations, including the Trans-Pacific Partnership (Correa 2006; Flynn et al.
2013).

Another route for lobbyists is directly targeting officials of intergovernmental organizations. In 2003, as WHO was preparing to release
new recommendations that no more than 10 percent of daily calories
should come from added sugars, the U.S.-based Sugar Association lobbied WHO officials and experts to withdraw the guidelines, and lobbied

U.S. government officials to use their influence at WHO to the same end (Boseley 2003; Cannon 2004). In 2014 the sugar industry protested again when WHO released updated draft recommendations, that limiting daily calories from added sugar to 5 percent would offer 'additional health benefits' (Nestle 2015). Following the publication of the World Bank's 1999 report *Curbing the Epidemic: Governments and the Economics of Tobacco Control* (CTE), advising governments on tobacco control, British American Tobacco (BAT) and Japan Tobacco International (JTI) attempted to establish a dialogue with World Bank officials as part of a strategy to minimize and discredit the report's findings. Despite the economic resources of these industries, it is notable that lobbying efforts do not necessarily prove decisive. WHO issued the 2003 and 2015 sugar guidelines, and the tobacco industry's outreach to the World Bank was reportedly rejected (Glantz, Mamudu and Hammond 2008).

Finally, corporations may lobby to weaken the impact of global norms at the national level. Following the adoption of the FCTC, WHO turned its focus to alcohol-related harms, first developing a resolution on the 'public health problems caused by harmful use of alcohol' in 2005, and then a Global Strategy to Reduce the Harmful Use of Alcohol in 2010 (Bakke and Endal 2010; WHO 2010). Examples of draft policy documents from multiple Sub-Saharan African countries suggest that, shortly after the 2005 WHA resolution, the industry-funded International Center for Alcohol Policies (ICAP) engaged as a 'partner' in the drafting of national alcohol policies in four countries. Bakke and Endal (2010) find the draft policies for Lesotho, Malawi, Uganda and Botswana—none of which had previously developed alcohol policies—to be 'almost identical in wording and structure' and 'likely to originate from the same source' (22). Each draft national policy focused on 'soft' preventative measures, such as educational campaigns, rather than binding regulatory measures such as taxation and marketing restrictions. Noting the timing of the publication of the draft policies, the authors suggest that ICAP and the alcohol industry made 'an attempt to establish policies on [the] continent before any WHO recommendations have a chance to influence the content of those policies' (Bakke and Endal 2010, 27). ICAP has also been involved in workshops focused on alcohol policy development in Vietnam and Papua New Guinea (Casswell 2013).

Developing a fuller picture of how lobbying influences global policy making remains challenging. In the United States, firms are required to disclose publicly key data about their lobbying activities, allowing for a minimum level of scrutiny and analysis. Few countries have transparency rules this extensive. In an analysis of eight European countries, the European Parliament, and the European Commission, Holman and Luneberg (2012) find that no countries require reporting on lobbying amounts for specific issues, while only two require disclosure of aggregate amounts. A recent report by Transparency International similarly found that just seven of nineteen European countries analysed had any regulation related to lobbying (Mulcahy 2015).

At the international level, there do not appear to be any lobbying disclosure requirements. WHO is barred from engaging with the tobacco and arms industries, but does not have similar policies for other industries. While WHO requires declarations of interest from experts serving on advisory committees, there are no requirements for industries to publicly disclose amounts spent on lobbying WHO officials, for example, or for participating in the WHA, where lobbyists have direct access to health officials of national delegations. Similarly, we did not find any information regarding lobbying disclosure requirements at the WTO (Eagleton 2006). Overall, weak or inconsistent transparency requirements across countries and internationally make understanding the influence of lobbying on global policy making difficult. Developing stronger and standardized disclosure requirements, at both national and global levels, would serve as a key source of knowledge related to lobbying practices and influence.

Public Communications

Businesses have strategically used public communications not only to advertise their products, but also to shift the narrative away from negative publicity, such as potentially harmful health impacts of their products. Public communications include the employment of public relations firms and mass media to highlight issues direct and peripheral to a firm's main business interests. For example, Tesler and Malone (2008) observe that, under an 'image makeover' undertaken by transnational tobacco company Philip Morris (PM), philanthropy considered of 'strategic value' focused on hunger, domestic violence and humanitarian aid aimed to 'foster a disconnect between people's views of cigarettes and the company that sold them' (Tesler and Malone 2008, 2125). BAT was similarly able to build trust and improve communications with the UK government by adopting a corporate social responsibility strategy that allowed them to engage with public officials on matters not seen as explicitly furthering their corporate interests (Fooks et al. 2011).

Communications strategies, focusing on personal choice and behaviour, shift the narrative of blame away from the company and toward the consumer. Such strategies have been frequently employed in the food and beverage sectors, where campaigns, such as Coca-Cola's 'Live Positively' initiative or Pepsi's 'Refresh Project', shift responsibility by the company, from providing healthy food to providing nutritional information. This approach emphasizes consumer choice, and thus responsibility for individuals to make appropriate decisions.

Since 2009, alcohol companies have substantially increased their funding for projects peripheral to advertising their main products. Babor and

Robaina (2013) note an industry-reported total of 408 CSR initiatives as of 2009, a more-than-tenfold increase compared with a decade earlier. These initiatives often focus on industry-related issues such as drunk driving campaigns, and largely aim to reduce excess drinking and youth alcohol consumption through education and media campaigns. Critics point to the lack of evidence behind such campaigns, suggesting that industry-led initiatives are undertaken as a countermeasure to stronger alcohol regulation (Freudenberg 2012; Hawkins and Holden 2013; Miller and Harkins 2010; Miller et al. 2011; Babor and Robaina 2013). The alcohol industry has circumvented stricter regulation through the introduction of voluntary standards, for example, such as voluntary advertising guidelines amid policy debates on more restrictive and binding measures (Sharma, Teret and Brownell 2010).

Finally, faced with criticism over the high prices they charge for medicines in LMICs, multinational pharmaceutical companies have sought to shift attention away from their pricing policies by consistently emphasizing in their public communications how weak health systems (rather than high prices) impede access to medicines (see, for example, IFPMA 2012).

Funding of Non-Profit Organizations as Front Groups

Corporations fund a substantial number of non-profit organizations operating at all levels of governance. Organizations that receive corporate funding can be loosely divided into two groups: organizations that carry out ostensibly public interest activities for the whole of society or a part of society, and organizations that may claim to carry out public interest activities but, in reality, operate to further private for-profit interests. The latter are sometimes called 'front' groups or 'astroturf' organizations to distinguish them from authentic 'grassroots' initiatives. In either case, accepting significant funds from corporate donors creates the risk of substantial influence upon, or conflicts of interest for, the non-profit organization.

The tobacco industry's use of funding to further its interests through non-profit organizations, including smokers' rights groups, retail organizations and think tanks, is well documented (Apollonio and Bero 2007). Philip Morris, with the help of public relations firm Burson Marsteller, effectively harnessed the 'voice' of grassroots activists with the establishment of the National Smokers' Alliance in the United States. A similar role is played by FOREST (Freedom Organisation for the Right to Enjoy Smoking Tobacco) in Europe, which advocates against stronger regulation (McDaniel et al. 2006). The International Tobacco Growers' Association (ITGA) supports tobacco farming, claiming to represent farmers while funded by large tobacco companies (Glantz, Mamudu and Hammond 2008). BAT similarly used front groups, including the European

Policy Centre, to argue that good governance in implementing the FCTC requires involvement of the industry as 'interested parties' (Smith et al. 2009).

Pharmaceutical companies have also funded patient-based front groups that advocate, with public and private insurance providers, to include company drugs in their coverage, or lobby for or against specific legislation (Brobeck and Mayer 2015). A *New York Times* investigation found that Novartis started a limited drug donation program for the drug Glivec® in several LMICs so that leukaemia patients would press their governments to begin paying for the drug once donations ended (Strom and Fleischer-Black 2003). In the food industry, the practice is believed so widespread that a watchdog group, the Center for Food Safety, issued a guide, 'The Best Public Relations Money Can Buy: A Guide to Food Industry Front Groups' (Simon 2013).

Finally, industry bodies themselves are sometimes treated as non-profit or civil society organizations (CSOs) and thus included in policy consultation processes. The GAPG and International Food and Beverage Alliance (IFBA), both industry bodies, attended consultations intended for CSOs leading up to the UN High-Level Meeting on Non-communicable Diseases (Cohen 2011). The U.S. delegation to the meeting included representatives of the Global Alcohol Consumers Group, Sanofi-Aventis and GlaxoSmithKline (Cohen 2011). The International Federation of Pharmaceutical Manufacturers Associations (IFPMA), which represents the multinational research-based pharmaceutical industry, is technically considered a non-profit organization and afforded the same type of 'official relationship' with the WHO as non-profits such as Doctors Without Borders. The draft WHO FENSA seeks to differentiate between industry groups like IFPMA and other non-profit entities because of concerns with the current policy. However, in the absence of disclosure requirements for non-profit organizations, regarding funding sources and amounts, it remains difficult to differentiate front groups from grassroots organizations.

Manipulating the Scientific Research Process

Manipulating the scientific process is a frequently used method by corporations to block, delay or weaken regulation, or to shift public focus away from a product's negative health effects. Attempts to counter government regulation with industry-funded research are evident across industries.

There is a lengthy and contentious debate, particularly in the clinical and biomedical sciences, regarding industry funding of research at universities and research institutes. The pharmaceutical industry has long funded academic research organizations that produce findings favourable to their products (Davidson 1986; Als-Nielsen et al. 2003; Lexchin et al. 2003; Goldacre 2012). Tobacco companies have funded research that questions existing scientific evidence on tobacco and health, recruiting scientists as consultants to publicly criticize the methodology and findings of studies (Muggli et al. 2001; Yach and Bialous 2001; Brandt 2007). Such 'junk science' can shift public attention away from the adverse health effects of products to other 'risks', or create doubt about independently funded science to delay behaviour change or stronger regulation. The tobacco industry funding of research on air quality to prevent public smoking bans (Muggli and Hurt 2003) and the food industry's funding of research on physical activity as prevention against obesity and diabetes are good examples of this strategy.

Scholars have also found similar industry attempts to manipulate science on alcohol-related harms. Three industry organizations in particular are frequent sources of funding—the European Foundation for Alcohol Research, Alcohol Beverage Medical Research Foundation, and the *Institut de Recherches Scientifiques sur le Boissons*. Such groups have challenged recent findings on alcohol's contribution to the global burden of disease (Casswell and Thamarangsi 2009). While researchers have identified some academics as recipients of industry funding, there is limited research on the impact of alcohol industry funding on potential conflicts of interest or bias (Babor and Robaina 2013). Meanwhile, industry-funded and university-affiliated research groups, such as the International Scientific Forum on Alcohol Research at Boston University, shift the narrative toward the promotion of measures focusing on individual responsibility for the moderate consumption of alcohol, possibly contributing to furthering the interests of the alcohol industry (Babor and Robaina 2013).

In addition, industry-funded scientists and research organizations can influence public policy by publicly interpreting or questioning existing evidence. Groups such as the Social Issues Research Centre (SIRC)—a think tank that has been criticized for its close ties to industry—have questioned the actual existence of an obesity 'epidemic'. Miller and Harkins (2010) suggest that the SIRC, which has received funding from the food, alcohol and sugar industries, has adopted a strategy of questioning scientific evidence to shift the conversation over published findings. Two types of influence can be observed: (a) influencing the evidence itself through the funding of research and scientists, and (b) wading into the public debate over what evidence may mean. In the above-mentioned example of the 2003 WHO sugar guidelines, the sugar lobby strongly criticized the scientific rigour of the guideline development process (Cannon 2004) (despite the fact that the Food and Agriculture Organization [FAO] and WHO came under scrutiny for concerns that the sugar industry, through the industry-funded International Life Sciences Institute, improperly influenced the selection of experts for the committee that developed the guidelines [BBC 2004]).

Receiving less attention in the existing literature is the participation of industry-funded public health experts in the production of non-clinical research affecting policy making, such as feasibility studies and evaluations of existing industry-funded health initiatives. Unlike clinical medicine, where a direct relationship between funding source and systemic bias in results has been demonstrated, we are unaware of meta-analyses examining potential bias when industry funds project evaluations, despite similar applicable risks.

DISCUSSION

This chapter reviews common strategies used by four industries—pharmaceuticals, tobacco, alcohol, and food and non-alcoholic beverages—to influence global health policy making through informal channels (see Table 6.1). Measures are needed at both the national and global levels, covering multiple industries, to protect policy-making processes from inappropriate influence. However, because informal channels are often not visible, gathering evidence regarding their use can be difficult. Information is relatively scarce on industry lobbying and funding to non-profit groups and scientific researchers, due to weak transparency and disclosure requirements. How can this type of influence best be governed? We briefly discuss each of the four strategies below and consider how greater transparency could aid in efforts to protect global health policy-making processes.

Lobbying

U.S. law requires corporations to report publicly on their lobbying activities towards U.S. officials. However, such policies do not exist in all countries, and very rarely at the global level. More widespread adoption of transparency and disclosure requirements by both national governments and international organizations would at least provide a clearer picture of where lobbying efforts are concentrated and the levels of financing involved.

Funding of Non-Profit Organizations

More stringent national requirements for non-profit organizations to disclose their sources of funding would clarify industry relationships, reveal potential conflicts of interest and facilitate better-informed consumption of research and recommendations from such organizations. While the United States requires non-profits to disclose the names of major funders through annual public reports, disclosing funding

Table 6.1.   Informal Influence of the Four Industries

	Pharmaceuticals	Tobacco	Alcohol	Food and non-alcoholic beverage
Lobbying	Lobbying US government on intellectual property issues (WTO, TRIPS-plus, TPP)	Lobbying World Bank on global tobacco report	Lobbying US government on WHO alcohol policy; Participating in domestic policymaking in developing countries	Lobbying WHO and US government to withdraw WHO sugar guidelines
Public communications	Emphasis on weak health systems in LMICs impeding access to medicines, rather than industry pricing policies	Strengthened public image through funding for hunger, domestic violence, humanitarian aid	Alcohol reduction behavioural campaigns	Healthy living behavioural campaigns
Funding of non-profit organizations	Patient groups lobbying for government purchase of certain drugs	National Smoker's Alliance; International Tobacco Grower's Association	Global Alcohol Producers Group	International Food and Beverage Association
Funding, dissemination and questioning of scientific research	Widespread funding of research institutes and scientists	Widespread funding of research institutes and scientists	European Foundation for Alcohol Research, Alcohol Beverage Medical Research Foundation, Institut de Recherches Scientifiques sur le Boissons	Social Issues Research Centre

amounts—as Coca Cola recently began doing—is voluntary (O'Connor 2015).

Manipulating the Scientific Research Process

Corporations should be required to disclose their funding for research, much as they are already required to disclose funding for lobbying. In addition, academic institutions and journal editors have an important role to play in enforcing rules regarding conflicts of interest and transparency of funding sources, for research. While most peer-reviewed journals require disclosure of potential conflicts, such disclosures are made at the discretion of the author, with significant variation in disclosure standards and requirements between publications. Better understanding of the ways in which corporations influence global health policy making beyond clinical research, to include the evaluation of non-clinical health initiatives funded by industry bodies, is urgently needed.

Public Communications

Whereas greater disclosure and transparency would be useful for counteracting the three strategies above, it is less clear that they would be effective for the public communication strategies described earlier. Sponsoring industries, after all, have a strategic interest in publicly associating their brands with health-oriented communications campaigns. Perhaps the most effective way of countering industry efforts to re-frame debates will simply be contestation of that re-framing by political leaders, NGOs and journalists.

CONCLUSION

We have focused our analysis on the informal channels that corporations use to influence global health policy making, and have argued that greater attention is needed to identify new ways to govern the use of such channels. Importantly, the WHO FENSA should be expanded in scope beyond formal means of corporate participation in WHO's norm-setting processes to take into account the strategies for informal channels of influence we have identified here. Other international organizations engaged in policy-making processes with health implications, should adopt similar safeguards against undue corporate influence. Such measures are also merited at the national level, although likely to be more difficult to implement across varying country contexts. Strengthened transparency and disclosure requirements at the national and global levels would serve an important role in shedding light on the many informal channels of influence and help to protect the policy-making process from improper influence.

NOTES

1. We use the term *global health* to refer to 'the health of the global population, with a focus on the dense relationships of interdependence that have arisen with globalization' (Frenk, Gómez-Dántes and Moon 2014).

2. While the debate around public versus private healthcare provision is one of the most contentious in public health, we excluded this issue from our analysis as it is well-covered elsewhere and tends to focus at the national level. We also excluded three other significant issues—labor conditions, climate change and environmental impacts of transnational businesses (TNBs)—largely because other scholars cover them in depth.

3. Author's calculations, based on GAPG disclosure forms provided by the Center for Responsive Politics (2015).

REFERENCES

Als-Nielsen, Bodil, Wendong Chen, Christian Gluud and Lise L. Kjaergard. 2003. 'Association of Funding and Conclusions in Randomized Drug Trials'. *JAMA* 290 (7): 921–28. doi:10.1001/jama.290.7.921.

Apollonio, Dorie E., and Lisa A. Bero. 2007. 'The Creation of Industry Front Groups: The Tobacco Industry and "Get Government Off Our Back"'. *American Journal of Public Health* 97 (3): 419–27. doi:10.2105/AJPH.2005.081117.

Babor, Thomas F., and Katherine Robaina. 2013. 'Public Health, Academic Medicine, and the Alcohol Industry's Corporate Social Responsibility Activities'. *American Journal of Public Health* 103 (2): 206–14. doi:10.2105/AJPH.2012.300847.

Bakke, Østein, and Dag Endal. 2010. 'Vested Interests in Addiction Research and Policy. Alcohol Policies Out of Context: Drinks Industry Supplanting Government Role in Alcohol Policies in Sub-Saharan Africa'. *Addiction* 105 (1): 22–28. doi:10.1111/j.1360-0443.2009.02695.x.

BBC News. 2004. 'UN Probes Sugar Industry Claims'. *BBC News*, 4 October. http://news.bbc.co.uk/1/hi/health/3726510.stm.

Boseley, Sarah. 2003. 'Sugar Industry Threatens to Scupper WHO'. *The Guardian*, 21 April. www.theguardian.com/society/2003/apr/21/usnews.food.

Brady, June Pauline. 2012. 'Marketing Breast Milk Substitutes: Problems and Perils throughout the World'. *Archives of Disease in Childhood* 97 (6): 529–32. doi:10.1136/archdischild-2011-301299.

Brandt, Allan M. 2007. *The Cigarette Century: The Rise, Fall, and Deadly Persistence of the Product That Defined America*. New York: Basic Books.

Brobeck, Stephen, and Robert N. Mayer, eds. 2015. *Watchdogs and Whistleblowers: A Reference Guide to Consumer Activism*. Santa Barbara, CA: ABC-CLIO.

Buse, Kent, and Gill Walt. 2000. 'Global Public-Private Partnerships: Part II—What Are the Health Issues for Global Governance?' *Bulletin of the World Health Organization* 78 (5): 699–709. doi:10.1111/j.1875-595X.2011.00034.x.

Buse, Kent, and Sonja Tanaka. 2011. 'Global Public-Private Health Partnerships: Lessons Learned from Ten Years of Experience and Evaluation'. *International Dental Journal* 61: 2–10.

Cannon, Geoffrey. 2004. 'Why the Bush Administration and the Global Sugar Industry Are Determined to Demolish the 2004 WHO Global Strategy on Diet, Physical Activity and Health'. *Public Health Nutrition* 7 (3): 369–80. http://dx.doi.org/10.1079/PHN2004625.

Casswell, Sally. 2013. 'Vested Interests in Addiction Research and Policy: Why Do We Not See the Corporate Interests of the Alcohol Industry as Clearly as We See Those of the Tobacco Industry?' *Addiction* 108 (4): 680–85. doi: 10.1111/add.12011.

Casswell, Sally, and Thaksaphon Thamarangsi. 2009. 'Reducing Harm from Alcohol: Call to Action'. *The Lancet* 373 (9682): 2247–57.

Center for Responsive Politics. n.d. 'Lobbying: Pharmaceuticals/Health Products Industry Profile'. www.opensecrets.org/lobby/indusclient.php?id=H04&year=2011.

———. 2015. 'Lobbying: Global Alcohol Producers Group: Issues'. www.opensecrets. org/lobby/clientissues_spec.php?id=D000051343&year=2015&spec=ALC.

Chan, Margaret. 2013. 'Opening Address at the 10th Global Conference on Health Promotion'. Lecture presented in Helsinki, Finland, 10 June. www.who.int/dg/ speeches/2013/health_promotion_20130610/en.

Cohen, Deborah. 2011. 'Will Industry Influence Derail UN Summit'. *BMJ* 343: d5328. doi: http://dx.doi.org/10.1136/bmj.d5328.

Corporate Europe Observatory. 2009. *Obscured by the Smoke—BAT's Deathly Lobbying Agenda in the EU*. http://stivoro.nl/wp-content/uploads/2012/docs/tabaksindustrie/ Obscured_by_the_Smoke%202009.pdf.

Correa, Carlos M. 2006. 'Implications of Bilateral Free Trade Agreements on Access to Medicines'. *Bulletin of the World Health Organization* 84 (5): 399–404.

Davidson, Richard A. 1986. 'Source of Funding and Outcome of Clinical Trials'. *Journal of General Internal Medicine* 1 (3): 155–58.

Eagleton, Dominic. 2006. *Under the Influence: Exposing Undue Corporate Influence over Policy-Making at the World Trade Organization*. Johannesburg: ActionAid International. www.actionaid.org.uk/sites/default/files/doc_lib/174_6_under_the_influence_ final.pdf.

Flynn, Sean M., Brook K. Baker, Margot E. Kaminski and Jimmy Koo. 2013. 'The U.S. Proposal for an Intellectual Property Chapter in the Trans-Pacific Partnership Agreement'. *American University International Law Review* 28 (1): 105–202. http:// dx.doi.org/10.2139/ssrn.2185402.

Fooks, Gary J., Anna B. Gilmore, Katherine E. Smith, Jeff Collin, Chris Holden and Kelley Lee. 2011. 'Corporate Social Responsibility and Access to Policy Élites: An Analysis of Tobacco'. *PloS Medicine* 8 (8): e1001076. doi:10.1371/journal.pmed.1001076.

Frenk, Julio, Octavio Gómez-Dántes and Suerie Moon. 2014. 'From Sovereignty to Solidarity: A Renewed Concept of Global Health for an Era of Complex Interdependence'. *The Lancet* 383 (9911): 94–97. doi:10.1016/S0140-6736(13)62561-1.

Freudenberg, Nicholas. 2012. 'The Manufacture of Lifestyle: The Role of Corporations in Unhealthy Living'. *Journal of Public Health Policy* 33 (2): 244–56.

Glantz, Stanton, Hadii M. Mamudu and Ross Hammond. 2008. 'Tobacco Industry Attempts to Counter the World Bank Report Curbing the Epidemic and Obstruct the WHO Framework Convention on Tobacco Control'. *Social Science & Medicine* 67 (11): 1690–99. doi:10.1016/j.socscimed.2008.09.062.

Goldacre, Ben. 2012. *Bad Pharma: How Drug Companies Mislead Doctors and Harm Patients*. New York: Faber and Faber.

Gopakumar, K. M., and Mirza Alas. 2015. 'No Consensus at World Health Assembly on Non-state Actors Engagement Framework'. *Third World Resurgence* 298 (9): 31–34.

Hawkins Benjamin, and Chris Holden. 2013. 'Framing the Alcohol Policy Debate: Industry Actors and the Regulation of the UK Beverage Alcohol Market'. *Critical Policy Studies* 7 (1): 53–71. doi:0.1080/19460171.2013.766023.

Heymann, David, Lincoln Chen, Keizo Takemi, David Fidler, Jordan Tappero, Mathew Thomas et al. 2015. 'Global Health Security: The Wider Lessons from the West African Ebola Virus Disease Epidemic'. *The Lancet* 385 (9980): 1884–901. http:// dx.doi.org/10.1016/S0140-6736(15)60858-3.

Holden, Chris, and Kelley Lee. 2009. 'Corporate Power and Social Policy: The Political Economy of the Transnational Tobacco Companies'. *Global Social Policy* 9 (3): 328–54. doi:10.1177/1468018109343638.

Holman, Craig, and William Luneburg. 2012. 'Lobbying and Transparency: A Comparative Analysis of Regulatory Reform'. *Interest Groups & Advocacy* 1 (1): 75–104. doi:10.1057/iga.2012.4.

Hurt, Richard D., Jon O. Ebbert, Monique E. Muggli, Nikki J. Lockhart and Channing R. Robertson. 2009. 'Open Doorway to Truth: Legacy of the Minnesota Tobacco Trial'. *Mayo Clinic Proceedings* 84 (5): 446–56. doi:10.1016/S0025-6196(11)60563-6.

International Federation of Pharmaceutical Manufacturers and Associations. 2012. *The Changing Landscape on Access to Medicines*. Geneva: IFPMA. www.ifpma.org/fileadmin/content/Publication/2012/ChangingLandscapes-Web.pdf.

Lee, Kelley, Devi Sridhar and Mayur Patel. 2009. 'Bridging the Divide: Global Governance of Trade and Health'. *The Lancet* 373 (9661): 416–22. http://dx.doi.org/10.1016/S0140-6736(08)61776-6.

Lexchin, Joel, Lisa A. Bero, Benjamin Djulbegovic and Otavio Clark. 2003. 'Pharmaceutical Industry Sponsorship and Research Outcome and Quality: Systematic Review'. *BMJ* 326 (7400): 1167–70. http://dx.doi.org/10.1136/bmj.326.7400.1167 .

McDaniel, Patricia A., Elizabeth A. Smith and Ruth E. Malone. 2006. 'Philip Morris's Project Sunrise: Weakening Tobacco Control by Working with It'. *Tobacco Control* 15 (3): 215–23. doi:10.1136/tc.2005.014977.

Miller, David, and Clarie Harkins. 2010. 'Corporate Strategy, Corporate Capture: Food and Alcohol Industry Lobbying and Public Health'. *Critical Social Policy* 30 (4): 564–89. doi:10.1177/0261018310376805.

Miller, Peter G., Florentine de Groot, Stephen McKenzie and Nicholas Droste. 2011. 'Vested Interests in Addiction Research and Policy: Alcohol Industry Use of Social Aspect Public Relations Organizations against Preventative Health Measures'. *Addiction* 106 (9): 1560–67. doi:10.1111/j.1360-0443.2011.03499.x.

Muggli, Monique E., Jean L. Forster, Richard D. Hurt and James L. Repace. 2001. 'The Smoke You Don't See: Uncovering Tobacco Industry Scientific Strategies Aimed against Environmental Tobacco Smoke Policies'. *American Journal of Public Health* 91 (9): 1419–23.

Muggli, Monique E., and Richard D. Hurt. 2003. 'Tobacco Industry Strategies to Undermine the 8th World Conference on Tobacco or Health'. *Tobacco Control* 12 (2): 195–202. doi:10.1136/tc.12.2.195.

Mulcahy, Suzanne. 2015. 'Lobbying in Europe: Hidden Influence, Privileged Access. Transparency International'. www.transparency.org/whatwedo/publication/lobbying_in_europe.

Nestle, Marion. 2015. 'World Health Organization: Eat Less Sugar'. *Food Politics* [blog], 10 March. www.foodpolitics.com/2015/03/world-health-organization-eat-less-sugar.

Ngo, Brittany. 2013. 'WHO Wrestles with Engagement of "Non-State Actors"'. *Intellectual Property Watch* [blog]. www.ip-watch.org/2013/06/25/who-wrestles-with-engagement-of-non-state-actors.

O'Connor, Anahad. 2015. 'Coke Discloses Millions in Grants for Health Research and Community Programs'. *New York Times* [blog], 22 September. http://well.blogs.nytimes.com/2015/09/22/coke-discloses-millions-in-grants-for-health-research-and-community-programs.

Ottersen, Ole P., Jashodhara Dasgupta, Chantal Blouin, Paulo Buss, Virasakdi Chongsuvivatwong, Julio Frenk et al. 2014. 'The Political Origins of Health Inequity: Prospects for Change'. *The Lancet* 383 (9917): 630–67. http://dx.doi.org/10.1016/S0140-6736(13)62407-1.

Saez, Catherine. 2014. 'WHO Board Tackles Reform, Engagement with Non-state Actors'. *Intellectual Property Watch* [blog], 24 January. www.ip-watch.org/2014/01/24/who-board-tackles-reform-engagement-with-non-state-actors.

Saez, Catherine, and William New. 2015. 'WHO Engagement with Non-state Actors: No Deal This Year, Work to Continue'. *Intellectual Property Watch* [blog], 26 May. www.ip-watch.org/2015/05/26/who-engagement-with-non-state-actors-no-deal-this-year-work-to-continue.

Sell, Susan. 2003. *Private Power, Public Law: The Globalization of Intellectual Property Rights*. Cambridge: Cambridge University Press.

Shaffer, Ellen R., and Joseph E. Brenner. 2004. 'International Trade Agreements: Hazards to Health?' *International Journal of Health Services* 34 (3): 467–81.

Sharma, Lisa L., Stephen P. Teret and Kelly D. Brownell. 2010. 'The Food Industry and Self-Regulation: Standards to Promote Success and to Avoid Public Health Failures'. *American Journal of Public Health* 100 (2): 240–46. doi:10.2105/AJPH.2009.160960.

Simon, M. 2013. 'Best Public Relations That Money Can Buy: A Guide to Food Industry Front Groups'. Center for Food Safety. www.centerforfoodsafety.org/files/front_groups_final_84531.pdf.

Smith, Katherine E., Anna B. Gilmore, Gary Fooks, Jeff Collin and Heide Weishaar. 2009. 'Tobacco Industry Attempts to Undermine Article 5.3 and the "Good Governance" Trap'. *Tobacco Control* 18 (6): 509–11. doi:10.1136/tc.2009.032300.

Strom, Stephanie, and Matt Fleischer-Black. 2003. 'Company's Vow to Donate Cancer Drug Falls Short'. *New York Times* 5 June. www.nytimes.com/2003/06/05/business/05DRUG.html?scp=1&sq=novartis%20strom%20fleischer%20bac&st=cse.

Tesler, Laura E., and Ruth E. Malone. 2008. 'Corporate Philanthropy, Lobbying, and Public Health Policy'. *American Journal of Public Health* 98 (12): 2123–33. doi:10.2105/AJPH.2007.128231.

World Health Organization. 2010. 'Global Strategy to Reduce the Harmful Use of Alcohol'. www.who.int/substance_abuse/alcstratenglishfinal.pdf.

———. 2015a. 'Framework of Engagement with Non-state Actors. WHA 68.9, Agenda item 11.2'. 26 May.

———. 2015b. *Global Health Expenditure Database*. Online database. http://apps.who.int/nha/database.

Yach, Derek, and Stella A. Bialous. 2001. 'Junking Science to Promote Tobacco'. *American Journal of Public Health* 91 (11): 1745–48.

SEVEN

How Corporations Shape Our Understanding of Problems with Gambling and Their Solutions

Rebecca Cassidy

In little more than one decade, global gambling revenue (the amount staked minus winning payouts) has more than doubled, from just over US$200 billion to US$450 billion (GBGC 2015). The origins of this remarkable expansion can be traced to the United States, where, during the 1970s, state governments were attracted to the potential tax revenue of regulated gambling. Previously, there had been no legal casinos in the United States outside Nevada. Today gambling is available in all states apart from Hawaii and Utah, and eighteen states have commercial land-based or riverboat casinos. In addition, so-called 'tribal' or 'Indian' 'gaming', protected since 1988, has grown into a US$28 billion industry (NIGC 2014). American corporations favour the softer term *gaming* over *gambling* and have worked hard to encourage legislators to use this term despite the confusion it causes. Between 1974 and 1994 the amount of money Americans legally wagered rose a staggering 2,800 percent, from US$17 billion to US$482 billion (Frontline 1996).

As the market for casino gambling in the United States approached saturation in the early 2000s, operators shifted their focus to Asia, which overtook North America as the largest regional market in 2010 (GBGC 2013). In Macau, home to the only legal casino gambling in China, gross revenue grew from less than US$1 billion in 2003 to US$46 billion by 2013. Despite a recent slowdown in growth, the regulated market in Macau is approximately seven times the size of Las Vegas (Riley 2014).

The impact of gambling expansion on global health is largely un-
known. Gamblers are a difficult-to-reach population, reticent about being
identified, and often guarded about their activities. As a result, research
often focuses on small numbers of self-selected subjects (treatment-seeking 'problem' gamblers) and rarely includes a longitudinal dimension
(Scholes-Balog et al. 2015). Despite these difficulties, studies in diverse
settings including Australia (Billi et al. 2014), the United States (Petry et
al. 2005) and South Korea (Park et al. 2010) suggest that people experiencing problems with gambling can suffer from a range of health issues
including increased rates of mental illness (Dowling et al. 2015), alcohol
and drug dependency (Petry et al. 2005) and elevated suicide rates (Petry
and Kiluck 2002).

Estimates of the social costs of gambling vary widely (Wynne and
Shaffer 2003, 120). In 1999, the Australian Productivity Commission suggested that the annual economic impact of a person experiencing a severe
problem with gambling ranged from AUS$6,000 to AUS$19,000 (1999,
9.10) while in the United States estimates vary from US$9,000 (Thompson
et al. 1997) to US$50,000 (Kindt 1995). It is also widely accepted that the
impact of problem gambling is not limited to individuals and that on
average, five to ten family members and friends are affected by each
person with gambling problems (Australian Productivity Commission
1999, 23).

Prior to regulation, gambling in Europe and North America was generally prohibited on moral grounds. When neoliberal ideologies gained
influence in the 1980s, state interventions to control private passions lost
legitimacy, and gambling was reframed as a leisure activity subject to
consumer freedom. A key element of this normalisation process has been
the creation of an abnormal category of behaviour called 'problem gambling' that effectively frees 'normal' gambling of negative associations
and provides corporations with a socially acceptable product to promote.

Based on data gathered from members of the gambling industries in
Europe, North America and Asia, this chapter describes how corporations seek to shape our understanding of gambling. It focuses on the
maintenance of two important tropes that underpin the current framing
of commercial gambling, 'responsible gambling' and 'problem gambling',
and the support by industry for research maintaining these ideas.

BACKGROUND

In 1996 the U.S. government created the National Gambling Impact Commission, with a budget of US$5 million, to assess the effects of the rapid
growth in gambling in the country. The same year, the American Gaming
Association, the trade organisation representing the land-based casino
industry, founded by former chairman of the Republican Party Frank

Fahrenkopf, created the National Centre for Responsible Gambling (NCRG). The role of the NCRG was to fund research to 'identify the risk factors for gambling disorders and determine methods for not only treating the disorder but preventing it, much like physicians can identify patients at risk from cardiovascular disease long before a heart attack' (NCRG website 2009, quoted in Schüll 2012, 261).

Anthropologist Natasha Schüll, who spent more than fifteen years conducting fieldwork in Las Vegas argues that

> by the mid-1990s, the gambling industry had already grasped (like the alcohol industry had some decades earlier) that a medical diagnosis linked to the excessive consumption of its product could serve to deflect attention away from the product's potentially problematic role in promoting that consumption, and onto the biological and psychological vulnerabilities of a small minority of its customers. (2012, 261)

The field of gambling studies developed alongside the commercial industry and is dominated by psychologists who identify, quantify and evaluate the treatment of individuals who have been harmed by gambling and, to a lesser extent, the impact of these experiences on their families and friends. Gambling that damages the health and well-being of individuals and their families is described as 'problem gambling' or 'pathological gambling', a more severe, clinically identifiable condition (Petry 2006). These approaches typically locate causal factors within individual behaviour, or physiological or psychological makeup, while largely overlooking structural factors such as the industry's role in society, social influences on individual choices, and the adequacy of regulation. Such framing is conducive to industry expansion, and lends legitimacy to gambling taxes as a source of government revenue (Hancock 2011; Kingma 2008).

METHODS

The concept of 'problem gambling' emerged during the 1980s, replacing the pejorative term *degenerate gambler*. It provides a medicalised framework for research (Reith 2007) that currently dominates gambling studies, which is traditionally housed within the discipline of psychology. Anthropologists, on the other hand, have investigated the diverse economic functions and symbolic meanings of gambling as a form of exchange. In the 1970s, Geertz described betting on cock fights in Bali as a competition for status between men in an extremely hierarchical society (Geertz 2005). In contrast, the hunting and gathering Hadza of Tanzania used gambling to reduce inequality, staking meat in order to create a distribution based on chance rather than differences in hunting ability (Woodburn 1982). Riches (1975) also found a moral obligation to gamble among Inuit communities whereby games helped to randomly distribute scarce commodities. Studies of commercial gambling in California (Hayano 1982) and Las Vegas (Schüll 2012) have similarly focused on the broader impacts of gambling as a means of distributing wealth and status.

Participant observation is fundamental to anthropological research into social processes. Bronislaw Malinowski (1922), credited with inventing participant observation in the 1920s, claimed that spending long periods of time with subjects enables anthropologists to compare what people say they do with what they actually do. This approach is particularly helpful in relation to gambling and other stigmatised activities. If anthropologists spend sufficient time in betting shops, casinos or bingo halls, people may begin to behave as they would before the anthropologist arrived. At the same time, anthropological fieldwork must be overt and all participants must provide informed consent. In practice this means that the knowledge created through participant observation is reflexive and dialogic, that is, it emerges from the relationships between the anthropologist and research participants.

This chapter is based on fieldwork with the people who produce and shape gambling. The majority of current research focuses on the consumption of gambling, and comparatively little is written about production issues such as the structure of the industry, what motivates employees, and how they view their work. The gambling industry is, in its own words, 'secretive, litigious and extremely well-funded' (North American casino executive 2012), and gaining access is very difficult. During the last nine years I have spent extended periods of time with gamblers in betting shops, casinos and bingo halls. I trained and worked as a cashier in betting shops and in social gaming studios in London, and at a mobile casino operator in Gibraltar.

These conventional ethnographic encounters were augmented by more disparate experiences at conferences, where key industry actors gather to express a collective identity. Between 2010 and 2015 I attended thirty industry conferences in London, Tokyo, Barcelona, Berlin, Dublin, Macau and Greece and listened to over a hundred presentations. Related research has included semi-structured interviews with 132 individuals, including traditional gambling operators, twenty newcomers to the gambling industry who had backgrounds in the media, console gaming, financial services and marketing, gaming lawyers, investors, politicians, regulators, journalists, researchers and treatment providers.

The gambling industry is heterogeneous: many people are interested in speaking openly with someone from outside their usual circle; others are guarded and view conversations with independent researchers as either a waste of time or a potential threat to commercial secrecy or reputation. I have anonymised the following quotes, providing only basic information that should not allow insiders to identify one another.

FINDINGS

In May 2014, Alan Feldman, chairman of the NCRG and senior vice president of public affairs for MGM Resorts International, addressed a conference in Japan, where casino gambling is currently banned. Earlier in the year, Japanese president Shinzo Abe had indicated that 'integrated resorts', featuring casinos similar to those found in Las Vegas and Singapore, would be legalised ahead of the 2020 Olympics as part of plans to kick start the economy. Media predicted that casinos could generate as much as US$40 billion annually, and become potentially the second-biggest market after Macau (Yamaguchi 2014). Asked to distinguish between problem gaming and responsible gaming, Feldman told the audience of Japanese legislators that 'we need to acknowledge the fact that there are people who are addicted to gambling, but their addiction is a brain issue, a brain disorder that is going to exist whether or not there is legalised gambling in the environment'.[1] He described responsible gambling as the universal solution to problems that may be associated with, but not 'caused' by, legal gambling, arguing that 'the notion of responsible gaming is very real, it's very identifiable, it's very consistent country to country in various parts of the world and it is something that is readily applicable here in Japan'. This distinction has been pivotal to industry expansion, emphasizing self-control of individual behaviour, and directing the discourse to a focus on treatment and education rather than limiting the supply or promotion of gambling.

Corporate actors present problems with gambling as an individual frailty that affects a minority of people. In 2011, for example, Neil Goulden, then chairman emeritus of the UK gambling corporation Gala Coral Group, and chairman of the GREaT Foundation (established to raise money from the industry to pay for research, education and treatment of gambling problems) told a UK House of Commons select committee that the problem gambler is

> obsessive, has a psychological problem and will bet on all forms of gambling. You are, therefore, dealing with the nature of the individual. They will often have drug problems, they will often have alcohol problems, they are predominantly smokers, and the person has a problem, because gambling in itself is not intrinsically addictive. (United Kingdom 2011)

Speaking more recently as chairman of the Association of British Bookmakers (ABB) and chair of the Responsible Gambling Trust (RGT), an industry-funded charity that 'funds education, prevention and treatment services and commissions research to broaden public understanding of gambling related harm' (Responsible Gambling Trust 2015), Goulden stated that there was 'very clear evidence that problem gambling is about the individual and not any specific gambling product or products'

(ABB 2013a). In the United States, the executive director of the NCRG told a *Salon* journalist that 'things are not addictive, they're just not. Addiction is a relationship between the object and a vulnerable person, and if you don't have that vulnerability, the odds are you won't get addicted. I play a slot machine for 10 minutes and I'm so bored I want to shoot myself' (quoted in Strickland 2008).

The corollary of problem gambling is 'responsible gambling', a concept based on the twin principles of informed choice and consumer freedom that emphasises education, minimal interventions and self-management and deemphasises restrictions on the supply of gambling that might impact on the rights of the 'normal' majority to consume freely. Striking parallels exist with positions adopted by the alcohol and tobacco industries. The recently created Senet Group (2015), which promotes responsible gambling in the UK, for instance, was modelled on the Portman Group, which promotes responsible drinking, and both industries support voluntary codes of practice, emphasise harm 'minimisation' (or 'reduction')—a concept initially used to counter punitive approaches to illicit drug use (McCambridge et al. 2014)—and establish charitable bodies in anticipation of regulatory changes. The RGT, for example, was established in the UK before the Gambling Act of 2005, while the Senet Group emerged before the release of the RGT's machine research in December 2014[2] and the general election in May 2015.

Similarity of approach is underpinned by the movement of key personnel across the alcohol, tobacco and gambling industries. Dirk Vennix, CEO of the ABB between 2011 and 2014 and former director of communications at the Tobacco Manufacturers Association between 2008 and 2011, recently noted that 'the two industries share many of the same contacts within government, and both have the same challenge—"facing a deluge of regulatory and taxation measures"' (Welbirg 2012, 18). In October 2014 Chris Searle, former chairman of the Portman Group, addressed an online gambling industry conference in Berlin, observing that

> frankly what has happened looks like a copy and paste job from the drinks industry. I think the gambling industry is 10 to 15 years behind the evolution of the drinks industry when it comes to social responsibility aspects. . . . What are the positive benefits of betting and gambling for society? They are not clearly merchandised and visible to the outsider. (quoted in Totally Gaming 2014)

Despite the fierce competition and deep distrust that exists between rival sectors, the UK gambling industry presents a relatively united front in its endorsement of responsible gambling. In 2013 the Association of British Bookmakers announced that 'we intend to create a step change in responsible gambling thinking based around informed choice by adult consumers' (ABB 2013b). For its part, the British Amusement Catering Trade Association (the UK trade association for amusement arcades and casinos) has noted that 'Social Responsibility is about caring for those few individuals who have a gambling addiction and need help' (BACTA 2016). In 2014 the Industry Group For Responsible Gambling, which comprises the ABB, BACTA, Bingo Association, National Casino Forum and Remote Gambling Association, came together to endorse this shared conception of 'responsible gambling' (Gaming Business 2014).

The industry has also been united in emphasising individual freedom. The online company Unibet, which describes itself as a 'leader in the European Moneytainment ® industry', describes responsibility as 'part of their corporate DNA' and defends the freedom of the 'normal' majority to gamble on its website, as well as the commercial right to operate across borders:

> For the vast majority of people, gambling—online and offline—is a fun and entertaining hobby or social activity. The questions to answer are: what do 98 per cent of gamblers get out of their gaming? What do they do right, that the minority does wrong? What good does it do them? What are the moral benefits for society as a whole? . . . When consumer protection at large is based upon an informed choice and self-responsibility, why should European consumers be denied and restricted in their choice to purchase services across borders? (Unibet 2015)

As one senior executive in the UK bookmaking industry argued:

> Education, fine. Whatever. We know it doesn't affect the bottom line. Messaging, fine, same thing. As long as it doesn't interfere too much with the punter you want to keep going . . . fine. Fewer machines? Lower stakes? Not fine. This is when you get serious. This is risky. Reducing the number of machines is a serious threat to my business. Step one: paint the opposition as 'Nanny staters'. Most of them are miserable, joyless little shits anyway, so that's easy. Step 2. Present yourself as a freedom loving, wealth creating hero. Easily done. (Male bookmaker, early forties, London, 2013)

Similarly, Steve Donoghue, industry consultant, secretariat of the Parliamentary All Party Betting & Gaming Group and former special advisor to the Culture, Media & Sport Select Committee Inquiry into the Gambling Act of 2005 said in 2013 that 'there's a party going on that the killjoys don't understand' (quoted by Bennett 2013). Such attitudes extend beyond the industry. In 2004 then UK culture secretary Tessa Jowell responded to criticism of the Gambling Act by saying that 'there's a whiff of snobbery in some of the opposition to new casinos. . . . They are entitled to those views, but they are not entitled to force them on others' (quoted in Kite 2004).

Similar approaches are found in the United States, where 'Promoting responsible gaming is part of the heritage and culture of Caesars' (Caesars 2014) and in Australia where in 2012, Clubs Australia launched a $2 million initiative to present themselves as the 'only body trying to help problem gamblers' at the website, partofthesolution.com.au.

While these views are normative, industry newcomers with back-grounds in mobile and online communications or financial services are sometimes more reflexive. An executive at a leading UK online operator mused that

> gambling operators talk about 'responsible gambling'—how much did they have to pay to get that phrase into the gambling jargon? 'Promot-ing responsible gambling'. Anyone who has read anything about mes-saging can see what a brilliant sleight of hand that was for the gam-bling industry. Well, just try out these two different approaches: Pre-venting problem gambling. Promoting responsible gambling. Which would you rather have? What about cigs? 'Preventing chain smoking' or 'Promoting moderate smoking': which would you sign up for?

Another executive involved in mobile gambling in the UK explained that

> when we came into his business we were absolutely flabbergasted that there was a built-in cushion for bad products. Problem gambling! When gambling goes wrong! (laughs) You know, you get this big let off. It says, 'Don't worry if people get addicted to your machine or your game—there are some real weirdos out there. What can you do? People are weak'. At a very basic level, it shifts responsibility from the indus-try to the consumer, and that is great for us, but not so great for you.

The efficacy of responsible gambling measures, often enshrined in codes of practice, has proven difficult to assess for want of baseline data and shared methodologies (Livingstone et al. 2014). However, a study of Australian clubs showed that

> responsible gambling practices have had little effect on the way the vast majority of respondents think about their gambling, feel about their gambling, how often they gamble, how long they gamble for and how much they spend. . . . Responsible gambling practices cannot be considered as being very effective for most problem gamblers or for most of those who are at risk. (Hing 2004, 42)

Corporate Influence of Gambling Research

There is profound disagreement within gambling studies about how relationships between corporations and researchers should be managed (Cassidy, Loussaourn and Pisac, 2014; Livingstone and Adams 2015). The RGT and NCRG favour a partnership model, and several senior research-ers accept industry research funding. In 2014 Alex Blaszczynski, editor of the journal *International Gambling Studies* (IGS), received AUS$1.2 million from the New South Wales clubs industry, which hosts the majority of Australia's controversial 'pokie' machines (Livingstone and Woolley 2007; Nicholls 2014). On the IGS website Blaszczynski states that

> I do not hold any ongoing position, receive ongoing or significant funding, and am not engaged in any business or organisation that creates a conflict of interest (real, perceived, actual or potential) in the work I would conduct as Editor of International Gambling Studies. (International Gambling Studies 2015)

He acknowledges, however, 'financial professional dealings with the gambling industry and various State and Federal governments' that include 'research grants from gambling corporations, governments, and research bodies within Australia, the United States and Canada', and 'compensation and reimbursement for expenses provided for some of this work' (International Gambling Studies 2015). Notwithstanding publisher guidelines (International Society of Addiction Journal Editors 2015), the grants, compensation and reimbursement are not quantified nor are their sources disclosed.

Mark Griffiths, arguably the leading UK figure in gambling studies, lists numerous grants and paid consultancies from gambling operators on four continents (Nottingham Trent 2015). Griffiths, with co-author Michael Auer (2015), recently defended the right of academics to work as consultants, arguing that 'research and consultancy are two very separate activities' with different aims and 'the real issue is whether doing consultancy with the gambling industry in any way impacts on independently funded and subsequently published gambling research'. Their position is that 'the gambling industry can benefit from our expertise and that there is nothing morally wrong in what we do. To us, this is totally separate from research activity'. Yet Auer has also described how he and Griffiths 'did one analysis with the data from Austrian Lotteries, who are the only internet gaming operator in Austria. In return for using our software, we used their data to publish scientific papers' (Auer 2013).

Interviews with researchers and members of the industry revealed varied and subtle forms of influence. As one veteran researcher working in the UK explained:

> The industry are very good, they can offer a very nice little perk. I was the recipient of quite a lot of corporate hospitality, very nice, thank you very much! They can do that so they are very good at getting people on their side by legitimate acceptable ways in this country or not. I mean I don't know if they cross the line, they probably do at times, like everybody else does.

Other researchers described more direct approaches. One academic, who had worked in both Australia and the UK, recalled how 'a professional organisation wanted to find out that the rate of problem gambling was less than 1 percent or something like that. My boss was offered a £10,000 bribe paid straight into his bank account. This bloke turned up in his Jaguar looking a bit like Arthur Daley off Minder'.

Relatedly, fears of legal action and intimidation can have a chilling effect on researchers and several left the field as a result:

> With the anxiety that I always felt about potentially upsetting the in-
> dustry and colleagues who were closely linked with them, I had
> enough. I didn't even finish writing up, because it was going to be too
> much. So no one ever told me not to publish, but in a sense I self-
> sabotaged. I was really scared about potentially annoying the industry
> and then getting my reputation trashed, because I saw that happen at
> [an event] and it really was horrible. So I had a choice, say everything is
> fine. In other words, lie. Or keep quiet and not expose myself to that
> critical attention. Wasn't very brave of me was it?

Another UK researcher described the actions of corporate lawyers who attended the launch of a new report:

> We ran some seminars and workshops to disseminate our findings and
> people came to those and attacked us—people from the industry pri-
> marily. . . . They tried to intimidate us indirectly in terms of what we
> published. And to discredit us in the eyes of other people. No one tried
> to shape directly what we wrote, but I didn't try to take the work
> forward after that.

This supports the opinion of an Australian researcher with more than twenty years' experience in the field who explained that 'most research is managed by never asking questions which are likely to produce embar-rassing results'. A gambling executive explained this strategy in more detail:

> People in the industry are just suspicious about research because, let's
> face it, the likelihood is that they already know if there's a problem and
> their job is to keep it quiet. If research comes up that we don't like then
> you either say it's not comparable, because it comes from somewhere
> else, or the offering is different, or regulation is different or whatever,
> or you look at the methodology and you say well it's only based on 50
> people so it's hardly representative, or you just get hold of some other
> research you've done already that says the opposite. It's not difficult.

Another UK-based industry veteran explained that he would just ignore bad news, before expressing his unhappiness to the charitable organisa-tions responsible:

> We just don't respond. Don't provide any oxygen, but behind the
> scenes we might give someone a bollocking for funding a bit of re-
> search. If we sit on a board we might show that we weren't very happy.
> When GamCare comes round cap in hand we might point out that we
> weren't very happy. Just the usual things that you would expect really.

CONCLUSION

Gambling studies is an emerging field and has yet to engage with the epistemological and ethical arguments that have taken place in alcohol or tobacco research. Anthropological research into how ideas about gambling problems are reproduced helps to explain the relative lack of reliable evidence in the area (Disley et al. 2011). Specifically, current approaches to analysis serve the interests of a powerful industry seeking to expand globally, and of governments keen to reap potential benefits in terms of employment or tax revenue. The common interest of the gambling industry and gambling studies researchers in perpetuating the idea of problem gambling as an individual shortcoming is a key element of how this discourse is framed, as is the willingness of researchers to accept industry funding (Orford 2012).

The impact on the research agenda, the range of methods used by researchers and the human geography of the field are profound. The research agenda remains focused on measuring and treating 'problem gamblers', and minimizing or reducing harm through education and self-management. The range of methods employed is narrow and mono-disciplinary, and the definition of accepted evidence is restricted to that which can be measured or counted, which is constrained by access issues (Young 2013). The result upon this fiercely politicised field is that broad questions about corporate influence and global health are marginalised. As commercial gambling expands into new markets globally, it is critical that effective ways to assess and counter its impacts on public health are devised. The intention of this chapter is to bring gambling studies into a wider conversation where it can benefit from insights developed in similar fields, and acknowledge the limitations of its rather singular approach to knowledge creation to date.

FUNDING

This chapter is based on fieldwork conducted as part of a project funded by the European Research Council under the European Union's Seventh Framework Programme (FP/2007-2013) / ERC Grant Agreement no. 263443.

NOTES

1. Speeches recorded while attending the conference in Tokyo.
2. For the full texts of the long-awaited machines research, see: http://www.responsiblegamblingtrust.org.uk/Research-Publications.

REFERENCES

ABB. 2013a. *Gaming Machines Policy Must Be Evidence Based*. www.politicshome.com/articles/opinion/association-british-bookmakers/gaming-machines-policy-must-be-evidence-based.

———. 2013b. *The ABB's Code for Responsible Gambling and Player Protection in Licenced Betting Offices in Great Britain*. www.abb.uk.com/wp-content/uploads/2014/09/ABB-code-for-responsible-gambling.pdf.

Auer, Michael. 2013. 'Mentor: Changing the Way We Play?' *Casino International*, April: 38–39

Australian Productivity Commission. 1999. *Australia's Gambling Industries, Report No. 10*. Canberra AusInfo.

BACTA. 2016. 'Social Responsibility'. Accessed 25 April 2016. www.bacta.org.uk/details.cfm?page=charity&section=social.

Bennett, Oliver. 2013. 'Fancy a Flutter?' *Management Today*, 29 May. www.managementtoday.co.uk/features/1182983/fancy-flutter-rise-middle-class-gambler.

Billi, Rosa, Christine A. Stone, Paul Marden and Kristal Yeung. 2014. *The Victorian Gambling Study: A Longitudinal Study of Gambling and Health in Victoria, 2008–2012*. Victoria, Australia: Victorian Responsible Gambling Foundation.

Brewster, Kerry. 2012. 'Clubs Australia Plans Pokies Reform Fight'. *ABC*, 14 June. www.abc.net.au/lateline/content/2012/s3525566.htm.

Caesars. 2014. 'Responsible Gaming'. http://caesarscorporate.com/about-caesars/responsible-gaming.

Cassidy, Rebecca, Claire Loussouarn and Andrea Pisac. 2014. *Fair Game: Producing Gambling Research*. London: Goldsmiths University of London.

Disley, Emma, Alexandra Pollitt, Deidre May Culley and Jennifer Rubin. 2011. *Map the Gap: A Critical Review of the Literature on Gambling-Related Harm*. RAND Corporation (TR-1013-RGF).

Dowling, Nicki A., Sean Cowlishaw, Alun C. Jackson, Stephanie S. Merkouris, Kate L. Francis and Darren R. Christensen. 2015. 'The Prevalence of Psychiatric Comorbidity in Treatment-Seeking Problem Gamblers: A Systematic Review and Meta-Analysis'. *Australian and New Zealand Journal of Psychiatry* 49 (6): 519–39. doi:10.1177/0004867415575774.

Frontline. 1996. 'Gambling Facts and Stats'. Accessed 12 May 2015. www.pbs.org/wgbh/pages/frontline/shows/gamble/etc/facts.html.

Gaming Business. 2014. 'Trade Associations Form New Responsible Gambling Group'. 21 March. www.igamingbusiness.com/news/trade-association-form-new-responsible-gambling-group.

GBGC. 2013. 'Global Gambling Spend Just US$ 82 Per Capita'. 23 April. Accessed 12 May 2015. www.gbgc.com/global-gambling-spend-just-us-82-per-capita.

———. 2015. 'Global Gambling Revenues Pass $450 Billion in 2014'. 30 April. Accessed 29 June 2015. www.gbgc.com/global-gambling-revenues-pass-us-450-billion-in-2014.

Geertz, Clifford. 2005. 'Deep Play: Notes on the Balinese Cockfight'. *Daedalus* 134 (4): 56–86.

Griffiths, Mark D., and Michael Auer. 2015. 'Research Funding in Gambling Studies: Some Further Observations'. *International Gambling Studies* 15 (1): 15–19. Accessed 29 June 2015. doi:10.1080/14459795.2014.1003576.

Hancock, Linda. 2011. *Regulatory Failure: The Case of Crown Casino*. Melbourne: Australian Scholarly Publishing.

Hayano, David M. 1982. *Poker Faces: The Life and Work of Professional Card Players*. Berkeley: University of California Press.

Hing, Nerilee. 2004. 'The Efficacy of Responsible Gambling Measures in NSW Clubs: The Gamblers' Perspective'. *Gambling Australia* 16 (1): 32–46.

International Gambling Studies. 2015. 'Editorial Board Conflict of Interest Declarations'. June. www.tandfonline.com/action/journalInformation?show=editorialBoa

rd&journalCode=rigs20&#.Vd2k4Zdd8-2.

International Society of Addiction Journal Editors. 2015. 'ISAJE Conflict of Interest Declaration'. www.parint.org/isajewebsite/conflict.htm.

Kindt, John W. 1995. 'U.S. National Security and the Strategic Economic Base: The Business/Economic Impacts of the Legalization of Gambling Activities'. *Saint Louis University Law Journal* 39: 567–84.

Kingma, Sytze F. 2008. 'The Liberalization and (Re)regulation of Dutch Gambling Markets: National Consequences of the Changing European Context'. *Regulation & Governance* 2 (4): 445–58. doi: 10.1111/j.1748-5991.2008.00045.x.

Kite, Melissa. 2004. '"Opponents of New Gambling Law Are Snobs", Says Tessa Jowell'. *The Telegraph*, 24 October. www.telegraph.co.uk/news/uknews/1474933/Opponents-of-new-gambling-law-are-snobs-says-Tessa-Jowell.html.

Livingstone, Charles, Angela Rintoul and Louis Francis. 2014. 'What Is the Evidence for Harm Minimisation Measures in Gambling Venues?' *Evidence Base* 2: 1–24. doi: 10.4225/50/558112A877C5D.

Livingstone, Charles, and Peter Adams. 2015. 'Clear Principles Are Needed for Integrity in Gambling Research'. *Addiction*, early view. doi: 10.1111/add.12913.

Livingstone, Charles, and Richard Woolley. 2007. 'Risky Business: A Few Provocations on the Regulation of Electronic Gaming Machines'. *International Gambling Studies* 7 (3): 343–58. doi: 10.1080/14459790701601810.

Malinowski, Bronislaw. 1992. *Argonauts of the Western Pacific: An Account of Native Enterprise and Adventure in the Archipelagos of Melanesian New Guinea*. London: Routledge & Kegan Paul Ltd.

McCambridge, Jim, Kypros Kypri, Collin Drummond and John Strang. 2014. 'Alcohol Harm Reduction: Corporate Capture of a Key Concept'. *PLoS Med* 11 (12): e1001767. doi:10.1371/journal.pmed.1001767.

Nicholls, Sean. 2014. 'Clubs Bet $1.2m on Gambling Research, Xenophon Claims "Stalling Tactic"'. *Sydney Morning Herald*, 21 May. www.smh.com.au/nsw/clubs-bet-12m-on-gambling-research-xenophon-claims-stalling-tactic-20140530-399ud.html#ixzz3lt1LlL7V.

NIGC. 2014. '2013 Indian Gaming Revenues Increased 0.5%'. www.nigc.gov/LinkClick.aspx?fileticket=E3BeULzk1cA%3d&tabid=1006.

Nottingham Trent University. 2015. 'Griffiths CV'. https://nottinghamtrent.academia.edu/MarkGriffiths/CurriculumVitae.

Orford, Jim. 2012. *An Unsafe Bet? The Dangerous Rise of Gambling and the Debate We Should Be Having*. Chichester: Wiley-Blackwell.

Park, Subin, Maeng Je Cho, Hong Jin Jeon et al. 2010. 'Prevalence, Clinical Correlations, Comorbidities, and Suicidal Tendencies in Pathological Korean Gamblers: Results from the Korean Epidemiologic Catchment Area Study'. *Soc Psychiatry Psychiatr Epidemiol* 45 (6): 621–29. doi:10.1007/s00127-009-0102-9. Epub 28 July 2009.

Petry, Nancy. 2006. 'Should the Scope of Addictive Behaviors Be Broadened to Include Pathological Gambling?' *Addiction* 101 (1): 152–60. doi: 10.1111/j.1360-0443.2006.01593.x.

Petry, Nancy, and Brian D. Kiluck. 2002. 'Suicidal Ideation and Suicide Attempts in Treatment-Seeking Pathological Gamblers'. *Journal of Nervous and Mental Disease* 190 (7): 462–69. doi:10.1097/01.NMD.0000022447.27689.96.

Petry, Nancy, Frederick Stinson and Bridget Grant. 2005. 'Comorbidity of DSM-IV Pathological Gambling and Psychiatric Disorders: Results from the National Epidemiologic Survey on Alcohol and Related Conditions'. *Journal of Clinical Psychiatry* 66: 564–74.

Reith, Gerda. 2007. 'Gambling and the Contradictions of Consumption: A Genealogy of the "Pathological" Subject'. *American Behavioral Scientist* 51 (1): 33–55, 41. doi: 0.1177/0002764207304856.

Responsible Gambling Trust. 2015. www.responsiblegamblingtrust.org.uk.

Riches, David. 1975. 'Cash, Credit and Gambling in a Modern Eskimo Economy'. *Journal of the Royal Anthropological Institute* 10: 21–33.

Riley, Charles. 2014. 'Macau's Gambling Industry Dwarfs Vegas'. *CNN Money*, 6 January. http://money.cnn.com/2014/01/06/news/macau-casino-gambling.

Scholes-Balog, Kristy E., Sheryl A. Hemphill, John W. Toumbourou and Nicki A. Dowling. 2015. 'Problem Gambling and Internalising Symptoms: A Longitudinal Analysis of Common and Specific Social Environmental Protective Factors'. *Addictive Behaviors* 46: 86–93. doi: 10.1016/j.addbeh.2015.03.011.

Schüll, Natasha D. 2012. *Addiction by Design: Machine Gambling in Las Vegas*. Princeton, NJ: Princeton University Press.

Senet Group. 2015. https://senetgroup.org.uk.

Strickland, Eliza. 2008. 'Gambling with Science: Determined to Defeat Lawsuits over Addiction, the Casino Industry Is Funding Research at a Harvard-Affiliated Lab'. *Salon*, 16 June. Accessed 12 May 2015. www.salon.com/2008/06/16/gambling_science.

Thompson, William, Ricardo Gazel and Dan Rickman. 1997. 'Social and Legal Costs of Compulsive Gambling'. *Gaming Law Review* 1: 81–89.

Totally Gaming. 2014. 'Gambling "Years Behind" Drinks Industry in Social Responsibility, Expert Warns'. 22 October. www.totallygaming.com/news/betting/gambling-years-behind-drinks-industry-social-responsibility-expert-warns.

Unibet. 2015. 'Responsible Gaming'. www.unibetgroupplc.com/corporate/templates/InformationPage.aspx?id=357.

United Kingdom Culture, Media and Sport Committee. 2011. 'Minutes of Evidence. HC 421'. 25 October. www.publications.parliament.uk/pa/cm201213/cmselect/cmcumeds/421/111025.htm.

Welbirg, Richard. 2012. 'Lobbying for Tobacco and Gambling'. *Public Affairs News*, 19 July.

Woodburn, James. 1982. 'Egalitarian Societies'. *Journal of the Royal Anthropological Institute* 17: 431–51.

Wynne, Harold, and Howard Shaffer. 2003. 'The Socioeconomic Impact of Gambling: The Whistler Symposium'. *Journal of Gambling Studies* 19 (2): 111–21. doi:10.1023/A:1023648230928.

Yamaguchi, Yuki. 2014. 'Caesars Ready to Invest $5 Billion in Japan Casino'. *Bloomberg*, 26 June. www.bloomberg.com/news/articles/2014-06-26/caesars-ready-to-invest-5-billion-in-japan-casino.

Young, Martin. 2013. 'Statistics, Scapegoats and Social Control: A Critique of Pathological Gambling Prevalence Research'. *Addictions Research and Theory* 21 (1): 1–11. doi:10.3109/16066359.2012.680079.

EIGHT

Corporate Manipulation of Global Health Policy

A Case Study of Asbestos

John Calvert

Few industries have had such an adverse impact on occupational health, and population health more widely, than asbestos. The World Health Organization (WHO), International Labour Organization (ILO), and numerous scientific and medical organizations have extensively documented the health effects of the deadly fibres, exposure to which can result in asbestosis, mesothelioma and other cancers. The WHO estimates that asbestos causes up to 107,000 deaths annually, with approximately 125 million people worldwide exposed to asbestos in their workplaces (WHO 2014). In light of the long latency period of cancer and other asbestos-related deaths (ARDs), and more than 200 million tonnes of asbestos now in our environment, it will be decades and perhaps centuries before total cumulative deaths are known.[1]

For much of the twentieth century, asbestos companies in high-income countries fought a determined, and very successful, rear-guard action to obscure the mineral's adverse health effects. They undermined the efforts of epidemiologists, physicians, public health officials, scientists, asbestos workers and their unions to ban its extraction and use. This history has been well-documented elsewhere (McCulloch and Tweedale 2008). How the industry migrated to markets in low- and middle-income countries (LMICs), where occupational and environmental health standards remain weak and poorly enforced, has received less attention. Industry output peaked in 1977 at 4.8 million metric tonnes (Mt) and remained above 4 million Mt until 1990 (USGS 2006, table 4). World output fell by over half during the years immediately following, fostering the hope that its use would rapidly decline. Since 1996, however, production has plateaued at approximately 2 million Mt. per year to 2014 (USGS 2015).[2] New investors, principally from Russia and Kazakhstan, have replaced those that abandoned the industry due to lawsuits, bankruptcies and bans in fifty-seven countries (Kazan-Allen 2014). The major producers today—based in Russia, China, Brazil and Kazakhstan—have maintained output by continuing domestic use and, except for China, expanding exports to LMICs (McCulloch and Tweedale 2008). Falling asbestos consumption in North America, Europe and Japan has been offset by the industry's expansion into new markets as widespread as India, Thailand, Iran and Cuba (USGS 2014). As Lemen (2014) writes, asbestos has become a truly global pandemic.

This chapter examines the role of corporations in this transition, focusing on how the industry has persuaded governments in both producing and consuming LMICs to ignore the regulations now in place in industrialized countries. It analyses how the industry has blocked the global health community's efforts to include asbestos in key international treaties governing environmental and occupational health. It argues that the restructured asbestos industry has learned much from the Canadian experience while making use of a familiar global network of lobbyists, consultants and manufacturers to sustain its interests.

METHODS

This chapter is based on a systematic review of the substantial secondary literature on asbestos and health, which spans science, medicine, epidemiology, occupational and environmental health, public health, public policy, economics, political science, law and international relations. It draws upon reports of government ministries and international organizations such as the WHO and ILO. In addition, it makes use of grey literature from advocacy organizations such as the International Ban Asbestos Secretariat (IBAS), Ban Asbestos Canada, trade union publications and documents from the asbestos industry itself. While drawing on insights from this multidisciplinary literature, this chapter adopts a political economy perspective to analyse the policy interaction between the industry, governments, workers and the public health community at both the national and global levels.

A key focus is the role of the Canadian-based Asbestos Institute (AI) (subsequently re-named the Chrysotile Institute) and its international counterparts. These organizations were responsible for coordinating the industry's research, lobbying and promotional activities over more than three decades. This chapter documents their activities through reviews of their own publications, analysis of government policies that reflected the industry's interests and the public proceedings—and decisions—of governments and various international agencies responsible for occupational and public health. In the process, it reveals the regrettable extent of the industry's role in shaping the public policy process both in Canada and internationally.

AN ECONOMICALLY PROBLEMATIC, YET HIGHLY PROFITABLE INDUSTRY

The migration of hazardous production processes (Baram 2009) and the marketing of harmful products, such as tobacco (Holden and Lee 2009), to less regulated jurisdictions has been a feature of economic globalization. Corporations relocate to countries offering lower environmental, labour, consumer protection, product liability and health standards, engaging in a 'race to the bottom' (Davies and Vadlamannati 2013). This transfer of activities no longer profitable in the industrialised world to LMICs, where production costs are lower, regulatory frameworks weaker, and governments permit environmental, health and social costs to be treated as externalities, has posed new challenges for protecting population health.

The global restructuring of the asbestos industry, however, cannot be explained by economic rationales alone. At first glance, the industry's economic survival is puzzling. The mineral's contribution to gross domestic product (GDP) is relatively small, even in major producing countries, compared to other natural resources or industrial products. With the exception of Kazakhstan, it is not a major source of foreign earnings. According to the UN's Comtrade database, in the five years to 2013, Russia, responsible for two-thirds of world exports, earned US$240 million on average annually. In contrast, its gas exports averaged slightly over US$60 billion annually in the same period according to the Bank of Russia. Asbestos bans in high-income countries have been followed by the introduction of many substitutes, most not significantly more expensive.

This chapter argues that explaining the industry's longevity lies not in asbestos' economic value, but in how corporations have influenced policy making globally and in LMICs. The more recent expansion of the industry in LMICs has followed a long history of deceptive practices in industrialised countries, during which time it shaped the economic and health policies of numerous governments. Initially, its success reflected the mineral's many uses and low cost. By the latter part of the twentieth century, however, the industry engaged in concerted efforts to obscure the mineral's adverse health impacts from workers, customers and the broader public (Tweedale 2000; McCulloch and Tweedale 2008). Through well-

Table 8.1. World Asbestos Production by Major Producing Country (metric tonnes)

Country	2009	2010	2011	2012	2013	2014
Brazil	288,452	302,257	306,321	304,569	307,000	291,000
Canada	150,000	100,000	50,000	nil	nil	nil
China	440,000	400,000	440,000	420,000	420,000	400,000
Kazakhstan	230,000	214,100	223,100	241,200	242,000	240,000
Russia	1,000,000	995,174	1,031,880	1,041,000	1,050,000	1,050,000
Total	2,110,000	2,010,000	2,050,000	2,010,000	2,020,000	1,980,000

Source: US Geological Survey Asbestos – 2013. Advance Release. Table 8, p. 8.7. and USGS. 2015. Mineral Commodity Summaries. p. 23.
Note: Table does not include production statistics from several other countries where no accurate data is available. However, their output is small.

targeted lobbying, inflated claims of economic benefits and dissemination of misinformation about the medical and scientific evidence, it succeeded in concealing the extent of the mineral's health harms (Braun et al. 2003; Ruff 2009; Rice 2011). The industry enlisted the support of a wide-ranging network of manufacturing companies that, by incorporating asbestos into their products, came to perceive a shared stake in the continued availability of the mineral and, therefore, common cause with keeping it on the market. American and European corporations—Johns-Manville, Raybestos, Grace, Eternit and Turner and Newall—established a web of over one hundred supportive trade and business organisations in countries worldwide, to promote its use and to defend it from growing opposition from health advocates (McCulloch and Tweedale 2008).

THE CANADIAN INDUSTRY'S AGENDA: CREATING NEW MARKETS FOR ASBESTOS IN LMICS

The exit of U.S. and European multinational corporations (MNCs) from production, over the final two decades of the twentieth century, left a major gap that Canada filled. Canadian companies, supported by provincial and federal governments, created new markets in LMICs. Canada provided the link between earlier MNCs and current producers in Russia, Kazakhstan, China and Brazil, offering lessons to them on international market expansion (Ruff 2009; Morris 2014). How the Canadian industry came to play this role offers important insights into current challenges to global governance of asbestos.

Canadian production began in 1878 in Thetford, Quebec. Due to its accessible surface deposits of chrysotile, Quebec became the industry's dominant producer, hosting ten of thirteen domestic mines (Kuyek 2003).

Canada produced 61.2 Mt of asbestos between 1900 and 2003, almost one-third of the world's total output, of which 77 percent was exported. Canadian production peaked at 1.7 million Mt in 1973 (USGS 2006, table 4).

Initially, the Canadian industry was largely foreign-owned and export-oriented. The largest producer was U.S.-based Johns-Manville, with Turner and Newall also a significant British investor. Proximity, combined with low production costs, made Quebec attractive for supplying the American market. Canada accounted for 94 percent of U.S. imports between 1910 and 2003 (USGS 2006; USGS 2012). Starting in the late 1970s, successful lawsuits by U.S. asbestos victims forced Johns-Manville, Raybestos, Grace and other American firms into chapter 11 bankruptcy proceedings. The U.S. MNCs abandoned Quebec. Domestic firms acquired ownership.

But the Quebec companies were provincially based and much smaller. They lacked the resources and global networks of the MNCs. However, the provincial government remained deeply committed to the industry. Consequently, the Parti Quebecois nationalised much of it between 1978 and 1982. Johns-Manville's operations were taken over by a local investor, J.M. Asbestos, in 1983 after the U.S. firm's bankruptcy (Robertson 1992). Nationalisation coincided with the rapid decline in shipments to the United States. Sales fell from 1.5 million Mt in 1977 to 665,000 Mt a decade later, with a continued fall thereafter (USGS 2005; USGS 2009). To survive and find new markets, the Quebec-based companies needed help (Sentes 2009). The Canadian and Quebec governments assisted them to expand sales to LMICs over the following three decades (Ruff 2009). By 2010, its last year of significant mining, over 90 percent of Quebec's production of 100,000 tonnes of asbestos went to LMICs, primarily in Asia (USGS 2014).

The companies also needed government support to counter the growing movement to ban production and consumption of the mineral globally. This also required Canada to continue to use the mineral domestically to show it was safe. From the early 1980s until production ceased, the Quebec and Canadian governments provided this support (Ruff 2015; Turcotte 2014). In 1984, the industry persuaded the two governments to fund the Asbestos Institute (AI) (renamed the Chrysotile Institute in 2004) to promote exports and defend the industry from health critics. The AI was modelled on the discredited Tobacco Institute, created in 1958 by American tobacco companies, and dissolved in 1998 as part of the Master Tobacco Settlement Agreement (Brandt 2007). By 2001 the two governments had provided the AI with over Cdn$54 million in direct subsidies (Ruff 2009; Rubin 2011). With the MNCs now gone, the AI became the industry's global marketing and promotional arm (McCulloch and Tweedale 2008; Kazan-Allen 2012).

The industry persuaded the Canadian government to lobby foreign governments and court potential customers in LMICs. Canada even linked some foreign aid to purchasing asbestos (Ruff 2009). The AI used the official Government of Canada insignia on its printed materials. Health Canada participated in conferences, such as the International Conference on Chrysotile in Montreal held in 2006, endorsing the industry's network of medical and scientific 'experts' to LMIC delegates. The government made appointments to the AI's board (Ruff 2009).

Like the MNCs, the AI funded 'research' to discredit evidence of the mineral's health harms (Egilman, Fehnel and Bohme 2003; Gray and Nolan 2011). Its sophisticated public relations campaign produced numerous pamphlets, such as the sixty-page 'Undeniable Facts about Chrysotile' and the 180-page 'Safe Use of Chrysotile Asbestos', to reassure LMIC manufacturers and their workers that asbestos was safe (AI 1993; AI n.d.). With 90 percent of asbestos used in building materials, the AI promoted its benefits as a reinforcing agent in concrete water pipes and corrugated boards, which could be produced cheaply with local cement and sand. It claimed asbestos-strengthened roofing could satisfy the housing needs of millions in LMICs, while asbestos-reinforced pipes could improve water and wastewater systems economically. The AI established a website to support these claims, posting papers written by industry-funded academics, such as David Bernstein and Jacques Dunnigan (Bernstein, Rogers and Smith 2004; Bernstein 2006; Dunnigan 2009; Bernstein et al. 2013), as well as proceedings of industry-sponsored conferences (Ruff 2009) It funded Corbett McDonald (Department of Environmental and Occupational Health, McGill University), who theorized that contamination of chrysotile by tremolite asbestos was responsible for ARDs (McDonald and McDonald 1997). The department's work, published in *Science*, the *New England Journal of Medicine* and *Lancet* from the 1970s to 1990s, created doubt about the extent of the mineral's harms. The industry still distributes these publications today.

As the adverse health evidence accumulated, the Quebec industry faced increasing pressure from organized labour, both in Canada (outside of Quebec) and globally, to ban asbestos. In response, the AI courted the unions representing Quebec's asbestos workers, and specifically, the United Steelworkers of America (USWA), to counter this pressure. Clement Godbout, Quebec director of the USWA, and later president of the Quebec Federation of Labour (QFL) (1993–1999), became a vocal industry advocate. Godbout became president of the AI in 2002 and chair of the International Chrysotile Association (ICA), the lobby group for the global asbestos industry (Calvert 2013).

Godbout strongly opposed demands of other Canadian and international unions for a ban. According to his biography, posted on the Chrysotile Institute's website, 'In the 1980's Mr. Godbout participated actively at the ILO Meetings of Experts on the regulation of the chrysotile mining industry, as well as drafting of the ILO code of Practice on Safety in the Use of Asbestos'. It continues: 'He was also consulted in the development of the ILO's Code of Practice 162 on the safe use of asbestos'. Quebec's asbestos unions built alliances with counterparts in other countries to prevent national labour union federations from supporting a ban (Cremers and Gehring 2013; Ruff and Calvert 2014). For three decades, the Quebec unions blocked Canadian construction, manufacturing and transportation unions from getting the Canadian Labour Congress (CLC) to support a ban, threatening its executive with Quebec disaffiliation if it permitted debate on anti-asbestos resolutions at its biennial conventions (CBC 2008). Fearing loss of one-third of its members, the CLC leadership complied until Quebec's industry closed down.

In the years following the exit of the MNCs, a new threat emerged: inclusion of occupational health and environmental restrictions in international treaties. In response, the industry persuaded the government to include the defence of asbestos in Canada's foreign policy (Ruff 2009; CBC 2009). Four initiatives stand out. The first was opposition to a proposed ban by the U.S. Environmental Protection Agency (EPA) announced in 1986 (Asbestos Ban and Phase-Out Rule, ABPR). Canadian opposition—in the form of representations by the federal and Quebec governments, and the AI in EPA hearings—reflected alarm at the potential loss of a US$72 million annual U.S. market, as well as impact on expanding LMIC sales. The AI claimed asbestos was safe. A ban would deny the U.S. economy asbestos' numerous benefits. The proposal also reflected anti-Canadian bias (Ruff and Calvert 2014). Canadian prime minister Brian Mulroney personally contacted U.S. president Ronald Reagan asking him to overrule the proposal (Kazan-Allen 2014). Quebec premier Robert Bourassa similarly lobbied U.S. officials (Galloway 2011). U.S. asbestos interests supported Canada's challenge. In 1991 a U.S. court struck down key parts of the EPA's proposed regulations (Ruff and Calvert 2014). According to IBAS, Canadian intervention facilitated an additional 300,000 tonnes of asbestos imports (Kazan-Allen 2011). The United States still does not ban asbestos.

Canada's second challenge was brought against France's 1996 Decree 96-1133, which banned asbestos imports, as an unfair trade measure under the WTO (Calvert 2013). The decree followed a major public health enquiry and bans adopted in Sweden, Norway, Denmark and Germany and would potentially trigger an EU-wide ban, which did not happen until 2005 (Parigot 2014). Canada argued that France's goal was to protect French firms producing asbestos substitutes, citing violations of three agreements—General Agreement of Tariffs and Trade 1994, the Agreement on Technical Barriers to Trade (TBT) and the Sanitary and the Phytosanitary Agreement (SBS). Article III:4 of the GATT required like imported products to be treated equally with similar domestic products (WTO Dispute DS135). However, in 2001, the WTO ruled against Canada's challenges and later rejected a Canadian appeal (Howse and Türk 2009).

A third notable action was preventing the listing of asbestos in the UN's Rotterdam Convention on the Prior Informed Consent Procedure for Certain Hazardous Chemicals and Pesticides in International Trade (Rotterdam). Signed in 1998 by 170 countries, it came into effect in 2004 (UNEP 2004). At the convention's second Conference of the Parties (COP2) in 2006, the review committee recommended listing chrysotile. This would not ban the asbestos trade, but would require exporters to notify importing countries of its hazards (Bitonti 2009). Canada led the opposition at the second, third and fourth COPs, supported by a handful of LMICs. At COP5 in 2012, Canada again anticipated support from Russia and several LMICs. Unexpectedly, these countries abstained. But, as decisions are by consensus, Canada's veto precluded listing (Ruff and Calvert 2014). By COP6 in 2013, Quebec's industry had closed. Canada abstained. However, learning from the Canadian example, Russia, Kazakhstan, India and several other countries opposed listing. In 2015, Russia again led opposition—supported by Kazakhstan, Kyrgyzstan and Zimbabwe—confirming its role as the industry new champion (Ruff 2015).

Finally, Canada defended asbestos at a 2007 meeting of the Basel Convention on Control of Transboundary Movements of Hazardous Wastes and Their Disposal called to ratify a UN Environment Programme Work Plan on managing asbestos-laden debris in disaster-prone areas. Following the 2004 Asia tsunami, the WHO proposed a permanent team of experts for emergency asbestos clean-up. It also recommended using substitutes in areas prone to earthquakes. Canada, supported by Russia and India, successfully opposed the proposal (Ruff and Calvert 2014).

Along with the above actions, Prime Minister Jean Chretien lobbied Chilean president Ricardo Lagos in 2001 not to ban the mineral. In 2006 Canada officially reminded South Africa of its WTO trade obligations to exert pressure, unsuccessfully, to drop a proposed ban. However, Canada successfully pressed Thailand and South Korea to remove warning labels on bags of asbestos (Ruff 2009).

To deflect criticism about exports to LMICs with weaker health and safety regulations, beginning in 1979, Canada endorsed 'controlled use' policy guidelines. In March 1997, the Quebec Minister of Natural Resources signed an agreement with Quebec's two major asbestos companies (J.M. Asbestos and LAB Chrysotile) affirming that Canada would not export to countries not following such guidelines. A decade later, the government claimed it was monitoring workplace safety practices, with Chrysotile Institute assistance in the eighty countries it claimed were importing Canadian asbestos (Mittelstaedt 2008; Mittelstaedt 2009; CBC 2009).

Faced with growing pressure for domestic restrictions, and export repercussions if Canada abandoned its 'controlled use' policy, in 2006 the federal government had Health Canada appoint an Expert Panel to support its position (Rubin 2011). The ministry consulted the industry, but not the public health community, and required panel members to sign confidentiality agreements (Stayner 2008).

In response to an NDP motion in Parliament to ban asbestos, Bloc Quebecois MP Andre Bellavance claimed the unreleased report endorsed the 'safe use of chrysotile'. The chair, Dr. Trevor Ogden, and the report's other lead scientist, Dr. Leslie Stayner, then wrote to Minister Clement on March 28, 2008, urging him to expedite the report's release. According to Stayner, its findings 'were being misrepresented for political purposes' (Stayner 2008). Quebec natural resources minister Christian Paradis, conservative MP for the asbestos region, also told the media the report supported 'controlled use'. Stayner replied that this was a 'total misrepresentation' (Schmidt 2011).

Overall, Canadian action succeeded in keeping the domestic and global asbestos markets open. But Quebec production steadily declined, due to exhaustion of surface deposits. Efforts by LAB Chrysotile to develop the Jeffrey underground mine in the late 1990s with government subsidies failed (Globe and Mail 2012). Production at the last working mine, Lac d'amiante du Canada, ceased in 2012. Remarkably, in 2012, industry interests persuaded Quebec's liberal government to offer to loan Cdn$58 million to any investor willing to reopen the mine. But the same year the Parti Quebecois, led by Pauline Maurais, won the provincial election and cancelled the loan offer, effectively ending all asbestos production (Ruff and Calvert 2014).

THE CANADIAN LEGACY ON THE GLOBAL GOVERNANCE OF ASBESTOS

While the Canadian asbestos industry ceased production in 2012, this chapter argues that it has left behind a deadly global health legacy. The exit of U.S. and European asbestos MNCs might have resulted in a corresponding demise in the mineral's production and use worldwide. However, the industry's success at persuading the Canadian and Quebec governments to champion its cause domestically and globally kept the asbestos trade alive. In addition to bridging the shift in production to new industry players and new markets in LMICs, Canadian-led policy actions sustained the policy influencing networks built by the MNCs, and extended their influence on global institutions (Rice 2011; Ruff and Mirabelli 2014). The ICA learned how to influence occupational health policies in LMICs and oppose efforts in key international environmental and occupational health bodies (Kazan-Allen 2003; McCulloch and Tweedale 2008). Several ICA spokespersons at Rotterdam 2015 were veterans of the Quebec industry. The ICA united the new asbestos exporters, led by

Russia, its new funder, with new manufacturers in India, Thailand, Viet Nam, Indonesia, Pakistan Iran, Mexico, Colombia and other LMICs.

India, the world's largest asbestos importer, now accounts for almost a quarter of global consumption, a dramatic increase from fifteen years ago (USGS 2014). Maintaining this market is key to the industry's future. Russia, Kazakhstan and Brazil, assisted by the ICA, have built an extensive network of Indian manufacturers who are now a major lobby for its continued use (Kazan-Allen 2007). In 2013, the ICA co-sponsored a major conference in New Delhi with the Asbestos Cement Products Manufacturers' Association (ACPMA) of India. Industry participants from Thailand, Russia, UK, the United States, Switzerland, Brazil, Viet Nam and the Ukraine also attended.

The ICA has also targeted LMICs considering new restrictions on asbestos. In 2011, it hired the Washington-based public relations firm APCO Worldwide, which had previously worked closely with the tobacco industry (Mombiot 2006), to lobby the Malaysian government to reject a proposed ban. Critics noted that the firm did not publicly disclose ICA funding (Kazan-Allen 2011). Malaysia still has no ban. Many other examples can be cited (Ruff and Mirabelli 2014).

Finally, the ICA continues to lobby successfully at Rotterdam. In 2015, it produced a glossy brochure containing correspondence between its

Table 8.2. World Asbestos Consumption 2011-2013 (metric tonnes)

Country	2011	2012	2013	Average 2011-2013
China	638,000	531,000	570,000	580,000
India	357,000	473,000	303,000	378,000
Russia	251,000	155,000	432,000	279,000
Brazil	185,000	168,000	181,000	178,000
Indonesia	124,000	162,000	156,000	147,000
Kazakhstan	156,000	5,000	67,000	76,000
Uzbekistan	17,000	104,000	81,000	67,000
Vietnam	80,000	79.000	58,000	72,000
Thailand	81,000	58,000	53,000	64,000
Sri Lanka	61,000	54,000	23,000	46,000
Ukraine	56,000	42,000	35,000	44,000
Colombia	20,000	25,000	16,000	20,500

Source: U.S. Geological Survey – Asbestos. 2014. Advance Release 2013. (numbers are rounded)
Note: Year to year fluctuations reflect varying dates of shipments and storage arrangements.

chairman, Jean-Marc Leblond, and the executive secretary of the Convention Rolf Payet, challenging the decision to revisit listing (ICA 2015). The brochure claimed that convention officials had been captured by the anti-asbestos lobby (ICA 2015). With Russia opposed, efforts to list chrysotile were once again defeated. Immediately after the decision, the ICA website was updated with a press release claiming the failure confirmed the mineral's safety (ICA 2015).

CONCLUSION

Asbestos is no longer used significantly in most high-income countries and fifty-seven countries now ban it. Leading medical and occupational health journals have called for a global ban. Stronger global governance of asbestos is now debated widely. In 2006, the ILO passed a resolution calling for the elimination of all future asbestos use. International labour federations—particularly the Building Workers' International (BWI)—have intensified their lobbying against asbestos (Cremers and Gehring 2013). There are increasingly effective victims' organizations in nineteen countries, including Indonesia, Hong Kong, Brazil and Argentina (IBAS 2015), partly reflecting the growing number of ARDs in LMICs (Association Nationale 2014). NGOs, such as IBAS and its counterparts in LIMCs, are now credible international players. Anti-asbestos NGOs now sponsor numerous conferences and lobby international meetings such as Rotterdam (IBAS 2015).The Collegium Ramazzini provides research for these campaigns. Even in Russia, a significant debate is emerging, despite the industry's influence on government (Kazan-Allen 2011). These are encouraging developments.

Despite these efforts, a global ban remains elusive. Asbestos has benefitted from the failure, globally, to establish an effective regulatory system. International environmental and health agreements remain unacceptably weak. They still rely on the good will, voluntary commitment and public responsibility of governments. Too often, this commitment is not there. Compounding this is the failure to fund the UN-affiliated environmental and occupational health agencies adequately. They lack the resources to support the needed research, education, advocacy and international diplomacy. And, too often, they are unduly influenced by the corporations and investors they regulate.

However, the failure to end the global asbestos trade is also a failure of political will by governments in developed countries. They do not see ending the global asbestos trade as a major priority and remain indifferent to its appalling health impacts LMICs—health impacts they no longer accept within their own borders. That they have the capacity is clear. To advance the interests of corporations, these same governments have established binding international trade rules, overseen by the WTO, to which all member countries must adhere. These rules have effective enforcement mechanisms through trade sanctions and investor-state dispute provisions.

When Ebola appeared to threaten population health in the United States, Europe and other high income countries in 2015, they quickly raised significant resources to fund vaccine research. They also implemented tough policy measures—some of which may not have been appropriate—to prevent its spread. Similarly, when they perceived threats to their national security, they allocated the military resources necessary to deal with such threats. But the same is not true for occupational and environmental health issues. They simply have not had the political commitment to do so.

Asbestos also underscores another weakness of the international regulatory system: the vulnerability of its institutions to strategic lobbying by corporations with narrow, but clearly focused economic interests. Where industries have the resources and determination to frustrate international regulatory initiatives, the institutions mandated to protect public health, human rights or labour conditions turn out to be exceedingly vulnerable. If there is a lesson here it is the urgent need to strengthen the mandate and resources of these institutions. The international health community must become a more effective countervailing force, capable of challenging corporate lobbying. And it must develop more effective ways to influence governments in both developed countries and LMICs to make occupational and environmental health the urgent priorities that they should be both domestically and internationally.

NOTES

1. The scientific and medical evidence is overwhelming that asbestos is a health hazard to all those who come in contact with it. This article takes as a given that the harms caused by asbestos are sufficiently well documented that there is no need to replicate the medical and scientific evidence here.

2. There are a number of data sources on the production and consumption of asbestos. The most widely cited is the U.S. Geological Survey (USGS), which contains statistics dating back to the end of the nineteenth century. This data base has been supervised by Robert Virta for many years. See http://minerals.usgs.gov/minerals/pubs/commodity/asbestos. The other major source is the UN's Comtrade Database on imports and exports of asbestos and asbestos products: http://comtrade.un.org.

REFERENCES

Asbestos Institute. n.d. 'Undeniable Facts About Chrysotile'. www.chrysotile.com/data/Undeniable_facts.pdf.
———. 1993. 'Safe Use of Chrysotile Asbestos'. September. www.chrysotile.com/data/Safety_use_Chryso-A_VF.pdf.

Association Nationale de Defense des Victimes de l'Amiante. 2014. 'International Day of Asbestos Victims; State of Science, State of the World'. www.andeva.fr/?Proceedings-of-the-symposium.

Baram, Michael. 2009. 'Globalization and Workplace Hazards in Developing Nations' *Safety Science* 47 (6): 756–66.

Bernstein, David. 2006. 'Chrysotile at a Turning Point: Results and Scientific Perspectives'. 23 May. www.chrysotile.com/data/conferences/Presentation_David_Bernstein.pdf.

Bernstein, David, Jacques Dunnigan, Thomas Hesterberg, Robert Brown, Juan Antonio Legaspi Velasco, Raul Barrera, John Hoskins and Allen Gibbs. 2013. 'Health Risk of Chrysotile Revisited'. *Critical Reviews in Toxicology* 43 (2): 154–83.

Bernstein, David, Rick Rogers and Paul Smith. 2004. 'The Biopersistence of Brazilian Chrysotile Following Inhalation'. *Inhalation Toxicology* 16 (11–12): 745–61.

Bitonti, Christopher. 2009. 'Exporting Ignorance: Canada's Opposition to the Regulation of the International Chrysotile Asbestos Trade under the Rotterdam Convention'. *Asper Review of International Business and Trade Law* 9: 171–99.

Brandt, Allan. 2007. *The Cigarette Century*. New York: Basic Books.

Braun, Lundy, Anna Greene, Marc Manseau, Raman Singhai, Sophie Kisling and Nancy Jacobs. 2003. 'Scientific Controversy and Asbestos: Making Disease Invisible'. *International Journal of Occupational and Environmental Health* 9 (3): 194–205.

Calvert, John. 2013. 'The End of Canada's Role as the Leading Global Advocate for the Production and Use of Asbestos'. In *The Long and Winding Road to an Asbestos Free Workplace*, edited by Jan Cremers, 59–76. Brussels: European Institute of Construction Labour Research.

Canadian Broadcasting Corporation (CBC). 2008. 'Canadian Labour Congress Delays Call for Ban on Asbestos Mining'. *CBC News*, 20 February.

———. 2009. 'Canada's Ugly Secret'. *CBC TV News*, 11 June.

Cremers, Jan, and Rolf Gehring, eds. 2013. *The Long and Winding Road to an Asbestos Free Workplace*. Brussels: European Institute for Construction Labour Research.

Davies, Ronald B., and Krishna Vadlamannati. 2013. 'A Race to the Bottom in Labour Standards? An Empirical Investigation'. *Journal of Development Economics* 103: 1–14.

Dunnigan, Jacques. 2009. 'Asbestos: The Cause of 100,000 Deaths Annually—Myth or Reality'. *Chrysotile Institute*. www.chrysotile.com/data/brochure_ICA_ang-f.pdf.

Egilman, David, Corey Fehnel and Susanna Rankin Bohme. 2003. 'Exposing the "Myth" of ABC, "Anything But Chrysotile": A Critique of the Canadian Asbestos Mining Industry and McGill University Chrysotile Studies'. *American Journal of Industrial Medicine* 44 (5): 540–57.

Galloway, Gloria. 2011. 'Documents Detail Mulroney-Era Efforts to Block US Asbestos Ban'. *Globe and Mail*, 18 October. www.theglobeandmail.com/news/politics/ottawa-notebook/documents-detail-mulroney-era-efforts-to-block-us-asbestos-ban/article619496.

Globe and Mail. 2012. 'Quebec Gives Jeffrey Asbestos Mine $58-Million Boost'. *Globe and Mail*, 29 June.

Gray, John, and Stephanie Nolen. 2011. 'Canada's Chronic Asbestos Problem'. *Globe and Mail*, 21 November. www.theglobeandmail.com/report-on-business/rob-magazine/canadas-chronic-asbestos-problem/article4184217/?page=all.

Holden, Chris, and Kelley Lee. 2009. 'Corporate Power and Social Policy: The Political Economy of the Transnational Tobacco Companies'. *Global Social Policy* 9 (3): 328–54.

Howse, Robert, and Elizabeth Türk. 2009. 'The WTO Impact on Internal Regulations—a Case Study of the Canada-EU Asbestos Dispute'. In *Trade and Human Health and Safety*, edited by G. C. Berman and P. Mavroidis, 77–117. Cambridge: Cambridge University Press.

International Ban Asbestos Secretariat (IBAS). 2015. 10 September. http://www.ibasecretariat.org.

International Chrysotile Association (ICA). 2015. 'Rotterdam Convention COP7 Meeting—2015'. http://chrysotileassociation.com/data/texte_sommaire_rotterdam _en.pdf.

Kazan-Allen, Laurie. 2003. 'The Asbestos War'. *International Journal of Occupational and Environmental Health* 9 (3): 173–93.

———. 2007. 'Killing the Future: Asbestos Use in Asia'. July. London: International Ban Asbestos Secretariat. http://worldasbestosreport.org/articles/killing_future/killing_the_future_asbestos_use_in_asia.pdf.

———. 2011. 'Russian Asbestos U-Turn International Ban Asbestos Secretariat'. 15 September. http://ibasecretariat.org/lka-russian-asbestos-u-turn.php.

———. 2012. 'The Rise and Fall of the Chrysotile Institute. International Ban Asbestos Secretariat'. 1 May. http://ibasecretariat.org/lka-rise-and-fall-of-chrysotile-institute.php.

———. 2014. 'Charting the Changing Pattern of Asbestos Production and Use 1950-2011'. In *International Day of Asbestos Victims; State of Science, State of the World,* edited by ANDEVA, 115–24. Paris: ANDEVA. www.andeva.fr/?Proceedings-of-the-symposium.

Kuyek, Joan. 2003. 'Asbestos Mining in Canada: A Brief Presented to the International Ban Asbestos Conference'. 13 September. Ottawa: Mining Watch Canada. www.miningwatch.ca/files/Asbestos_Mining_in_Canada_0.pdf.

Lemen, Richard. 2014. 'Epidemic to Pandemic: Asbestos in Our World'. In *International Day of Asbestos Victims; State of Science, State of the World,* edited by ANDEVA, 3–34. Paris: ANDEVA. www.andeva.fr/?Proceedings-of-the-symposium.

McCulloch, Jock, and Geoffrey Tweedale. 2008. *Defending the Indefensible: The Global Asbestos Industry and Its Fight for Survival.* New York: Oxford University Press.

McDonald, Corbett J., and A. D. McDonald. 1997. 'Chrysotile, Tremolite and Carcinogenicity'. *Annals of Occupational Hygiene* 41 (6): 699–705.

Mittelstaedt, Martin. 2008. 'Medical Journal Blasts Ottawa over Asbestos'. *Globe and Mail,* 19 October.

———. 2009. 'Government Trying to Protect Quebec Industry, Scientist Alleges'. *Globe and Mail,* 22 April.

Mombiot, George. 2006. 'The Denial Industry'. *Guardian,* 19 September. www.theguardian.com/environment/2006/sep/19/ethicalliving.g2.

Morris, Jim. 2014. 'Exporting an Epidemic: Human Toll Reaches Millions as Asbestos Industry Expands Worldwide'. www.publicintegrity.org/2010/07/21/3401/exporting-epidemic.

Parigot, Michel. 2014. 'Asbestos and the World Trade Organization'. In *International Day of Asbestos Victims; State of Science, State of the World,* edited by ANDEVA, 163–72. http://issuu.com/lindareinstein/docs/book_andeva_uk_jiva2014final.

Rice, James. 2011. 'The Global Reorganization and Revitalization of the Asbestos Industry 1970—2007'. *International Journal of Health Services* 41 (2).

Robertson, David. 1992. 'Mazarin to Buy Quebec's Stake in Asbestos Mines'. *The Northern Miner* 78 (28).

Rubin, Ken. 2011. 'Research Data on Asbestos Exposure Hidden'. 17 May. www.kenrubin.ca/articles/research-data-on-asbestos-exposure-hidden.pdf.

Ruff, Kathleen. 2009. 'Exporting Harm: How Canada Markets Asbestos to the Developing World'. Ottawa: The Rideau Institute. www.rightoncanada.ca/?p=248.

———. 2015. 'Scientific Journals and Conflict of Interest Disclosure: What Progress Has Been Made?' *Environmental Health* 14: 45. doi:10.1186/s12940-015-0035-6.

Ruff, Kathleen, and John Calvert. 2014. 'Rejecting Science-Based Evidence and International Co-operation: Canada's Foreign Policy on Asbestos under the Harper Government'. *Canadian Foreign Policy Journal* 20 (2): 131–45.

Schmidt, Sarah. 2011. 'Canada: Telling Lies about Asbestos'. *Montreal Gazette,* 28 March.

Sentes, Kyla. 2009. 'Oh, Canada—We Stand on Guard for Asbestos'. *Canadian Foreign Policy* 15 (3): 30–49.

Stayner, L. 2008. 'Canada, Chrysotile and Cancer: Health Canada's Asbestos International Panel Report'. *Journal of Occupational and Environmental Medicine* 50 (12).

Turcotte, Fernand. 2014. 'Asbestos and Health Risks in Quebec'. *International Day of Asbestos Victims. op. cit.*, chapter 3.

Tweedale, Geoffrey. 2000. *Magic Mineral to Killer Dust: Turner-Newall and the Asbestos Hazard.* New York: Oxford University Press.

United Nations Environment Program (UNEP). 2004. 'Report of the Conference of the Parties to the Rotterdam Convention on the Prior Informed Consent Procedure for Certain Hazardous Chemicals and Pesticides in International Trade on the Work of Its First Meeting'. Geneva, 22 October. "www.unido.org/fileadmin/user_media/Services/Environmental_Management/GUDDIS/Legal_Frameworks/rotterdam_convention.pdf.

USGS. 2005. *Mineral Commodity Profiles—Asbestos.* Circular 1255—KK. Reston, Virginia. www.usgs.gov.

———. 2006. *Worldwide Asbestos Supply and Consumption Trends from 1900 to 2003.* U.S. Geological Survey (Mineral Industry Surveys). Circular 1298.

———. 2009. *World Asbestos Consumption from 2003 through 2007.* U.S. Geological Survey (Mineral Industry Surveys). July.

———. 2012. *Mineral Commodity Summaries: Asbestos.* U.S. Geological Survey. January.

———. 2014. *2013 Mineral Yearbook (Advance Release).* U.S. Geological Survey. October.

———. 2015. *Mineral Commodity Summaries.* January.

World Health Organization. 2014. 'Asbestos: Elimination of Asbestos Related Diseases'. Fact Sheet no. 343, July. www.who.int/mediacentre/factsheets/fs343/en.

WTO Dispute DS135. 1998. 'European Communities—Measures Affecting Asbestos and Products Containing Asbestos'. May 28. Geneva:. www.wto.org/english/tratop_e/dispu_e/cases_e/ds135_e.htm.

NINE

The Entrenchment of the Public-Private Partnership Paradigm

Michael Stevenson

Public-private partnerships (PPPs) are governance arrangements whereby private for-profit entities voluntarily assume a degree of responsibility for enabling access to goods or services that have historically been associated exclusively with non-profit or government entities (Reich 2002, 1). As collaborative arrangements aimed at addressing health and social problems, PPPs are controversial in part because they provide private actors with opportunities to shape public policy making (Buse and Harmer 2007, 267). While the profit-seeking purpose of business is traditionally seen as distinctive from, and even in opposition with, the public good (Birn 2014, e8), the PPP paradigm has allowed business to become an equal partner with the public and the third sector (non-profits and non-governmental organisations [NGOs]) in framing and managing efforts to mitigate particular adverse effects of broader social inequalities (Ruggie 2004).

The first PPPs concerned with improving health in developing country contexts were forged in the late 1970s to bridge gaps between public, private and third-sector organisations perceived to be limiting the development and uptake of new low-cost contraceptive options (Stevenson 2014). By the 1990s, PPPs were embraced at the global level as a means of compensating for the difficulties experienced by states and markets in developing essential health technologies for populations with limited purchasing power (Moran and Stevenson 2013). By the end of the first decade of the new millennium, the argument that for-profit entities must be formally involved in the development and management of frameworks focused on mitigating the adverse health effects of global poverty and inequality had become entrenched within global governance (Moran and Stevenson 2014).

PPPs constitute governance innovation in global efforts to develop, finance, produce and disseminate essential health technologies and health-related public goods. Yet they are controversial for providing corporations—which, in many cases, have long ignored the needs of poor and marginalised populations—with opportunities to assume a managerial role in initiatives aimed at improving the welfare of these same groups. Moreover, early successes in the application of the partnership paradigm to product development have served to reinforce the problematic logic that technological innovations can provide solutions to problems with deep political determinants. There are also real concerns that PPPs are indirectly serving to erode the capacity and authority of the specialised agencies of the United Nations (UN) system and of governments and public sector agencies in low- and middle-income countries (LMICs). PPPs present new coordination, legitimacy and accountability challenges in already-crowded policy-making arenas. Nevertheless, this chapter argues that there is evidence that numerous global health partnerships are fulfilling their intended purpose, and that the paradigm is now deeply entrenched within global health governance.

METHODS

Data for this chapter are derived from a secondary analysis of published materials relating to public-private partnerships focused on population health issues. These include peer-reviewed articles, book chapters and monographs, print media and NGO reports, identified via searches of Google Scholar. This material was supplemented by key informant interviews with two of PATH's three co-founders (Richard Mahoney and Gordon Perkin), which were conducted in a manner consistent with the oral history method (Ritchie 2014), a research methodology that gives subjects considerable control over the direction of the interview. It is particularly useful in soliciting explanations for the actions of individuals/groups in instances where archival documents showcasing decision making are not readily available.

BACKGROUND

A small, tightly knit group of American not-for-profit organisations have featured prominently in the development of the PPP paradigm within global health governance. The partnership era arguably began with the formation in 1977 of the Seattle-based non-governmental organisation Program for Appropriate Technology in Health (PATH), which was established to connect investing partners, product manufacturers and distribution networks in order to improve access to health products for targeted populations. PATH's efforts initially focused on reproductive health technologies, but were broadened when it became apparent that gaps also existed in other areas of primary care and prevention, such as immunisations (R. Mahoney, personal communication, 4 December 2014; G. Perkin, personal communication, 8 July 2014). Although largely ignored by scholars of global health politics, PATH's successes in working with industry to develop low-cost, culturally appropriate health technologies provided substance to the narrative, championed by the U.S. Agency for International Development and the Bill and Melinda Gates Foundation (BMGF), that private-sector efficiency and resources are critical for improving public health in poor countries (Mahoney and Maynard 1999, 647).

By the 1980s, the ascendency of neoliberal economic philosophy and policy led to marked declines in overseas development aid, and decreased spending on health by governments of LMICs, resulting in reduced capacity on the part of development organisations sustained by public funds. Together, these trends increased the relevance of organisations operating at the public-private interface, which were willing to bring private sector resources to bear on public health challenges (Moran and Stevenson 2013). This was particularly true for the development of essential medicines and health technologies. Costs associated with meeting newly harmonised quality assurance standards for pharmaceuticals saw the majority of national governments pass responsibility for developing and producing preventative, diagnostic and therapeutic agents to industry, which had few incentives to invest in products for low income populations (Mahoney, Pablos-Mendez and Ramachandran 2004, 788). This resulted in stagnation in research and development related to deleterious diseases, widespread lack of access to existing essential products (such as anti-retrovirals for HIV) due to excessive costs, and an international patent-regime that largely prevented generic drug development. There was also mounting pressure on states, the UN system, and the pharmaceutical industry, to find a governance solution to address these challenges (Ollila 2005).

Against this backdrop, the Rockefeller Foundation expanded PATH's approach by establishing the International AIDS Vaccine Initiative (IAVI), a stand-alone organisation created to coordinate public and private sector research, with the goal of developing a vaccine for HIV/AIDS (Widdus and White 2004). Established in 1996, IAVI was the first of a series of disease-specific funding pools used to subsidise capital-intensive, high-risk research undertaken by large pharmaceutical corporations intended to benefit the world's poorest populations (Wheeler and Berkley 2001). The irony was that public funds were now being used to overcome market failures created, in part, by states ceding responsibility for developing and manufacturing such essential technologies to corporations. By the time the Gates Foundation was launched in 1999, PPPs had become the primary strategy for incentivising technical innovation in the face of market failure, and for transferring proprietary technologies to parties intent on strengthening access to these technologies in poor countries (Moran and Stevenson 2013). The BMGF, the world's largest philanthropic foundation and most significant non-state funder of global health initiatives, has, since its inception, focused on catalysing the development of new high-risk and high-impact health technologies. The foundation focuses on expanding the scale and scope of public-private partnering for global health innovation (Birn 2005).

With the creation of the BMGF-enabled Global Alliance for Vaccine and Immunisation (GAVI) in 2000, public-private cooperation for global health moved beyond product development to innovative financing and political advocacy (Mahoney, Ramachandran and Xu 2000). Political receptivity for public-private financing for global health was reinforced in 2002 with the establishment of the Global Fund to Fight AIDS, Tuberculosis and Malaria (GFATM), created to galvanise financial and political support for combating HIV/AIDS, malaria and TB (Attaran and Sachs 2001; Stevenson 2014, 160). The majority of overseas development aid specifically earmarked for vaccines, malaria, TB and HIV/AIDS is now channelled through these two global health financing partnerships. The primary utility of these mechanisms is thus mobilising and distributing health-targeted capital for use in developing country contexts (Atun et al. 2012).

PPPs inspired by PATH, and supported by the Rockefeller and Gates foundations, have been cited as evidence of the viability of increasing public-private cooperation by scholars such as John Ruggie and Jeffrey Sachs. As assistant secretary general for strategic planning at the UN from 1997 to 2001, Ruggie oversaw the creation and institutionalisation of both the Global Compact and the Millennium Development Goals (MDGs). Both were engineered around the PPP paradigm, and were intended to bring renewed focus and resources to longstanding UN goals related to social and environmental stewardship and poverty reduction (Smith 2009, 202; Stevenson 2014, 160–61). As a normative framework guiding international development, the MDGs institutionalised several key PPP logics: first, that the innovative capacity of the private sector must be tapped to respond to health challenges affecting the world's poor (Mahoney and Maynard 1999, 647); second, that the partnership paradigm is the most appropriate means for achieving this (Sachs 2001); and finally, that business and public sector institutions should be afforded equal levels of responsibility in the development and management of strategies oriented towards reducing global health disparities (Reich 2002).

DISCUSSION

Diverging Perspectives on PPPs in Global Health Governance

Two very different views exist on the utility of PPPs for global health, which reflect ideological discord regarding the theory and practice of global health governance, and the paradoxical role of business in the creation and resolution of health inequities. Proponents of PPPs argue that the approach offers a neat solution to a pervasive shortage of government resources (Nelson 2002), and represents a vehicle for business to establish greater social legitimacy (Ruggie 2013). They further reject the idea that PPPs act as Trojan horses through which corporations threaten to capture public sectors interests, instead portraying them as mechanisms that enable the private sector and the market economy as a whole to supplement the efforts of public authorities to address problems that no single actor is deemed capable of solving autonomously (Ruggie 2004).

Critics, by contrast, argue that by giving equal weight to the public good and the interests of unaccountable corporations (Richter 2003), PPPs serve to institutionalize the voices of private entities within public policy-making arenas (Buse and Harmer 2007, 267). This in turn erodes the public-private distinction (Utting 2000), distorts public policy objectives (Bull, Boas and McNeill 2004), reduces transparency of process (Forman and Segaar 2006) and undermines the ability of governments and international organisations to credibly claim that they act in the public interest (Utting 2000), resulting in the erosion of public sector legitimacy (Cutler 2002, 34).

While PPPs have proven to be an effective means of bringing together diverse and relevant actors to attempt to address challenges facing the world's most marginalised populations, there is clear variation in the extent to which they succeed in doing so. Instances of failure—for example, related to the use of social marketing to promote condom use—have been linked to a reliance on business strategies that lack consideration for community perspectives and/or larger structural determinants of the diseases that such partnerships were forged to address (Pfeiffer 2004).

Moreover, the sustainability of the model must also be questioned, as PPPs typically require enablers such as the BMGF to function as organisers, and to provide the seed money necessary to get them off the ground. This is then leveraged to attain greater operating capital, which usually comes from the public purse, as opposed to corporate resources (Moran 2011). Corporate reticence to invest its own capital is not surprising, as doing so is inherently in conflict with their organisational purpose, particularly the fiduciary responsibility to maximise profits (Friedman 1970). Partnerships such as the Mectizan Donation Program, which for over three decades has seen Merck work with African governments around the free distribution of its anti-parasitic drug used in the treatment of Onchocerciasis (Collins 2004), are atypical. This is because from the paradigm's inception, it has been standard practice for the organizers of partnerships to take the business needs of participating firms into consideration (Reich 2002). Yet other PPPs, such as nutrition and food security initiatives involving multinational food and beverage companies with histories of targeting poor populations for products high in sugar, salt and saturated fats (Grier and Kumanyika 2010) are viewed simply as calculated strategies aimed at silencing legitimate criticisms that their business models are, in fact, perpetuating health inequalities (Stuckler and Nestle 2012).

Given the Gates Foundation's role as chief contemporary supporter of global health partnerships, it is not surprising that critics view BMGF as inadvertently working against those governments and public sector agencies that it claims to help, by ensuring public funds are directed to corporations without guarantees of benefit to the public good (Birn 2014). McGoey (2014), for example, argues that BMGF's support for the advance purchase agreement model is a case in point. The strategy of earmarking a specific amount of capital to entice industry to develop new products for poor populations, which would then be bought in bulk at fixed prices, perversely limits government's ability to negotiate with multinational pharmaceutical companies for lowest possible prices. This seemingly reinforces existing arguments that the foundation's ultimate function is to strengthen U.S. economic power through the provision of new markets for American firms (Parmar 2012).

PPPs Are Entrenched, but to What Effect?

The entrenchment of the PPP paradigm in global health governance has had three key impacts. First, viewed collectively, PPPs constitute the creation of a new global approach for developing, financing, producing, and disseminating essential health products and services. GAVI and the Global Fund stand out for creating important political commitments to immunisation and efforts to reduce the incidence of HIV/AIDS, malaria and tuberculosis, three leading causes of morbidity and mortality. Both partnerships have been credited with playing a key role in the advancement of the MDGs, particularly goal 4, reducing child mortality rates, and goal 6, combatting HIV/AIDS, malaria and other major diseases (GAVI 2010, 12; Moran and Stevenson 2014).

But questions remain as to why this form of governance has found acceptance in an unjust global economic system. Magnusson (2010) argues that partnerships cannot be seen as being politically neutral because they largely accept the rules of the global economy. Product development partnerships, for example, often confer intellectual property rights to participating pharmaceutical companies (Wheeler and Berkley

2001), despite many of these same firms attempting to limit LMICs from superseding drug patents in the face of legitimate public health emergencies, which, in theory at least, is allowable, under the flexibility provision of the Agreement on Trade-Related Aspects of Intellectual Property Rights (Asante and Zwi 2007).

Because of the considerable financial support that the BMGF provides to global health partnerships, PPPs are inherently linked with 'philanthrocapitalism', which is premised on the assumption that applying the traditional business model to social problems will bring about positive social change (Edwards 2008). Critics, however, see the foundation's embrace of this logic as indirectly shutting out other viable organisational models (Buse and Naylor 2009). It has also been accused of disingenuousness, given that its tax-sheltered endowment has indirectly benefited from corporate exploitation of those the organisation aspires to help, such as those adversely affected by Shell's socially and ecologically damaging extraction operations in the Niger Delta (Piller, Sanders and Dixon 2007).

The second implication of the entrenchment of PPPs is that technological interventions are being prioritised as solutions to problems that have deep political and social determinants. Such reliance on product development as a means to improving health suggests global health leaders have forgotten the abject failure of the World Health Organization's (WHO) Global Malaria Eradication Program (MEP). The program, a poorly thought-out attempt to eliminate mosquito vectors through the spraying of DDT, despite a lack of evidence that it was effective in large-scale prevention (Litsios 2007, 53), did little to address anemic health systems in the countries in which it operated from 1951 until 1964 (Staples 2006, 179).

To be sure, technology plays a critical role in the mitigation and treatment of many pressing global health challenges. Vaccination, for example, is among the most cost-effective means of reducing morbidity and mortality in both rich and poor countries (Ozawa et al. 2012), and remains a cornerstone of preventative medicine. Moreover, technology can also be critical to efforts to mitigate, at least in the short term, the adverse effects of political determinants of health not being met, as is the case of oral rehydration therapy in contexts where governments cannot ensure access to safe drinking water (Connolly et al. 2004). The potential benefits of involving corporations such as Monsanto and Pioneer, which hold valuable intellectual property, into partnerships with states and communities may ultimately prove to be crucial for strengthening agriculture across Sub-Saharan Africa in the face of prolonged drought or flooding associated with climate change (Paarlberg 2008).

Yet there is also merit to the charge that supporters of PPPs focused on improving health indicators in low-income countries are relying on technological innovations at the expense of public sector capacity building across the global South. Ensuring product uptake and delivery in turn crowds out other viable and less resource-intensive options (Birn 2005). Further, while technological innovation can assist in controlling communicable diseases, which is the focus of the majority of current partnerships (Shiffman 2006), it is less applicable to mitigating the risks of chronic non-communicable diseases (NCDs). This has particular implications for LMICs, which account for almost three-quarters, or 28 million deaths, of NCD-attributable global mortality (World Health Organization 2014). The question then becomes whether PPPs can help public authorities function as regulators and educators, for example in efforts to limit access to tobacco among minors, or reduce levels of sodium, sugar and saturated fats in foods consumed by the general population (Magnusson 2010, 491).

The third implication of the entrenchment of PPPs is that acceptance of the partnership paradigm is indirectly illuminating multiple crises facing the specialised agencies of the UN system, and more specifically the WHO. Critics argue that narrowly focused partnerships convened by unelected private actors are undermining the authority of WHO (Ollila 2005; Williams and Rushton 2011, 18), thus usurping authority from the one organisation mandated by the world's states to coordinate international efforts to control disease (McNeil 2008). There is merit to these charges. The MDG program has provided legitimacy to the idea of giving corporations agenda-setting power equal to that enjoyed by public authorities in efforts to reduce global health disparities, despite their established role in creating those same disparities (Reich 2002). However, through its acceptance and promotion of the MDGs, the UN has lent credence to the basic argument that gave rise to the PPP paradigm in first place, which is that it is essential to draw upon the innovative capacity of business if solutions to the world's greatest health are to be developed and sustained (Mahoney and Maynard 1999).

CONCLUSION

In less than two decades, PPPs have evolved from a novel innovation to a seemingly permanent fixture on the landscape of global health governance. Organisations such as PATH and the BMGF continue to be well-positioned to influence the public-private interface, and have enabled and championed corporate involvement in efforts to reduce global health disparities and strengthen public health in LMICs.

If PPPs are entrenched, their impact on global health governance remains contested. By developing and lobbying for alternative governance mechanisms outside of traditional multilateral arenas, PATH and the Rockefeller and Gates foundations either have worked to undermine the legitimacy of WHO (McCoy and McGoey 2011, 156), or have endeavoured to compensate for its deficiencies, depending on which of two opposing perspectives one assumes to be correct.

There is evidence to support both perspectives. Partnerships are indeed creating previously unanticipated coordination and accountability problems in already-crowded policy-making spaces. However, the decline of WHO authority in the neoliberal era is in no small part the result of political and fiscal constraints that have been imposed on it by donor states, as well as by its own antiquated governance structures that limit its ability to cooperate with non-state actors in pursuit of common goals.

Legitimate concerns persist: affording business a formal role in the development and management of frameworks focused on mitigating the adverse health effects of global poverty and inequality serves to deflect attention from corporations' role in creating such problems, and invites potential conflicts of interest. Yet sustained support from both donors and beneficiaries suggests the paradigm will remain an important organisational model for the indeterminate future. At the very least, PPPs have provided both proponents and detractors of global capitalism with a new way of conceptualising the role of business in society.

REFERENCES

Asante, Augustine D., and Anthony B. Zwi. 2007. 'Public-Private Partnerships and Global Health Equity: Prospects and Challenges'. *Indian Journal of Medical Ethics* 4 (4): 176–80.

Attaran, Amir, and Jeffrey Sachs. 2001. 'Defining and Refining International Donor Support for Combating the AIDS Pandemic'. *The Lancet* 357 (9249): 57–61. doi:http://dx.doi.org/10.1016/S0140-6736(00)03576-5.

Atun, Rifat, Felicia Marie Knaul, Yoko Akachi and Julio Frenk. 2012. 'Innovative Financing for Health: What Is Truly Innovative?' *The Lancet* 380 (9858): 2044–49. doi:10.1016/S0140-6736(12)61460-3.

Birn, Anne-Emanuelle. 2005. 'Gates's Grandest Challenge: Transcending Technology as Public Health Ideology'. *The Lancet* 366 (9484): 514–19. http://dx.doi.org/10.1016/S0140-6736(05)66479-3.

———. 2014. 'Philanthrocapitalism, Past and Present: The Rockefeller Foundation, the Gates Foundation, and the Setting(s) of the International/Global Health Agenda'. *Hypothesis* 12 (1): e8. doi: 10.5779/hypothesis.v12i1.229.

Bull, Benedicte, Martin Boas and Desmond McNeill. 2004. 'Private Sector Influence in the Multilateral System'. *Global Governance* 10 (4): 481–98.

Buse, Kent, and Andrew Harmer. 2007. 'Seven Habits of Highly Effective Global Public–Private Health Partnerships: Practice and Potential'. *Social Science and Medicine* 64: 259–71. doi:10.1016/j.socscimed.2006.09.001.

Buse, Kent, and Chris Naylor, 2009. 'Commercial Health Governance'. In *Making Sense of Global Health Governance: A Policy Perspective*, edited by Kent Buse, Wolfgang Hein and Nick Drager, 187–208. Basingstoke, UK: Palgrave Macmillan.

Collins, Kimberly Layne. 2004. 'Profitable Gifts: A History of the Merck Mectizan Donation Program and Its Implications for International Health'. *Perspectives in Biology and Medicine* 47 (1): 100–109. doi: 10.1353/pbm.2004.0004.

Connolly, Máire A., Michelle Gayer, Michael J. Ryan, Peter Salama, Paul Spiegel and David L. Heymann. 2004. 'Communicable Diseases in Complex Emergencies: Impact and Challenges'. *The Lancet* 364 (9449): 1974–83. http://dx.doi.org/10.1016/S0140-6736(04)17481-3.

Cutler, A. Claire. 2002. 'Private International Regimes and Interfirm Cooperation'. In *The Emergence of Private Authority in Global Governance*, edited by Rodey Bruce Hall and Thomas J. Biersteker, 23–40. Cambridge: Cambridge University Press.

Edwards, Michael. 2008. *Just Another Emperor? The Myths and Realities of Philanthrocapitalism*. New York: Demos and The Young Foundation.

Forman, Shepard, and Derk Segaar. 2006. 'New Coalitions for Global Governance: The Changing Dynamics of Multilateralism'. *Global Governance* 12 (2): 205–25.

Friedman, Milton. 1970. 'The Social Responsibility of Business Is to Increase Its Profits'. *New York Times Magazine* 13: 32–33.

Global Alliance for Vaccines and Immunization. 2010. *GAVI Alliance Progress Report 2010*. Geneva: GAVI Alliance.

Grier, Sonya A., and Shiriki Kumanyika. 2010. 'Targeted Marketing and Public Health'. *Annual Review of Public Health* 31: 349–69. doi: 10.1146/annurev.publhealth.012809.103607.

Litsios, Socrates. 2007. 'Selskar Gunn and Paul Russell of the Rockefeller Foundation: A Contrast in Styles'. In *Philanthropic Foundations and the Globalization of Scientific Medicine and Public Health*, edited by Benjamin B. Page and David A. Valone, 44–55. Lanham, MD: University Press of America.

Magnusson, Roger S. 2010. 'Global Health Governance and the Challenge of Chronic, Non-communicable Disease'. *The Journal of Law, Medicine & Ethics* 38 (3): 490–507. doi: 10.1111/j.1748-720X.2010.00508.x.

Mahoney, Richard T., and James Maynard. 1999. 'The Introduction of New Vaccines into Developing Countries'. *Vaccine* 17 (7–8): 646–52. doi:10.1016/S0264-410X(98)00246-1.

Mahoney, Richard. T., A. Pablos-Mendez and Sujatha Ramachandran. 2004. 'The Introduction of New Vaccines into Developing Countries: III. The Role of Intellectual Property'. *Vaccine* 22 (5): 786–92. doi:10.1016/j.vaccine.2003.04.001.

Mahoney, Richard. T., Sujatha Ramachandran and Zhi-Yi Xu. 2000. 'The Introduction of New Vaccines into Developing Countries II. Vaccine Financing'. *Vaccine* 18 (24): 2625–35.

McCoy, David, and Lindsey McGoey. 2011. 'Global Health and the Gates Foundation: In Perspective'. In *Partnerships and Foundations in Global Health Governance*, edited by Simon Rushton and Owain Williams, 143–63. New York: Palgrave Macmillan.

McGoey, Linsey. 2014. 'The Philanthropic State: Market–State Hybrids in the Philanthrocapitalist Turn'. *Third World Quarterly* 35 (1): 109–25. doi:10.1080/01436597.2014.868989.

McNeil, Donald G. 2008. 'WHO Official Criticizes Gates Foundation 'Cartel' on Malaria Research'. *New York Times*, 18 February. Accessed 6 March 2015. www.nytimes.com/2008/02/18/health/18iht-gates.1.10134837.html.

Moran, Michael. 2011. 'Private Foundations and Global Health Partnerships: Philanthropists and "Partnership Brokerage"'. In *Partnerships and Foundations in Global Health Governance*, edited by Simon Rushton and Owain Williams, 137–40. New York: Palgrave Macmillan.

Moran, Michael, and Michael Stevenson. 2013. 'Illumination and Innovation: What Philanthropic Foundations Bring to Global Health Governance'. *Global Society* 27 (2): 117–37.

———. 2014. 'Partnerships and the MDGs: Challenges of Reforming Global Health Governance'. In *The Handbook of Global Health Policy*, edited by Garrett Brown, Gavin Yamey and Sarah Wamala. West Sussex, UK: John Wiley & Sons.

Nelson, Jane. 2002. *Building Partnerships: Cooperation between the United Nations System and the Private Sector*. New York: United Nations.

Ollila, Eeva. 2005. 'Global Health Priorities–Priorities of the Wealthy?' *Globalization and Health* 1 (6). doi:10.1186/1744-8603-1-6.

Ozawa, Sachiko, Andrew Mirelman, Meghan L. Stack, Damian G. Walker and Orin S. Levine. 2012. 'Cost-Effectiveness and Economic Benefits of Vaccines in Low- and Middle-Income Countries: A Systematic Review'. *Vaccine* 31 (1): 96–108. doi:10.1016/j.vaccine.2012.10.103.

Paarlberg, Robert. 2008. *Starved for Science: How Biotechnology Is Being Kept Out of Africa*. Cambridge: Harvard University Press.

Parmar, Inderjeet. 2012. *Foundations of the American Century: The Ford, Carnegie, and Rockefeller Foundations in the Rise of American Power*. New York: Columbia University Press.

Pfeiffer, James. 2004. 'Condom Social Marketing, Pentecostalism, and Structural Adjustment in Mozambique: A Clash of AIDS Prevention Messages'. *Medical Anthropology Quarterly* 18 (1): 77–103. doi: 10.1525/maq.2004.18.1.77.

Piller, Charles, Edmund Sanders and Robyn Dixon. 2007. 'Dark Cloud over Good Works of Gates Foundation'. *Los Angeles Times*, 7 January. Accessed 8 January 2007. www.latimes.com/news/nationworld/nation/la-nagatesx07jan07,0,6827615.story?coll=la-home.

Reich, Michael, ed. 2002. *Public-Private Partnerships for Health*. Cambridge: Harvard University Press.

Richter, Judith. 2003. *'We the Peoples' or 'We the Corporations': Critical Reflections on UN-Business Partnerships*. Geneva: IBFAN-GIFA.

Ritchie, Donald A. 2014. *Doing Oral History*. Oxford: Oxford University Press.

Ruggie, J. G. 2004. 'Reconstituting the Global Public Domain: Issues, Actors and Practices'. *European Journal of International Relations* 10 (4): 499–531.

———. 2013. *Just Business: Multinational Corporations and Human Rights (Norton Global Ethics Series)*. New York: W.W. Norton.

Sachs, Jeffrey. 2001. 'Thinking Boldly'. *Bulletin of the World Health Organization* 79 (8): 772.

Shiffman, Jeremy. 2006. 'Donor Funding Priorities for Communicable Disease Control in the Developing World'. *Health Policy and Planning* 21 (6): 411–20. doi: 10.1093/heapol/czl028.

Smith, Richard. 2009. 'Global Health Governance and Global Public Goods'. In *Making Sense of Global Health Governance: A Policy Perspective*, edited by Kent Buse, Wolfgang Heine and Nick Drager, 122–36. New York: Palgrave MacMillan.

Staples, Amy. 2006. *The Birth of Development: How the World Bank, Food and Agriculture Organization, and World Health Organization Changed the World, 1945–1965*. Kent: Kent State University Press.

Stevenson, Michael. 2014. 'Agency through Adaptation: Explaining the Rockefeller and Gates Foundation's Influence in the Governance of Global Health and Agricultural Development'. PhD diss., University of Waterloo.

Stuckler, David, and Marion Nestle. 2012. 'Big Food, Food Systems, and Global Health'. *PLoS Medicine* 9 (6): 678. doi:10.1371/journal.pmed.1001242.

Utting, Peter. 2000. *UN-Business Partnerships: Whose Agenda Counts?* Geneva: UNRISD.

Wheeler, Craig, and Seth Berkley. 2001. 'Initial Lessons from Public-Private Partnerships in Drug and Vaccine Development'. *Bulletin of the World Health Organization* 79 (8): 728–34. http://dx.doi.org/10.1590/S0042-96862001000800008.

Widdus, Roy, and Katherine White. 2004. *Combating Diseases Associated with Poverty*. Switzerland: Initiatives for Public-Private Partnerships for Health and Global Forum for Health Research.

Williams, Owain David, and Simon Rushton. 2011. 'Private Actors in Global Health Governance'. In *Partnerships and Foundations in Global Health Governance*, edited by Simon Rushton and Owain Williams, 1–28. New York: Palgrave Macmillan.

World Health Organization. 2014. *Global Status Report on Non-communicable Diseases*. Geneva: WHO.

TEN

Trade and Investment Agreements

The Empowerment of Pharmaceutical and Tobacco Corporations

Ashley Schram and Ronald Labonte

Over the past two decades, states have been negotiating a progressively larger and more complex web of trade and investment agreements (TIAs) with profound implications for public health. This has prompted calls for greater policy coherence between TIAs and public health from non-state actors (Blouin 2007; Lee et al. 2009). One avenue through which we can better understand how such agreements have the capacity to empower corporations in global health governance (GHG) are intellectual property rights (IPRs), which threaten access to medicines and tobacco control, along with the investor-state dispute settlement (ISDS) mechanisms that enforce these provisions.

Each year millions of people around the world die from illnesses that are treatable or preventable with existing medicines that are unaffordable (Bird 2009). Efforts to redress this situation through GHG arrangements, such as the Global Fund and UNITAID, have directly challenged market-driven supply of such medicines. The cost of antiretroviral (ARV) therapy for human immunodeficiency virus (HIV), for example, decreased from US$10,000 per person when on patent, to US$100 per person when made available generically (Kapczynski 2015). By contrast, tobacco use presents one of the greatest threats to public health in human history, killing approximately 6 million people annually, including more than 600,000 non-smokers exposed to second-hand smoke (World Health Organization 2014). Global expansion of transnational tobacco companies

(TTCs) into emerging economies has markedly shifted the burden of to-bacco morbidity and mortality to low- or middle-income countries, where nearly 80 percent of the world's 1 billion smokers now reside (World Health Organization 2014). Effective governance, to regulate this addictive and lethal substance, and to prevent its adverse health, eco-nomic, environmental and societal impacts (Mackey et al. 2013), has been the focus of efforts under the WHO Framework Convention on Tobacco Control (FCTC).

To counter these GHG efforts, pharmaceutical companies and TTCs, seeking to expand their markets worldwide, have positioned IPRs as a priority trade issue (Bird 2009). Within IPR-related chapters of TIAs, pharmaceutical companies have pursued provisions that extend the time period their products are protected under patents, thus delaying the en-try of more affordable generic drugs into the market, keeping prices high-er, longer, for patients. Similarly, TTCs request that states place in these chapters stronger trademark protections to prevent packaging regula-tions that restrict the use of logos, graphics and other exclusive design elements. In this way, stronger protections for patents and trademarks within IPRs chapters draw tighter boundaries around the available policy space for GHG.

The upholding of these protections is substantially enhanced by the inclusion of ISDS mechanisms in a growing number of agreements. This mechanism creates the right of an investor from one country (home state), who invests in another country (host state), with both agreeing to ISDS, to bring a matter to an arbitral tribunal if there is a perceived violation of investor rights granted. ISDS was originally intended to pro-mote foreign investment from capital-exporting states into low-income economies, offering protection from illegal seizure of their investments by the host state. However, ISDS cases are increasingly initiated against high-income countries (increasing from historical average of 28 percent to 40 percent in 2014) (United Nations Conference on Trade and Develop-ment 2015). Jurisdictions with relatively stable and reliable legal systems are being challenged, not for *direct* expropriation and illegal seizure of property, but for the introduction of regulations construed as violating investor rights. Fair and equitable treatment (FET), a common investor right that can be evoked in an ISDS claim, has been a successful 'catch-all' clause used by investors when other claims have failed (Bernasconi-Os-terwalder et al. 2012).

The recent trend towards the exercise of rights, afforded under a growing number of TIAs, by private investors has raised concerns about the undue empowering of corporations in GHG (Friel et al. 2013; Stuckler and Nestle 2012; Weishaar et al. 2012). Such concerns are illustrated in this chapter through an examination of two key case studies: Eli Lilly's attempt to oppose Canadian patent law, and Philip Morris's attempt to thwart Australian legislation on the standardised packaging of tobacco products. In both cases, corporations have invoked arbitral mechanisms, provided for in TIAs, to sue a host government, alleging infringement of their IPRs, in response to the adoption of domestic health policy measures. A review of these cases will exemplify how corporations have so far utilised TIAs to gain influence in GHG. The focus of this analysis will be on the ISDS channel—that is, access to litigation that can award financial compensation. In doing so, ISDS decisions have the capacity to influence future decision making on public health policy far beyond states party to a dispute. This chapter will also examine how these industries have attempted to influence ongoing negotiations, lobbying for greater IPR protections that affect the flow of medicines and health-harmful commodities (e.g., tobacco), threatening to further restrict future policy space for GHG.

METHODS

To analyse paths of influence by corporations in GHG through TIAs, we conducted a narrative review. Narrative review attempts to draw holistic conclusions on a topic based on summaries of primary studies, along with the reviewers' own experiential knowledge (Campbell Collaboration 2001; Kirkevold 1997). Results focus on qualitative meanings with the opportunity for self-knowledge and reflective practice (Jones 2004). For primary studies on the arbitral disputes and their implications for GHG, we searched Google Scholar using search terms including *Australia, plain packag*, dispute settlement, Philip Morris, ISDS, Canada, patent law, promise of the patent, promise doctrine, Eli Lilly,* and *global health governance* combined with Boolean terms. Using the same search terms, we also conducted a search of the grey literature and available primary documents of relevant ISDS proceedings.

The authors also drew heavily on their ongoing work examining pathways between TIAs and health, including access to medicines and tobacco control. Conceptual and theoretical constructs applied in the aforementioned work, specifically new constitutionalism, provided a framework from which to examine the role of corporations in TIAs as a pathway to GHG. The pattern of increased rights for investors internationally has been described as a type of new constitutionalism, wherein there has been a restructuring of the state, in part through constitutional and legal means, expanding the power and influence of the market and 'locking-in' rules and regulations protecting neoliberal patterns of accumulation (Gill and Cutler 2014). Underlying this process of new constitutionalism is hegemonic preservation, driven in part by economic elites (including large corporations) seeking to lock in their policy preferences through judicial empowerment against the interests of underrepresented groups that may threaten their existing arrangements and to which majoritarian decision-making arenas may be more favourable (Hirschl 2004). It has been suggested that new constitutionalism has emerged as 'a de facto governance structure for the global political economy, one that is premised upon both domestic and constitutional transformation as well as "progressive liberalisation" of the global political economy' (Gill and Cutler 2014, 13–14).

This analysis highlights the elements of these theoretical constructs present in the two cases to help understand how corporations can utilise and direct structures within TIAs to influence GHG. Specifically, we will describe evidence for an enhanced role of the judiciary, moving controversial policy issues from political domains to arbitral tribunals; attempts at broad interpretations of investment provisions in an attempt to find in favour of investors and influence future case law; conflicts of interest among frequently appointed arbitrators' relationships with corporations; and finally corporate lobbying during the negotiation of new agreements to enhance current IPR protections and restrict future policy space.

ELI LILLY VERSUS CANADA

Pharmaceutical giant Eli Lilly's claim filed against Canada on 2 November 2012 set historical precedent as the first time a patent-holding pharmaceutical company invoked an ISDS mechanism under a U.S. trade agreement on IPR grounds (Stastna 2013). Eli Lilly announced it would utilise the ISDS mechanism in the North American Free Trade Agreement (NAFTA) to sue the Canadian government for US$100 million dollars for revoking it patent on Straterra®, a drug used to treat chronic attention-deficit hyperactivity disorder (ADHD) (Trew 2013). Their case was previously heard in 2012 by the Canadian Federal Court of Appeal, which ruled that a short-term study (a twenty-one-person three-week study finding a 30 percent greater reduction of ADHD in eleven of twenty-one patients), not disclosed in the patent as required, still would not be sufficient to support Lilly's claim that the drug would be an effective long-term treatment of ADHD (Baker 2013). Eli Lilly later increased the value of their NAFTA lawsuit to US$500 million, adding the invalidation of its patent on Zyprexa®, an anti-psychotic drug (Trew 2013). The Canadian government in its statement of defence suggested that 'Eli Lilly . . . is a disappointed litigant. Having lost two patent cases before the Canadian courts, it now seeks to have this Tribunal misapply NAFTA Chapter Eleven and transform itself into a supranational court of appeal from reasoned, principled, and procedurally just domestic court decisions' (Government of Canada 2014).

The case hinges on Canada's patent utility standard known as the promise doctrine. International standards generally require that an invention must be novel, not obvious, and useful or capable of industrial application to be awarded a patent (McDermid 2015). The Canadian promise doctrine goes beyond this, requiring that the promised utility either be demonstrated, or be based on a *sound prediction,* at the time of filing, and that the evidence for the basis of the predicted utility must be disclosed in the original patent application (McDermid 2015). The Canadian standard reinforces the integrity of the patent system such that, in exchange for a monopoly on a product, the inventor must have sound evidence for their claims at the time of filing. As the U.S. Supreme Court has equally noted, 'A patent is not a hunting licence. It is not a reward for the search, but compensation for its successful conclusion' (Gold and Shortt 2014, 4).

Eli Lilly's case is built on the alleged violation of three investor rights. First, they are claiming a violation of the FET standard by arguing that the promise doctrine was introduced into Canadian patent law after receiving its patents, thus breaching their legitimate expectations of a stable business and legal environment. However, legal analyses have demonstrated the promise doctrine throughout Canadian patent law going back to 1959 (Gold and Shortt 2014; Government of Canada 2014), well before the 1990s, when Eli Lilly filed the patents in question. Second, Eli Lilly alleges its profits were indirectly expropriated, asserting that the promise doctrine violates three other international treaty obligations that Canada has a positive obligation to uphold—the Trade-Related Aspects of Intellectual Property Rights (TRIPS) Agreement, the Patent Cooperation Treaty (PCT) and the Paris Convention for the Protection of Industrial Property Convention. Perplexingly, one of the agreements referenced (the WTO TRIPS agreement) was not operative at the time NAFTA was signed, while the remaining two agreements (on patent cooperation and protection of industrial property) do not contain any relevant provisions on substantive patenting standards (Baker 2013).

Finally, Eli Lilly's most convoluted claim is that the promise doctrine violates its right to national treatment, a standard requiring countries to provide foreign investors with treatment that is no less favourable than the treatment provided to domestic companies in like circumstances. Since both international and domestic companies must adhere to the promise doctrine, common sense suggests that there could be no violation of national treatment. However, Eli Lilly has devised an unusual interpretation of this standard, contending that, because this standard is not required by the foreign applicants' own national jurisdictions or international rules, it disadvantages foreign nationals who are not used to contending with such requirements (Baker 2013).

Eli Lilly's litigation against Canada is still underway with the hearing set to conclude in June 2016 (Procedural Order No. 1 2014). While a review of their claims ranges from unconventional to baffling, the ISDS system gives three arbitrators the power to interpret these provisions without any binding precedent, who have historically been shown to provide expansive, investor-friendly interpretations, and be caught in a number of undisclosed conflicts of interest (Eberhardt and Olivet 2012). In the Eli Lilly case one of the three arbitrators, Albert Jan van den Berg, is a member of an 'elite 15'[1] of investment arbitrators, repeatedly appointed by investors. Van den Berg has supported contradictory outcomes in two cases against Argentina where the facts and reasoning of defence of both lawsuits were almost identical. His impartiality was questioned by Argentina, although this challenge was rejected (Eberhardt and Olivet 2012, 40). If Eli Lilly is successful in their claim for compensation, it would leave Canada especially vulnerable to future litigation from other pharmaceutical companies that have had patents invalidated because of the promise doctrine, who may not have previously felt they had a case worth pursuing.

Implications of Eli Lilly Challenge for Global Health Governance

The Canadian Supreme Court upheld the revocation of two of Eli Lilly's patents on the grounds that they did not adhere to the domestic patent law of a sovereign state. Dissatisfied with this outcome, Eli Lilly turned to an international arbitral tribunal system in 2012 according to which three privately appointed arbitrators will rule on whether Canadian patent law is compliant with NAFTA's investor protections. Within the international investment arbitration system, this 'elite 15' have decided 55 percent of all investment disputes, and 75 percent of all disputes valued at around US$4 billion. Many of these elite arbitrators have sat on corporate boards, and concerns about their true independence have been raised. Individuals, for example, could be motivated to find in favour of an investor to elicit future appointments (Eberhardt and Olivet 2012). In 2014 the panel that ordered Russia to pay damages in excess of US$50 billion to Yukos Oil (Davies et al. 2014), the largest arbitral award thus far, was entirely comprised of 'elite 15' arbitrators, with another 'elite 15' arbitrator representing the investor. Although the tribunal does not have the authority to overturn Canadian law, it can award financial compensation large enough to make it prohibitive to enforce in the future.

While precedent is not de jure in these courts, it is often implemented de facto. If the tribunal were to support Eli Lilly's reinterpretation of the national treatment standard, the decision would enter into existing case law and become available for reference in future litigation. Obliging countries to compensate pharmaceutical companies for upholding national patenting standards that are more stringent than familiar international standards undermines national sovereignty and provides corporations with new channels into influencing domestic policy, particularly in areas where they may have previously lacked enough political influence to develop more industry-friendly and capital-accumulating standards. Canada's promise doctrine attempts to deter speculative patenting. Patent law in other countries, such as India, is intended to deter pharmaceutical companies from renewing patent protections (and thus higher prices) on new uses of existing or known drugs that do not increase therapeutic efficacy (Kapczynski 2015). Protecting the patenting system from exploitation by pharmaceutical companies, including unsubstantiated utility or so-called evergreening,[2] is recognized as vital to achieving affordable access to medicines. If Eli Lilly proves to be successful, it may weaken Canada and India's ability to uphold these elevated standards and deter other states from introducing similar measures.

THE TOBACCO INDUSTRY VERSUS AUSTRALIAN STANDARDISED PACKING LAW

Previous international trade disputes concerning tobacco products (see, for example, *1990 Thailand—Restrictions on Importation of and Internal Taxes in Cigarettes* or *2011 United States—Measures Affecting the Production and Sale of Clove Cigarettes*) have largely centred on quotas or tariffs. Challenges to Australia's standardised packaging legislation is indicative of a new era of disputes premised on whether *social and environmental policies* unduly restrict tobacco-related trade and investment (Levin 2012). In December 2012 Australia became the first country to require all tobacco products supplied in the country to be sold in standardised packaging (Australian Government Department of Health 2014a). The legislation covers all facets of cigarette packaging including the specified position, font, size and colour product of the brand name, while the use of any trademarks is prohibited (Australian Government Department of Health 2014b). The focus of the challenge to this legislation has been that the ban on the use of trademarks (protected under intellectual property) interferes with consumer capacity to differentiate brands, thus violating basic expectations of TTCs and damaging the value of their investment (Lo 2012).

Analogous to the Eli Lilly case, TTCs[3] were dissatisfied with the Australian High Court ruling in favour of the government on constitutional grounds (Fletcher 2013; Liberman 2013). In determining whether Australia had acquisitioned the property of tobacco companies, in denying the use of their brand logos, the court ruling differentiated between 'taking', which involves *deprivation* of property, and 'acquiring', which involves *receiving* of property (Fletcher 2013). Since the right to use the trademarks in question was not received by Australia or a third party, it was ruled that there was a taking, but not an acquisition. TTCs attempted to make the case that Australia obtained benefits of a 'proprietary' nature, such as giving the state *advertising space* on packaging to deliver their own health messages, which the companies likened to requiring Coca-Cola products to carry the message, 'Pay your taxes on time' (Liberman 2013). TTCs also suggested that the Australian government obtained benefits, such as the fulfilment of its legislative objectives under the FCTC, and reduced healthcare expenditure as fewer people smoked (Fletcher 2013; Liberman 2013). While this outcome was a victory for public health, its significance has been described as 'somewhat peripheral to the global showdown regarding tobacco control that has yet to fully unfold' (Fooks and Gilmore 2013, 24).

This 'global showdown' commenced with Philip Morris Asia (PMA) challenging Australia's plain packaging legislation under the 1993 Agreement between the Government of Australia and the Government of Hong Kong for the Promotion and Protection of Investment (Australian Government Attorney-General's Department 2015). Notably, PMA acquired PM Australia after the legislation was announced to gain standing to this bilateral agreement, a phenomenon referred to as *forum-shopping* (Van Harten and Loughlin 2006). PMA's case will utilise, among others, two of the core investor rights in investment treaties, namely, FET and the right to compensation in the case of expropriation (Australian Government Attorney-General's Department 2015). Previous dispositions have revealed substantial discrepancies in panel interpretations, and a lack of precedent has resulted in contradictory decisions and resultant ongoing uncertainty for countries about the compliancy of their regulations (Bernasconi-Osterwalder et al. 2012). Two of the three arbitrators on the panel, Professor Gabrielle Kaufmann-Kohler and Dr. Karl-Heinz Böckstiegel, are among the 'elite 15' of investment arbitrators (Eberhardt and Olivet 2012). Kaufmann-Kohler was recently chastised by a review committee for failing to disclose her role as a corporate board member of the Swiss Bank UBS, the single largest shareholder in Vivendi, and a shareholder in EDF, companies that appointed her as their arbitrator in two claims against Argentina in 2004. Although her impartiality was challenged by Argentina, their claim for annulment was denied. Böckstiegel, on the other hand, has been known to portray 'states as the biblical Goliath, the gigantic warrior who terrorises the kingdom, and companies with the underdog David' (Eberhardt and Olivet 2012, 40). The case remains in its preliminary stages as of July 2015.

Implications of Standardised Tobacco Packaging for Global Health Governance

Lencucha (2010) outlines three major implications, of the outcomes of litigation against standardised packaging, for the role of corporations and state sovereignty in GHG. First, it will set an important precedent about the interplay of health and economic agreements. What should be prioritised is a state's sovereignty to enact legitimate public health regulatory objectives or a state's responsibility to protect the rights of an investor including from a change in the domestic regulatory environment regardless of the intentions of said policies. Second, this case has important implications for the types of tobacco control measures supported by the FCTC that states may feel confident about introducing without sanction by another international authority, specifically whether standardised packaging will be considered compliant with investor protection commitments. Third, important conclusions will be drawn about the extent to which global tobacco control legislation (i.e., FCTC), as international law and a normative commitment, is able to legitimise government regulatory action over trade and investment obligations (Lencucha 2010; Liberman 2013). This will be particularly important given the lack of consensus during FCTC negotiations, and amid industry lobbying, which resulted in compromise language that avoided specifying the pre-eminence of either trade or health policy (Mamudu et al. 2011). Moreover, there will be wider implications for the future utility of international frameworks for the control of alcohol misuse and unhealthy diets, currently under development, in future trade and investment disputes.

Another important outcome of ISDS proceedings against tobacco control under TIAs is regulatory chill. This occurs when a government reduces the severity of, delays implementation of, or abandons a regulation altogether to avoid a potential trade or investment dispute, the associated legal costs and financial penalties. Because the amount of compensation in investment arbitrations is not linked to a country's ability to pay, regulatory chill is likely to have greater impact on low- and middle-income countries (LMICs) (Fooks and Gilmore 2013). For example, in 2010 PMI (annual revenue US$77 billion) launched an ISDS challenge against Uruguay (annual GDP US$50 billion) (Lencucha 2010; Levin 2012), prompting the reaction that 'the cost of defending this case, and the risk of being held liable, would intimidate all but the most wealthy, sophisticated countries into inaction' (Kennedy 2014, 626). In a two-year span, TTCs threatened Namibia, Togo and Uganda with lawsuits that the companies suggested would cost these governments millions of dollars to defend, leading them to drop new tobacco control laws (Seccombe 2014). Moreover, LMICs are not the only target of this strategy. It is believed that Canada abandoned standardised packaging measures in the 1990s due to a legal threat from RJR-MacDonald, BAT and other tobacco companies (Lo 2012; Mackey et al. 2013; Porterfield and Byrnes 2011).

A NEW FRONT? THE TRANS-PACIFIC PARTNERSHIP AGREEMENT

One of the most comprehensive TIAs being negotiated to date is known as the Trans-Pacific Partnership (TPP) agreement. This agreement, among twelve Pacific Rim countries (including Australia and Canada), has been described as a bill of rights for transnational companies whose representatives serve as official advisors (estimated at six hundred), and actively lobby to extend IPR protections and investment rights (Fooks and Gilmore 2013). The TPP has been described as 'the worst-ever agreement in terms of access to medicine', with proposed investor protections projected to raise health care costs to patients, companies and governments in all TPP member states by trillions of dollars if adopted (Rehle 2015).

In relation to the case studies addressed in this chapter, the IPR chapter leaked in 2015 revealed that U.S. negotiators have advocated the position of transnational pharmaceutical companies on every issue (Rehle 2015). In the negotiations, the pharmaceutical and biotechnology industries are pushing for a twelve-year exclusivity period for biotech medicines or 'biologics', which include most new cancer drugs, along with many other medicines and vaccines (Gleeson, Lopert and Moir 2014). The draft reveals options of zero, five, eight or twelve years of exclusivity. In the United States, biologics currently have twelve years of exclusivity, although the White House budget has repeatedly proposed reducing this to seven years. The U.S. government estimates that, over a ten-year period, this would save the federal health program US$3 billion, while patients would save tens of billions of US$. Despite domestically opposing a twelve-year exclusivity period, if the U.S. government successfully negotiates the same in the TPP, this would result in longer and wider-ranging patent protections for medicines, higher prices for such medicines, and ultimately reduced affordability.

On tobacco control, PMI publicly released its objectives for the TPP, requesting 'harmonisation of legitimate, science-based regulations', inclusion of ISDS mechanisms, and a comprehensive TRIPS-plus IPR chapter, including a 'high standard of protection for trademarks' (Fooks and Gilmore 2013). Increased protections for trademarks are not a surprising request, given their focal role in the ongoing litigation reviewed above. Importantly, all of PMI's requests have been reflected in leaked drafts of relevant TPP chapters (Fooks and Gilmore 2013). This suggests that the United States is proposing clearer language on positive rights for trademarks in the TPP (McGrady 2013) that would support tobacco industry arguments of the right to *use* their trademarks, rather than simply the right to register and exclude others from using them. There are also proposed provisions that may give the tobacco industry new rights to use their trademarks with a place name, including geographic areas such as Marlboro or Salem, building in a new layer of trademark protection (Shaffer and Brenner 2013). A draft of the investment chapter suggests broad language around expropriation, including ambiguous language protecting 'reasonable investment-backed expectations'. If adopted, tobacco companies would be able to argue that the ability to use their trademarks was a reasonable expectation at the time of investment (Shaffer and Brenner 2013).

The TPP is also anticipated to permit corporations increased access to the health policy process through the development of a national coordinating body (NCB). The NCB would have the power to review regulatory measures for compliance with 'good regulatory practices', increase involvement of non-health ministries with alternative priorities in the development of health regulations, and improve collaboration between governments and stakeholders (including industry) (Fooks and Gilmore 2013). 'The TPP is an RTA unlike any of its predecessors. It is a misnomer to call it a trade agreement: The TPP will be more like an investment treaty, designed to increase economic integration and arguably shifting the balance of policy-making power firmly in favour of corporate interests' (Friel et al. 2013, 2).

CONCLUSION

This chapter's examination of international trade and investment litigation demonstrates how such agreements have the capacity to empower corporations to challenge legitimate public health objectives globally. Such cases can directly interfere with the provision of affordable care for all, or weaken public health regulatory capacity. Neither of the ISDS cases reviewed here had been concluded as of October 2015. The decisions will have profound implications for GHG efforts to date to strengthen access to medicines and tobacco control, and will influence the direction of future national and global health policy responses. These cases are but two examples alongside attempts by corporations to influence a new generation of trade and investment agreements with the potential to further strengthen IPR and investor rights in their favour. The outcome of these cases will set new precedents about the boundaries that TIAs can place around future public health regulatory space, as well as legitimise the role of corporate actors in GHG.

NOTES

1. 'A group of fifteen arbitrators that have captured the decision making in 55 percent of the total investment treaty cases known today. This elite fifteen have the heaviest caseload as arbitrators in investment treaty disputes, handle most of the biggest cases in terms of amounts demanded by the corporations and have been repeatedly ranked as top arbitrators by well-known surveys' (Eberhardt and Olivet 2012, 38).

2. 'Evergreening is achieved by seeking extra patents on variations of the original drug—new forms of release, new dosages, new combinations or variations, or new forms. Big pharma refers to this as "lifecycle management". Even if the patent is dubious, the company can earn more from the higher prices than it pays in legal fees to keep the dubious patent alive' (Moir and Gleeson 2014).

3. Japan Tobacco International (JTI), British American Tobacco (BAT), Australasia Ltd, Imperial Tobacco and Philip Morris International (PMI).

REFERENCES

Australian Government Attorney-General's Department. 2015. 'Tobacco Plain Packaging—Investor-State Arbitration'. www.ag.gov.au/tobaccoplainpackaging.

Australian Government Department of Health. 2014a. 'Introduction of Tobacco Plain Packaging in Australia'. www.health.gov.au/internet/main/publishing.nsf/Content/tobacco-plain.

———. 2014b. 'Tobacco Plain Packaging—Your Guide'. www.health.gov.au/internet/main/publishing.nsf/Content/tppbook.

Baker, Brook. 2013. 'Corporate Power Unbound: Investor-State Arbitration of IP Monopolies on Medicines—Eli Lilly and the TPP'. *PIJIP Research Paper Series*, May. http://digitalcommons.wcl.american.edu/research/36.

Bernasconi-Osterwalder, Nathalie, Aaron Cosbey, Lise Johnson and Damon Vis-Dunbar. 2012. 'Investment Treaties & Why They Matter to Sustainable Development: Questions and Answers'. *International Institute for Sustainable Development*. www.iisd.org/sites/default/files/pdf/2011/investment_treaties_why_they_matter_sd.pdf.

Bird, Robert C. 2009. 'Developing Nations and the Compulsory License: Maximizing Access to Essential Medicines while Minimizing Investment Side Effects'. *The Journal of Law, Medicine & Ethics* 37: 209–21. doi:10.1111/j.1748-720X.2009.00366.x.

Blouin, Chantal. 2007. 'Trade Policy and Health: From Conflicting Interests to Policy Coherence'. *Bulletin of the World Health Organization* 85: 169–73. doi:10.2471/BLT.06.037143.

Campbell Collaboration. 2001. 'Campbell Collaboration Guidelines'. www.campbellcollaboration.org.

Davies, Megan, Jack Stubbs and Thomas Escritt. 2014. 'Court Orders Russia to Pay $50 Billion for Seizing Yukos Assets'. *Reuters*, 29 July. www.reuters.com/article/2014/07/29/us-russia-yukos-idUSKBN0FW0TP20140729.

Eberhardt, Pia, and Cecilia Olivet. 2012. 'Profiting from Injustice: How Law Firms, Arbitrators and Financiers Are Fuelling an Investment Arbitration Boom'. *Corporate Europe Observatory and the Transnational Institute*. www.tni.org/briefing/profiting-injustice.

Fletcher, Daniel. 2013. 'JT International SA v Commonwealth: Tobacco Plain Packaging'. *Sydney L. Rev.* 35: 827–43.

Fooks, Gary, and Anna B. Gilmore. 2013. 'International Trade Law, Plain Packaging and Tobacco Industry Political Activity: The Trans-Pacific Partnership'. *Tobacco Control*: 1–9. doi:10.1136/tobaccocontrol-2012-050869.

Friel, Sharon, Deborah Gleeson, Anne-Marie Thow, Ronald Labonte, David Stuckler, Adrian Kay and Wendy Snowdon. 2013. 'A New Generation of Trade Policy: Potential Risks to Diet-Related Health from the Trans Pacific Partnership Agreement'. *Global Health* 9. doi:10.1186/1744-8603-9-46.

Gill, Stephen, and A. Claire Cutler. 2014. *New Constitutionalism and World Order*. Cambridge: Cambridge University Press.

Gleeson, Deborah, Ruth Lopert and Hazel Moir. 2014. 'TPP Proposals Would Cost $215 Million More for Medicines per Year'. *Australian Fair Trade and Investment Network*. http://aftinet.org.au/cms/node/907.

Gold, E. Richard, and Michael Shortt. 2014. 'The Promise of the Patent in Canada and Around the World'. *Canadian Intellectual Property Review* 30: 35–81.

Government of Canada. 2014. 'Eli Lilly and Company v. Government of Canada: Government of Canada Statement of Defence'. *Foreign Affairs, Trade and Development Canada*. www.international.gc.ca/trade-agreements-accords-commerciaux/topics-domaines/disp-diff/eli-statement-declaration.aspx?lang=eng.

Hirschl, Ran. 2004. 'The Political Origins of the New Constitutionalism'. *Indiana Journal of Global Legal Studies* 11: 71–108.

Jones, Kip. 2004. 'Mission Drift in Qualitative Research, or Moving toward a Systematic Review of Qualitative Studies, Moving Back to a More Systematic Narrative Review'. *Qualitative Report* 9: 95–112.

Kapczynski, Amy. 2015. 'The Trans-Pacific Partnership—Is It Bad for Your Health?' *New England Journal of Medicine* 373: 201–3. doi:10.1056/NEJMp1506158.

Kennedy, Mary Scott. 2014. 'Australia's Tobacco Plain Packaging Act: Convergence of Public Health and Global Trade'. *North Carolina Journal of International Law & Commercial Regulation* 39: 591–629.

Kirkevold, Marit. 1997. 'Integrative Nursing Research—an Important Strategy to Further the Development of Nursing Science and Nursing Practice'. *Journal of Advanced Nursing* 25: 977–84.

Lee, Kelley, Devi Sridhar and Mayur Patel. 2009. 'Bridging the Divide: Global Governance of Trade and Health'. *The Lancet* 373: 416–22. http://dx.doi.org/10.1016/S0140-6736(08)61776-6.

Lencucha, Raphael. 2010. 'Philip Morris versus Uruguay: Health Governance Challenged'. *The Lancet* 376: 852–53. doi:10.1016/S0140-6736(10)61256-1.

Levin, Myron. 2012. 'Tobacco Industry Uses Trade Pacts to Try to Snuff Out Anti-Smoking Laws'. *NBC News*, 29 November. http://investigations.nbcnews.com/_news/2012/11/29/15519194-tobacco-industry-uses-trade-pacts-to-try-to-snuff-out-anti-smoking-laws.

Liberman, Jonathan. 2013. 'Plainly Constitutional: The Upholding of Plain Tobacco Packaging by the High Court of Australia'. *Am. JL & Med.* 39: 361–81.

Lo, Chang-fa. 2012. 'External Regime Coherence: WTO/BIT and Public Health Tension as an Illustration'. *Asian Journal of WTO and International Health Law and Policy* 7: 263.

Mackey, Tim K., Bryan A. Liang and Thomas E. Novotny. 2013. 'Evolution of Tobacco Labeling and Packaging: International Legal Considerations and Health Governance'. *American Journal of Public Health* 103: e39–43. doi:10.2105/AJPH.2012.301029.

Mamudu, Hadii M., Riss Hammond and Stanton Glantz. 2011. 'International Trade versus Public Health during the FCTC Negotiations, 1999-2003'. *Tobacco Control* 20: e3. doi:10.1136/tc.2009.035352.

McDermid, John. 2015. 'A NAFTA Challenge to Canada's Patent Utility Doctrine Is Necessary: Patents & Patent Law'. *IPWatchdog.com: Patents & Patent Law*. www.ipwatchdog.com/2014/06/11/a-nafta-challenge-to-canadas-patent-utility-doctrine-is-necessary/id=49994.

McGrady, Benn. 2013. 'Plain Packaging, Tobacco Trademarks and Geographical Indications in the TPP'. *Trade, Investment and Health*, 15 November. www.oneillinstitutetradeblog.org/plain-packaging-tobacco-trademarks-geographical-indications-tpp.

Moir, Hazel, and Deborah Gleeson. 2014. 'Explainer: Evergreening and How Big Pharma Keeps Drug Prices High'. *The Conversation*, 5 November. http://theconversation.com/explainer-evergreening-and-how-big-pharma-keeps-drug-prices-high-33623.

Porterfield, Matthew C., and Christopher R. Byrnes. 2011. 'Philip Morris v. Uruguay: Will Investor-State Arbitration Send Restrictions on Tobacco Marketing Up in Smoke?' *Investment Treaty News* 1: 3–5.

'Procedural Order No. 1'. 2014. *Foreign Affairs, Trade and Development Canada*. www.international.gc.ca/trade-agreements-accords-commerciaux/assets/pdfs/disp-diff/eli-04.pdf#page=1&zoom=auto,-73,792.

Rehle, Michaela. 2015. 'Leaked TPP Document Shows US Favoring Big Pharma'. *Reuters*, 1 July. http://rt.com/usa/271084-tpp-leak-big-pharma.

Seccombe, Mike. 2014. 'Big Tobacco's Plan to Stub Out Plain Packaging'. *The Saturday Paper*, 8 March. www.thesaturdaypaper.com.au/opinion/topic/2014/03/08/big-tobaccos-plan-stub-out-plain-packaging/1394197200.

Shaffer, Ellen, and Joe Brenner. 2013. 'Intellectual Property Chapter of Trans-Pacific Partnership Trade Agreement, Tobacco, and Public Health'. *Center for Policy Analy-*

144 Ashley Schram and Ronald Labonte

sis on Trade and Health. www.cpath.org/sitebuildercontent/sitebuilderfiles/
TPP_IP_TobaccoNov25_2013.pdf.
Stastna, Kazi. 2013. 'Eli Lilly Files $500M NAFTA Suit against Canada over Drug
Patents'. CBC News, 13 September. www.cbc.ca/1.1829854.
Stuckler, David, and Marion Nestle. 2012. 'Big Food, Food Systems, and Global
Health'. PLoS Medicine 9: e1001242. doi:10.1371/journal.pmed.1001242.
Trew, Stuart. 2013. 'Eli Lilly Adds $400 Million to NAFTA Lawsuit against Canada's
Patent Norms'. The Council of Canadians, 17 July. http://canadians.org/content/eli-
lilly-adds-400-million-nafta-lawsuit-against-canadas-patent-norms.
United Nations Conference on Trade and Development. 2015. 'Recent Trends in IIAS
and ISDS'. United Nations Conference on Trade and Development. http://unctad.org/en/
PublicationsLibrary/webdiaepcb2015d1_en.pdf.
Van Harten, Gus, and Martin Loughlin. 2006. 'Investment Treaty Arbitration as a
Species of Global Administrative Law'. European Journal of International Law 17:
121–50. doi:10.1093/ejil/chi159.
Weishaar, Heide, Jeff Collin, Katherine Smith, Thilo Grüning, Sema Mandal and Anna
Gilmore. 2012. 'Global Health Governance and the Commercial Sector: A Documen-
tary Analysis of Tobacco Company Strategies to Influence the WHO Framework
Convention on Tobacco Control'. PLoS Medicine 9: e1001249. doi:10.1371/jour-
nal.pmed.1001249.
World Health Organization. 2014. 'Tobacco Fact Sheet No 339'. WHO, May.
www.who.int/mediacentre/factsheets/fs339/en.

ELEVEN

Health Policy, Corporate Influence and Multi-Level Governance

The Case of Alcohol Policy in the European Union

Chris Holden and Benjamin Hawkins

A key feature of contemporary political organisation is the development of 'multi-level governance' (MLG) structures, often associated with global processes of economic liberalisation. Hirst and Thompson (1999, 268–69), for example, note that 'politics is becoming more polycentric, with states as merely one level in a complex system of overlapping and often competing agencies of governance'. While such structures can most clearly be seen in the case of the European Union (EU), they are also present in other regions, as well as globally. The concept of MLG is important for understanding how health policy is made and implemented because the existence of multiple decision-making forums permits 'venue shifting', a process whereby political actors seek to divert decision making to those forums in which they are more likely to exert influence and thus achieve favourable policy outcomes. Transnational corporations (TNCs) have a higher capacity to engage in venue shifting due to their size, resources and the number of countries in which they operate.

Previous research has found that TNCs pursue sophisticated political strategies that may operate simultaneously at different levels of governance, with substantial implications for health policy. Greer et al. (2008) found that, in the health sector, interest groups that are important at the member state level also bring significant resources to bear at the EU level. Indeed, according to Coen (2007, 336), health was the fastest-growing lobbying sector within EU institutions in the first decade of the millennium. In the food sector, corporations were able to outmanoeuvre public health advocates on the issue of labelling by reframing the issue according to their preferences and by dominating lobbying coalitions within the European Parliament (Kurzer and Cooper 2013). Pharmaceutical firms have played a key role in developing intellectual property rights policy in Europe by using EU-level litigation strategies (Bouwen and McCown 2007, 435).

In this chapter, we take an approach rooted in the disciplines of political science and policy studies. We use the concept of MLG to analyse and explain recent developments within European alcohol policy and to demonstrate some of the implications of MLG structures for health policy making. We focus on alcohol policy because developments in this field at the state, sub-state and EU levels allow us to illustrate how levels of policy making can overlap and facilitate venue shifting. The next section outlines the key concepts of MLG and venue shifting in more depth, identifies the political structures to which they relate, and discusses the importance of these for health policy. The subsequent section briefly explains the methodology by which we apply the MLG concept to analyse the alcohol sector as a case study. We then examine how processes of devolution in Scotland and political integration within the EU have affected alcohol policy in the UK. In doing so, we aim to contribute to a fuller understanding of the implications of MLG systems for health policy more broadly.

MULTI-LEVEL GOVERNANCE AND POLICY MAKING

The concept of MLG first developed out of attempts to understand the EU as a system of policy making. Notable in the EU system is the way in which regulation and policy making occur not only at the national state level, but also at the supranational (EU), sub-national and local levels (Marks et al. 1996; Hooghe and Marks 2001). The EU is a highly complex polity comprised of five principle institutions: the European Council, composed of heads of state and government at which the highest level political decisions are taken; the Council of the European Union, representing member state governments in specific policy areas (e.g., health); the European Commission, which proposes legislation and undertakes various executive functions; the European Parliament, elected by European citizens; and the Court of Justice of the European Union (CJEU), which encompasses the 'European Court of Justice' and rules on issues of EU law and the compatibility of national law with this. Within the European Commission, different sub-divisions, known as Directorates General (DGs), focus on specific policy areas such as health or transport. The EU treaties designate policy areas that are exclusive EU-level competencies, those that are national-level competencies and those that are shared competencies between the EU and its member states. Stephenson (2013, 817) describes the MLG concept as 'a simplified notion of what is pluralistic and highly dispersed policy-making activity, where multiple actors (individuals and institutions) participate, at various political levels, from the supranational to sub-national or local'.

The involvement of sub-national units of political organisation in EU policy making has been a particular theme of the MLG literature. Many states have federal constitutional structures that designate considerable powers to sub-national units of government. Many non-federal states have also undergone processes of devolution or decentralisation in recent decades. In the UK, for example, significant powers have been devolved to assemblies and executives in Scotland, Wales and Northern Ireland, including responsibilities for public health. In the multi-level polity of the EU, these sub-state units can relate to EU-level institutions in new and direct ways that go beyond simple intergovernmental bargaining between member state governments.

The EU is not the only world-regional governance structure, although it is the most developed. Many regions in the world are undergoing some process of integration, although these are usually based on attempts to facilitate trade integration through liberalisation, rather than to construct new political structures of the EU kind. Nevertheless, the increasing number of regional formations, and their growing entwinement with cross-regional and global governance processes, gives the MLG concept relevance beyond the borders of the EU. In the case of the EU, the European Commission often directly represents member states in multilateral institutions that influence health policy at the EU and member state levels. For example, the commission has played a significant role in tobacco control, not only within the EU, but also on behalf of member states during negotiation of the World Health Organisation's Framework Convention on Tobacco Control (Mamudu and Studlar 2009). EU member states are also represented by the commission within the World Trade Organisation (WTO) (Knodt 2004), which again has substantial implications for health policy.

In their pursuit of policy influence, actors may have different capacities to pursue their interests via various levels of policy making. Large firms generally have more capacity to influence policy in multi-level systems than citizens' groups because of their greater resources. Such resources include not just financial means but also information, knowledge and expertise (Dur and Mateo 2012), as well as reputation and organisational capacity (Coen 2007). Information, knowledge and expertise are particularly important because they constitute 'access goods'—that is, they allow firms to access policy-making forums in return for the information and expertise that they command with regard to particular markets or industrial sectors (Bouwen 2002). As a result, large corporations have generally been invited by EU institutions, particularly the European

Commission, to become 'insiders' in the policy process, with a number of forums set up specifically for the purpose of drawing upon the expertise of such firms (Coen 1997). Interest representation in the EU system has thus been characterised as a system of 'elite pluralism', in which membership of the elite group is competitive and confers strategic advantages on participants (Coen 1997, 98).

Large corporations operate simultaneously at different levels of policy making and utilise multiple channels of access to EU-level institutions, not just for the purpose of immediate policy influence, but in order to build their reputations and credibility as providers of 'reliable, issue-specific and pan-European information' (Coen 2007, 339). This places them in a position to influence policy over the long term and to develop strategic relationships with key decision-making actors. Having recourse to a variety of political channels also minimises the uncertainty caused by the possibility that any given channel may fail to yield the expected insider status. European policy making 'displays a new interest behaviour logic based on the sophisticated and simultaneous usage of a number of political channels by firms' (Coen 1997, 106). However, only resource-rich organisations are likely to be able to monitor and attempt to influence policy via all available channels and at all relevant levels of governance (Dur and Mateo 2012, 972). Within the European Commission, for example, public health non-governmental organisations (NGOs) tend to focus their EU-level lobbying on the DG for health (DG Sanco), rather than other DGs that may also have a significant impact on health, such as DG Trade. Thus, while corporations have established relationships with multiple politically influential DGs, NGOs' contacts tend to be limited to those most closely related to their specific remit.

The expenditure of resources to maintain a profile and develop relationships with policy actors at multiple levels, and via a variety of channels, is cost-effective for large firms because it increases opportunities to influence policy over the long term. As Coen (2007, 339) writes, in relation to the European Commission, large firms may 'discount the cost of participation in one channel against improved access to the Commission via another channel'. Consequently, access to EU institutions, and to the Commission in particular, is biased towards business interests, which have 'a comparative advantage in terms of organizational capacity, financial resources, expertise and information' (Coen 2007, 335). TNCs may also be able to navigate and utilise multi-level structures more strategically than other actors as a result of their everyday orientation towards the transnational coordination of activities across a range of national states and regulatory jurisdictions (Holden and Lee 2011).

The multiplicity of policy-making forums creates opportunities for political actors to engage in venue shifting (or even 'venue construction'), that is, to act strategically in choosing (or even creating) particular venues through which they can best pursue their interests (Baumgartner and

Jones 1991; Mazey and Richardson 2006). This is especially the case if we take into account corporations' strategic use of different venues and levels over time (Coen 2007, 340). Where one level or 'venue' of policy making does not produce the desired results, actors may attempt to shift the issue to another venue where they are more likely to get the result that they want. Such venue-shifting activities also often involve the redefinition of the 'policy image' (Baumgartner and Jones 1991), what in other contexts has been referred to as issue 'framing' (Hawkins and Holden 2013), in terms amenable to their political objectives. While citizen's groups can also sometimes successfully shift an issue to a venue where they can have more influence, away from closed and non-transparent forums, there is a cost involved in attempting to do so. As Baumgartner and Jones (1991, 1071) note in the context of U.S. politics:

> Strategic manipulation of image involves a sophisticated understanding of the policy process and requires resources not controlled by all. Many venues require the mastery of specialized language and the understanding of complicated concepts. Courts, regulatory agencies, and congressional committees all require the presentation of policy proposals in specialized and arcane language, and all have complicated rules of formal agenda access. Hence, agenda entrance barriers will favour those able to master these rules or pay for specialists who do. Even with many venues, there remain substantial barriers to entry into the pluralist heaven.

One specific form of venue shifting involves recourse to litigation at either the national or European levels. As Coen (2007, 340) notes, the assertion of the European Court of Justice's (ECJ) primacy over national law 'gives rise to new "veto points"' that interest groups may use to attempt to 'block and redefine laws at the end of the policy process'. However, this process of vetoing laws can also be a way of shaping them. As Bouwen and McCown (2007, 426) write, the highly prescriptive nature of ECJ rulings that override national laws means that interest groups that successfully litigate 'not only effect the removal of national rules, on the basis of EU law, but also shape the form of future legislation'. As with multi-level lobbying strategies generally, successful EU litigation requires the maintenance of focus on complex issues over long periods of time, and thus favours organisations, such as large corporations, that have the necessary organisational capacity and resources (Bouwen and McCown 2007, 427).

METHODOLOGY

We employ the MLG concept to analyse the alcohol sector, in order to understand how the dual processes of devolution and supranational integration can impact on public health policy making. We use two main sources for this analysis. First, we draw upon the findings of a study on the role of alcohol corporations in the policy-making process during the development of alcohol pricing policies in Scotland and the United Kingdom. For this study, we undertook thirty-five qualitative interviews with policy actors in Edinburgh and London, and analyzed submissions by the alcohol industry and other actors to the Scottish government's 2008 public consultation on alcohol policy (see Holden et al. 2012; McCambridge et al. 2013; and McCambridge et al. 2014 for a fuller discussion of the methodology). Interviews were conducted with respondents from alcohol companies and trade associations, policy makers including Members of Parliament (MPs) and Members of the Scottish Parliament (MSPs), and public health advocates. The aim was to understand how industry actors, acting unilaterally or in collaboration with others (e.g., through trade associations), attempted to influence policy, at what points in the policy process they did so, and the degree of success they enjoyed in accessing decision makers. Key themes and issues were identified from the interviews through a process of thematic coding using Nvivo software. This process allowed us to understand alcohol policy making at the state and sub-state level as well as the important interplay among decision making at each level. Second, we analyse EU-level alcohol policy via an examination of relevant EU and UK policy documents and direct correspondence with key participants in EU-level decision-making forums. By analysing the role of corporations in EU-level alcohol policy alongside their role in UK and Scottish policy, we aim to contribute to a better understanding of the implications of MLG systems for health policy more broadly.

DEVOLUTION AND ALCOHOL POLICY IN THE EUROPEAN UNION

Alcohol policy within the EU remains principally the responsibility of member states. In practice, however, the picture is more complicated, since member states with federal structures or significant levels of devolution may cede responsibility to sub-state units of government. These sub-state units may have responsibility for public health, but not necessarily for every area of policy that impacts upon public health or which is necessary to protect and advance it, nor for every area of policy that pertains to the sale and consumption of alcohol. Furthermore, the EU itself has an alcohol strategy which is designed to complement the policies of member states and which interacts with them. Additionally, other important areas of EU law, such as competition and trade law, may impact upon, constrain or otherwise have implications for public health.

The EU-level Alcohol Strategy (EC 2006) was first adopted by the European Commission in 2006. The strategy identified five priority themes for action for the period to 2012, which were seen as relevant to all member states, and for which action at EU level would add value (EC 2006):

- Protect young people, children and the unborn child;
- Reduce injuries and death from alcohol-related road accidents;
- Prevent alcohol-related harm among adults and reduce the negative impact on the workplace;
- Inform, educate and raise awareness on the impact of harmful and hazardous alcohol consumption, and on appropriate consumption patterns; and
- Develop and maintain a common evidence base at EU level.

Following intense lobbying by alcohol corporations, proposals for mandatory health warnings on all alcoholic drinks were omitted from the strategy (Baumberg and Anderson 2007; Gornall 2014a).

As of 2015, discussions were underway on the possibility of a new alcohol strategy (CNAPA 2014a). In the interim an 'action plan on youth drinking and heavy episodic drinking' had been agreed for the period 2014–2016 (CNAPA 2014b), a focus that reflects the preferences of industry actors for targeting specific groups seen to be at risk, rather than the whole-population approach favoured by public health advocates and supported by the evidence base (Babor et al. 2010; Gornall 2014a). While considered complementary to action at the member-state level, the EU-level strategy has significant implications for national-level discourse and practice on alcohol policy, as do other elements of EU policy and law.

The EU Alcohol Strategy consists of actions at three levels: measures implemented by member states at national level, coordination of national policies at EU level and actions by the Commission, including facilitating cooperation with stakeholders (Zamparutti et al. 2012, 5). Two EU-level institutional forums were set up to facilitate implementation of the strategy: the Committee on National Alcohol Policy and Action (CNAPA) and the European Alcohol and Health Forum (EAHF). CNAPA is composed of delegates of member states, mainly public health officials, and coordinates action between the member states. A key role of CNAPA is to share information about national-level policy between member states, to identify best practice and to hold discussions on thematic issues. While there has been some progress on this, with policies in other member states used as examples in national policy discussions, for example, CNAPA's contribution in the area of pricing policies has been limited (Zamparutti et al. 2012, 9–10).

The EAHF is designed to facilitate stakeholder actions to reduce alcohol-related harm. Members are composed of both corporations and NGOs, and include EU-level umbrella groups, national and sub-national organisations and individual corporations. The EAHF works on the basis of partnership with private corporations, encouraging them to behave in a socially responsible manner. Member organisations are encouraged to pledge voluntary action to address at least one of the forum's priorities, and to report annually on the implementation of their actions. In 2012, EAHF had sixty-eight members, with twenty-six of these being NGOs and health organisations, and twenty-eight production and sales organisations. Roughly half of the total members were organisations operating at the EU level (Zamparutti et al. 2012, 16). Commitments made by corporations tend to be concentrated in the areas of responsible commercial communications and sales, and education programmes on the effects of harmful drinking and on responsible patterns of consumption, and have led to the expansion of self-regulatory systems (Zamparutti et al. 2012, 16–21). However, self-regulatory systems have been criticised as ineffective (Baggott 2006; Babor et al. 2010; McCambridge et al. 2013), and may serve as a strategy by corporate actors to ward off effective mandatory regulation (Hawkins et al. 2012; Hawkins and Holden 2013; Gornall 2014a).

This commitment to 'partnership', and self-regulatory initiatives at the EU level, it is argued here, reflects alcohol corporations' favoured policy prescriptions and their attempts to shape the policy agenda. The framing of policy debates in these terms reinforces their attempts to promote self-regulation at the national level, allowing the industry to point to EU-level policy norms to buttress their claims for a similar approach within member states. The 'public health responsibility deal' in the UK, for example, which includes a number of alcohol corporations, was a key initiative of the 2010–2015 Conservative-led Coalition government, but has attracted much criticism from public health advocates (Gilmore et al. 2011; Hawkins et al. 2012). Here we see the apparent coordination of corporate activity at EU and national levels in an attempt to normalise a discourse of partnership and voluntary action at both levels.

The international research consensus suggests that self-regulatory initiatives and a focus on marketing and education alone are not effective in substantially reducing alcohol-related harm (Babor et al. 2010). The evidence shows that an effective and comprehensive alcohol harm-reduction strategy should also involve measures such as those on price, along with restrictions on the availability of alcohol and advertising (Babor et al. 2010). While such measures were not covered within the EU's alcohol strategy, there has been increasing attention to price-based measures within member states. This has particularly been the case in Scotland since the Scottish National Party (SNP) became the largest party in the Scottish Parliament in 2007 and formed a Scottish government. The SNP's goal was to introduce a minimum unit price (MUP) for alcohol in order to raise the price of the cheapest forms of alcoholic beverages. One reason for the Scottish government deciding to pursue this goal by setting an MUP was that it did not have authority over taxation policy within the devolution settlement that was then operating, with this authority instead being reserved to the UK government as a whole.

The Scottish government's initial attempt to introduce MUP via the Alcohol Etc. (Scotland) Bill (2010) was defeated because the SNP did not command an overall majority within the Scottish Parliament. During the run up to the Bill's introduction, alcohol corporations mobilised to oppose the adoption of MUP, utilising a range of influencing tactics including direct lobbying of government ministers, civil servants and MSPs (Holden and Hawkins 2013; Hawkins and Holden 2014). Media campaigns were also initiated in an attempt to challenge the Scottish government's framing of the alcohol problem as one requiring a whole-population approach, and to promote instead a frame that focused on problematic drinkers requiring individually-targeted interventions (Hawkins and Holden, 2013). While not all corporations in the alcohol sector have identical interests, and some were even prepared to accept MUP, those opposing the measure proved to be more vocal (Holden et al. 2012). In an apparent attempt at venue shifting, some alcohol corporations argued that the issue should be addressed via taxation, which was not a competence of the Scottish government, and that the UK government in Westminster was thus the appropriate forum for the making of alcohol pricing policy (Holden and Hawkins 2013, 260). The Conservative-led Westminster government was at the same time considering alcohol pricing policies, but was understood to be more likely to adopt the prohibition of alcohol sales below duty plus value added tax (VAT)—provisions that would have set a much lower floor price. Indeed, econometric modelling suggests that such a policy would be largely ineffective in reducing alcohol related harms (Brennan 2014).

When the alcohol corporations opposing MUP realised that they would be unable to convince the Scottish government to back down from its proposals, given that the SNP did not command an overall majority in the Scottish Parliament, they switched their lobbying attention to opposition MSPs who subsequently voted down the proposed measure (Holden and Hawkins 2013, 265; Gornall 2014b). However, the subsequent achievement by the SNP of an overall majority in 2011 allowed them to reintroduce and then pass MUP legislation.

A key motivation for the opposition of some alcohol corporations to MUP in Scotland appears to be that they feared it would impact on their sales in other parts of the world (Holden and Hawkins 2013). Many alcohol corporations are large transnational businesses (Jernigan 2009; Hawkins et al. 2016) and are thus seeking to expand sales in emerging markets such as China, amid intensified global competition (*The Economist* 2011; Ipsos 2013). Corporations seemed particularly afraid of 'policy contagion', whereby unfavourable policies are transferred from one jurisdiction to another. The potential domino effect, should a policy demonstrate effectiveness, also meant that regulation at home would make it more difficult to resist regulation in overseas markets. These concerns led some corporations to enlist the support of overseas governments and trade associations in lobbying the Scottish government (Holden and Hawkins 2013, 264) and the European Commission (Gornall 2014b). This demonstrates how MLG can potentially be both an asset and a problem for corporations. Whilst MLG affords corporations scope for venue shifting, devolved administrations can be policy innovators, providing a positive example of policy change that other jurisdictions may then adopt (Keating 2009, 280).

When opponents in the alcohol industry were ultimately unsuccessful in blocking the adoption of MUP via lobbying, their strategy shifted again to additional venues, namely the Scottish and European courts, in an attempt to 'veto' the legislation. The Scotch Whisky Association (SWA) lodged a complaint with the European Commission in July 2012, and then filed a petition for judicial review with the Scottish Court of Session. While the Scottish Court did not accept the SWA's complaint, it referred the case to the ECJ in April 2014. The case, which has not been resolved as of 2015, principally revolves around whether MUP is compatible with the EU's rules on the free movement of goods, and whether or not the objective of the policy could be achieved by any other means less restrictive of trade (BBC 2013; Baumberg and Anderson 2008).

EU-level alcohol policy is presently relatively limited, relying on most measures to be formulated and implemented at the member state level. However, we have shown how actions at the level of EU institutions, which are often highly susceptible to corporate influence, can have an impact on policy at other levels. The development of a discourse of 'partnership' and self-regulation at the EU level helps to inform and reinforce a framing of the alcohol problem, and of appropriate solutions, that are focused on actions that suit industry interests, but that the evidence suggests will not be effective. When the devolved Scottish government attempted to introduce an innovative policy in the form of MUP, supported by robust evidence of its likely effectiveness, alcohol corporations attempted to derail this via extensive lobbying and ultimately by attempting to 'veto' it through recourse to EU-level law.

CONCLUSION

This chapter argues that MLG structures render policy making more complex and consequently provide corporations with opportunities for venue shifting. Within the EU, corporations are able to affect health policy in a number of ways including participation in stakeholder structures at EU, member state and other levels; lobbying at state, sub-state and supranational levels; and litigation at both national and EU levels. This case study of alcohol policy in the EU has shown how corporations can employ multiple strategies, sometimes simultaneously and sometimes in a sequential fashion, shifting from one form of attempted policy influence to another when the first was unsuccessful. Alcohol corporations can be seen to have attempted to set the agenda via the EAHF in order to promote a discourse of partnership and self-regulation. They also pursued coordinated multi-level lobbying at the devolved (Scottish), UK and EU levels in an attempt to defeat MUP. The ultimate resort to EU-level litigation, in an attempt to veto MUP, is important for the precedent that it may set, and, even if unsuccessful, will have played a role in substantially delaying legislation with the potential to improve public health. Importantly, the corporations concerned seem to have taken these actions because they deem MUP to have implications not only for their UK and European markets, but also for their global strategies, as they seek to expand in emerging markets.

The multi-level strategizing identified in the case of alcohol policy in the EU has implications for other areas of health policy, as well as for MLG structures in other regions and globally. MLG can make it difficult for governments, and other actors at any particular level of governance, to monitor or regulate corporate activity. Importantly, there may be no effective counterweight within the wider policy community to corporate attempts to shape policy agendas and determine the forums in which decisions are taken. NGOs and public health advocates may lack the necessary resources to operate effectively at multiple levels in comparative ways. The result can be that governments and public health actors are outflanked as policy is shifted from one political or jurisdictional level to another. The substantial resources commanded by TNCs, and their ability to utilise MLG structures strategically to influence public policy, can thus be seen as a potential threat to the protection of public interests in the making and implementation of effective public health policy.

REFERENCES

Babor, Thomas, Raul Caetano, Sally Casswell, Griffith Edwards, Norman Giesbrecht, Kathryn Graham, Jowel W. Grube, Linda Hill, Harold Holder, Ross Homel, Michael Livingston, Esa Osterberg, Jurgen Rehm, Robin Room and Ingeborg Rossow. 2010. *Alcohol, No Ordinary Commodity: Research & Public Policy.* Oxford: Oxford University Press.

Baggott, Robb. 2006. *Alcohol Strategy and the Drinks Industry: A Partnership for Prevention?* York: Joseph Rowntree Foundation.

Baumberg, Ben, and Peter Anderson. 2007. 'The European Strategy on Alcohol: A Landmark and a Lesson'. *Alcohol & Alcoholism* 42 (1): 1–2.

———. 2008. 'Health, Alcohol and EU Law: Understanding the Impact of European Single Market Law on Alcohol Policies'. *European Journal of Public Health* 18 (4): 392–98.

Baumgartner, Frank R., and Bryan D. Jones. 1991. 'Agenda Dynamics and Policy Subsystems'. *The Journal of Politics* 53 (4): 1044–74.

BBC. 2013. 'Minimum Alcohol Pricing: Summary of the European Commission Position'. *BBC News*, 25 July. Accessed 13 February 2015. www.bbc.co.uk/news/uk-scotland-scotland-politics-23433466.

Bouwen, Pieter. 2002. 'Corporate Lobbying in the European Union: The Logic of Access'. *Journal of European Public Policy* 9 (3): 365–90.

Bouwen, Pieter, and Margaret McCown. 2007. 'Lobbying versus Litigation: Political and Legal Strategies of Interest Representation in the European Union'. *Journal of European Public Policy* 14 (3): 422–43.

Brennan, Alan, Yang Meng, John Holmes, Daniel Hill-McManus and Petra S. Meier. 2014. 'Potential Benefits of Minimum Unit Pricing for Alcohol versus a Ban on Below Cost Selling in England 2014: Modelling Study'. *British Medical Journal* 349: g5452.

CNAPA. 2014a. *CNAPA Scoping Paper: Member States Call on the European Commission for a New and Comprehensive Strategy to Tackle Harmful Use of Alcohol and Alcohol Related Harm*. Brussels: Committee for National Alcohol Policy and Action.

———. 2014b. *Action Plan on Youth Drinking and on Heavy Episodic Drinking (Binge Drinking)*. Brussels: Committee for National Alcohol Policy and Action.

Coen, David. 1997. 'The Evolution of the Large Firm as a Political Actor in the European Union'. *Journal of European Public Policy* 4 (1): 91–108.

———. 2007. 'Empirical and Theoretical Studies in EU Lobbying'. *Journal of European Public Policy* 14 (3): 333–45.

Dur, Andreas, and Gemma Mateo. 2012. 'Who Lobbies the European Union? National Interest Groups in a Multilevel Polity'. *Journal of European Public Policy* 19 (7): 969–87.

EC. 2006. *An EU Strategy to Support Member States in Reducing Alcohol Related Harm*. Brussels: Commission of the European Communities.

Gilmore, Anna, Emily Savell and Jeff Collin. 2011. 'Public Health, Corporations and the New Responsibility Deal: Promoting Partnerships with Vectors of Disease?' *Journal of Public Health*, 33 (1): 2–4.

Gornall, Jonathan. 2014a. 'Europe Under the Influence'. *British Medical Journal* 348: g1166.

———. 2014b. 'Under the Influence: Scotland's Battle over Alcohol Pricing'. *British Medical Journal* 348: g1274.

Greer, Scott L., Elize Massard de Fonseca and Christopher Adolph. 2008. 'Mobilizing Bias in Europe: Lobbies, Democracy and EU Health Policy-Making'. *European Union Politics* 9 (3): 403–33.

Hawkins, Benjamin, and Chris Holden. 2013. 'Framing the Alcohol Policy Debate: Industry Actors and the Regulation of the UK Beverage Alcohol Market'. *Critical Policy Studies* 7 (1): 53–71.

———. 2014. '"Water Dripping on Stone"? Industry Lobbying and UK Alcohol Policy'. *Policy & Politics* 42 (1): 55–70.

Hawkins, Benjamin, Chris Holden, Jappe Eckhardt and Kelley Lee. 2016. 'Reassessing Policy Paradigms: A Comparison of the Global Tobacco and Alcohol Industries'. *Global Public Health*, DOI: 10.1080/17441692.2016.

Hawkins, Benjamin, Chris Holden and Jim McCambridge. 2012. 'Alcohol Industry Influence on U.K. Alcohol Policy: A New Research Agenda for Public Health'. *Critical Public Health* 22 (3): 297–305.

Hirst, Paul, and Grahame Thompson. 1999. *Globalization in Question*, 2nd ed. Cambridge: Polity Press.

Holden, Chris, and Benjamin Hawkins. 2013. '"Whisky Gloss": The Alcohol Industry, Devolution and Policy Communities in Scotland'. *Public Policy & Administration* 28 (3): 253–73.

Holden, Chris, Benjamin Hawkins and Jim McCambridge. 2012. 'Cleavages and Co-operation in the UK Alcohol Industry: A Qualitative Study'. *BMC Public Health* 12: 483.

Holden, Chris, and Kelley Lee. 2011. '"A Major Lobbying Effort to Change and Unify the Excise Structure in Six Central American Countries": How British American Tobacco Influenced Tax and Tariff Rates in the Central American Common Market'. *Globalization and Health* 7: 15.

Hooghe, Liesbet, and Gary Marks. 2001. *Multilevel Governance and European Integration.* Oxford: Rowman & Littlefield.

Ipsos. 2013. 'Drinking to the Future: Trends in the Spirits Industry'. March. Accessed 6 March 2015. www.ipsos.com/sites/ipsos.com/files/Drinking-to-the-Future-Trends-in-the-Spirits-Industry.pdf.

Jernigan, David H. 2009. 'The Global Alcohol Industry: An Overview'. *Addiction* 104 (1): 6–12.

Keating, Michael. 2009. 'Spatial Rescaling, Devolution and the Future of Social Welfare'. In *Social Policy Review 21,* edited by Kirstein Rummery, Ian Greener and Chris Holden, 269–84. Bristol: Policy Press.

Knodt, Michele. 2004. 'International Embeddednes of European Multi-Level Governance'. *Journal of European Public Policy* 11 (4): 701–19.

Kurzer, Paulette, and Alice Cooper. 2013. 'Biased or Not? Organised Interests and the Case of EU Food Information Labeling'. *Journal of European Public Policy* 20 (5): 722–40.

Mamudu, Hadii M., and Donley T. Studlar. 2009. 'Multilevel Governance and Shared Sovereignty: European Union, Member States, and the FCTC'. *Governance* 22 (1): 73–97.

Marks, Gary, Liesbet Hooghe and Kermit Blank. 1996. 'European Integration since the 1980s: State-Centric Versus Multi-Level Governance'. *Journal of Common Market Studies* 34 (3): 343–78.

Mazey, Sonia, and Jeremy Richardson. 2006. 'Interest Groups and EU Policy-Making: Organisational Logic and Venue Shopping'. In *European Union: Power and Policy-Making,* 3rd ed., edited by Jeremy Richardson. Abingdon: Routledge.

McCambridge, Jim, Benjamin Hawkins and Chris Holden. 2013. 'Industry Use of Evidence to Influence Alcohol Policy: A Case Study of Submissions to the 2008 Scottish Government Consultation'. *PLoS Medicine* 10 (4): e1001431.

———. 2014. 'The Challenge Corporate Lobbying Poses to Reducing Society's Alcohol Problems: Insights from UK Evidence on Minimum Unit Pricing'. *Addiction* 109 (2): 199–205.

Stephenson, Paul. 2013. 'Twenty Years of Multi-Level Governance: "Where Does It Come From? What Is It? Where Is It Going?"' *Journal of European Public Policy* 20 (6): 817–37.

The Economist. 2011. 'Diageo's Deals: Replenishing the Drinks Cabinet?' *The Economist,* 3 May.

Zamparutti, Tony, Guillerno Hernandez and Kamila Bolt. 2012. *Assessment of the Added Value of the EU Strategy to Support Member States in Reducing Alcohol-Related Harm.* Brussels: DG Health and Consumers.

TWELVE

Tobacco Industry Strategies to Influence Global Governance

Ross MacKenzie and Kelley Lee

As smoking prevalence declines in the traditional markets of Western Europe and North America, transnational tobacco companies (TTCs) have responded by moving into low- and middle-income countries (LMICs). Asia's large populations, growing affluence and high smoking rates (Euromonitor International 2015a) have made it a particularly attractive target for commercial expansion. Previous studies have focused on TTC entry into selected Asian markets through strategies related to marketing, advertising and promotion; corporate social responsibility (CSR) initiatives; and illicit trade (Lee, Ling and Glantz 2012). There has been limited comparative analysis of these strategies across countries in the region to date, and this is particularly true of the extent to which industry expansion has influenced global efforts to strengthen tobacco control.

This chapter presents a comparative political economy analysis of TTC strategies to influence health governance in Cambodia, China and Thailand, three countries that have in common an impending public health crisis based on current levels of tobacco consumption (table 12.1). It specifically concentrates on attempts by the tobacco industry to influence official support in these countries for the Framework Convention on Tobacco Control (FCTC), the first international treaty to be negotiated under the auspices of the World Health Organization (WHO). An international legal instrument that requires ratifying parties to enact regulation on a range of tobacco control issues including promotion, taxation, and illegal trade (WHO 2015a), the FCTC is recognised as a key development in global health governance and represents an explicit threat to the operations of the global tobacco industry.

All three countries ratified the FCTC soon after its adoption by the World Health Assembly in 2003 (United Nations 2015), but subsequent commitment to implementation has varied enormously. Cambodia ratified the agreement in 2005 but has made modest progress in meeting FCTC minimum commitments. China was initially unsupportive of the treaty process, opposing many measures under negotiation but, perhaps surprisingly, ratified in 2005. Conflicts of interest related to the national tobacco monopoly have been blamed for weak implementation to date (Wan et al. 2011). By contrast, the Thai government was an early champion of the FCTC, ratifying in 2004, and has remained a strong advocate and participant in the process. Implementation of many of the treaty's key requirements, including taxation increases and graphic health warnings, has built on the country's previously strong policy record.

This chapter argues that tobacco industry influence on the policy process has played an important part in explaining the divergent attitudes toward the FCTC displayed across the three countries and that degree of influence is explained by the respective political and economic systems and the tobacco market structure within each country.

ANALYTICAL FRAMEWORK AND METHODS

This comparative political economy analysis of tobacco industry influence on the FCTC process in three Asian countries applies Holden and Lee's (2009) conceptualisation of the dynamic relationship between the structural and agency power of TTCs. *Structural power* derives from state reliance on corporate investment, production, employment and taxation.

Table 12.1.   Smoking Prevalence and Annual Tobacco Deaths in Three Asian Countries

	Smoking Prevalence Adult Males 15+ years (2012)	Smoking Prevalence Adult Females 15+ years (2012)	Annual Mortality From Tobacco-Related Diseases (rank among risk factors)
Cambodia	39.1%	3.4%	10 400 (3)
China	68%	3.2%	1 200 000 (1)
Thailand	46.6%	2.6%	74 000 (2)

Source: WHO 2015; Tobacco Atlas, 5th edition; Chen, Zhengming, Richard Peto, Maigeng Zhou et al. for the China Kadoorie Biobank (CKB) collaborative group. 2015. "Contrasting male and female trends in tobacco-attributed mortality in China: evidence from successive nationwide prospective cohort studies." *The Lancet* 386: 1447-1456.

The rise of the transnational corporation and global value chains has significantly enhanced corporate structural power and compelled many national governments to ensure their domestic markets are 'investor-friendly' by reducing corporate taxation rates and modifying social programmes (Crotty, Epstein and Kelly 1998). Holden and Lee (2009) argue that TTCs derive structural power from supply chains and interrelated activities across a large number of markets, a process that has been significantly enhanced by global expansion and restructuring of the industry since the 1970s.

Agency power refers to direct and indirect attempts to influence policy through political engagement and institutional participation; a third aspect, corporate provision of essential goods and services has limited applicability to specific analysis of the tobacco industry given the inherently deleterious effects of its products (Farnsworth and Holden 2006). Political engagement includes corporate membership in networks that include political elites, lobbying, donations to political parties and research funding in order to influence debates. *Institutional participation* refers to more direct participation in policy-making processes, generally through association with government policy bodies and agencies. With specific reference to TTCs, Holden and Lee (2009) theorise that structural and agency power 'have existed in a dynamic relationship', and this analytical framework is used to explain the influence of the tobacco industry in the three case study countries. It draws on secondary data sources from government, business and nongovernmental organisations, as well scholarly articles on industry activities in the three countries based on internal corporate documents.

DISCUSSION: STRUCTURAL POWER AND THE TOBACCO INDUSTRY

TTC strategies have reflected opportunities and obstacles arising from the respective political and economic systems of the three countries. Distinctive governmental organisation has resulted in divergent market conditions, and has shaped the capacity of TTCs to participate in the policy process.

Cambodia

Having emerged from decades of civil war and Vietnamese occupation in the early 1990s, Cambodia's political system has evolved into a 'competitive authoritarian regime' (Levitsky and Way 2010) in which political competition exists, but is skewed by one-party dominance of the electoral system, state resources and media. The Cambodian People's Party (CPP) controls a political system characterised by nepotism, corruption, frequent violence, a loyal military and party control of the national Constitutional Council and the court system (Gainsborough 2012; Peou 2011). It is dominated by a political and economic power élite comprised of party loyalists who have benefitted from sweeping economic liberalisation, through which they have accumulated vast holdings in natural resources, property development and other sectors (Hughes 2007).

The Cambodian government's adoption of far-reaching economic liberalisation in the 1990s attracted tobacco industry attention and investment. British American Tobacco (BAT), active in the country from the 1930s until the exodus of foreign interests during the Khmer Rouge regime in the mid-1970s, was quick to recognise that the country's desperate need for foreign investment meant that the potentially lucrative Cambodia market be exploited at 'very preferential terms' (Manning 1991). Motivated by the young and growing population, weak tobacco control regulation, an opportunity to gain an advantage over rival Philip Morris (PM) (which was precluded from the market by a U.S. trade embargo) and Cambodia's key role in regional contraband networks (MacKenzie et al. 2004; Collin et al. 2004), BAT entered into negotiations with state officials. In 1996, the government agreed to a joint venture arrangement that stipulated that BAT would hold a 51 percent majority share, and enjoy additional financial inducements (MacKenzie et al. 2004). By 2015, British American Tobacco Cambodia (BATC) controlled 40 percent of Cambodia's cigarette market,[1] and its success has led BAT's chief executive for Southeast Asia to describe the company as 'almost a role model of what we would like to do everywhere' (John 2000).

BATC has made significant investments in manufacturing infrastructure and employment, and taxation of its operation contributes to government revenue. Positive portrayal of these contributions to economic growth and social reconstruction, endorsed by government officials and the local media (MacKenzie et al. 2004), has provided the company with an apparent role in health policy formulation (MacKenzie and Collin 2016). BATC's general manager Arend Ng neatly summarised this situation during a speech at the company's tenth anniversary celebration in 2006, which was attended by leading government officials. Ng underlined BATC's important place in national economic recovery and noted that as a 'leading international company and a model investor in the Kingdom of Cambodia', it was essential that the 'industry is adequately and sensibly regulated and that these regulations are suitability enforced' to ensure profitability (BATC 2007b).

China

China is a socialist state under one-party rule, and the Communist Party of China (CPC) continues to assert its influence over aspects of society that it considers to be politically significant. It has, since the 1980s, gradually relinquished control over many components of the economy to market forces resulting in what Gore has described as a system of state capitalism that includes both state-owned enterprises and private companies in which the government exercises significant influence through majority or minority ownership (Du 2014; Gore 2015). Resultant economic growth, fuelled by the dual engines of a huge domestic economy and export markets, made China the world's second largest economy in 2014, measured by gross domestic product. Accession to the World Trade Organization (WTO) in 2001 further underlined its integration within the world economy.

BAT dominated the Chinese market from the early twentieth century until nationalisation of the industry in the 1950s, which locked TTCs out of the market. Hopes that China's 'open door policy' in the late 1970s would lift restrictions on the world's largest cigarette market (Novotny 2006) were disappointed. The China National Tobacco Corporation (CNTC), which is administrated by the State Tobacco Monopoly Administration (STMA), controls tobacco leaf cultivation, the production and distribution of cigarettes and other tobacco products, and a limited import and export trade. As the world's largest tobacco company, the CNTC accounts for around 43 percent of global production, and contributes between 7–11 percent of central government revenue (Hu et al. 2008). Continuing restrictions on FDI and imports have meant that TTCs remain minor players in the market. In 2013, PM, BAT and JTI accounted for 1.2 percent of legal domestic sales (Euromonitor International 2015b), and joint ventures have been limited to licensing and technology transfer agreements (Tong et al. 2008; He, Takuc and Yano 2013).

Thailand

Politics in Thailand have been described as a 'heady mix of pluralism and structural corruption, leading to a remarkably open but somewhat dysfunctional system' (Chantornvong and McCargo 2001). The fragility of the country's constitutional monarchy system of government is reflected by the nineteen military coups between 1932 and 2014. Stability persists only through reverence for the monarchy, fear of the military, and the strength of the civil service, but is increasingly threatened by growing popular unrest, polarisation and intolerance (Ghoshal 2015). Thailand is a newly industrialising and middle-income country, and has experienced steady economic growth since the 1970s, due to a strategy of integration with the global economy that includes attracting foreign direct investment (FDI), diversification, joint ventures and export-led growth. This approach has made Thailand the second largest economy in Southeast Asia, although heavy reliance on exports has left the country vulnerable to regional and global economic downturns.

TTCs also faced a monopoly market in Thailand, where the Thailand Tobacco Monopoly (TTM) controlled all aspects of production and sales, apart from a small volume of duty-free import sales, until 1990. Thailand's refusal to lift restrictions on cigarette imports in the 1980s led U.S.-based manufacturers PM, Brown & Williamson and RJ Reynolds (RJR) to petition the U.S. Trade Representative (USTR) to act on their behalf. Following inconclusive deliberations, the dispute was referred to General Agreement on Tariffs and Trade (GATT) arbitration, which ruled that Thailand was obliged to open its market to imports as a party to GATT (MacKenzie and Collin 2012). Importantly, it also found that tobacco control legislation was acceptable if applied equally to TTCs and the TTM (Chaloupka and Laixuthai 1996). Enactment of the Tobacco Products Control Act and the Nonsmokers' Rights Protection Act in 1992, and subsequent regulation, has meant that Thailand escaped the extensive degree of TTC brand promotion experienced by Japan, Taiwan and Korea following market opening in those countries (Lee, Ling and Glantz 2012).

Despite Thailand's comprehensive tobacco control agenda, TTCs have made significant, if initially slow, inroads into the Thai market. Increases in market share—from 0.6 percent of sales in 1990 to 31.8 percent in 2011—are due almost entirely to PMI, which controls 90 percent of import sales (28.7 percent of total) (Euromonitor International 2015c). Government commitment to tobacco control and the TTM's continued, though declining, dominance of the market, have precluded PMI and competitor corporations from establishing a commercial and policy presence similar to that created by BAT in neighbouring Cambodia. The TTM's status as one of Thailand's most profitable state-owned enterprises (Thailand Ministry of Finance 2015; Thailand Tobacco Monopoly 2016) would suggest an opportunity for accumulating structural power, but Thai government structure separates Ministry of Finance administration of the monopoly from the National Committee for the Control of Tobacco Use, ensuring a crucial distance is maintained between the interests of commerce and health (Hogg, Hill and Collin 2015).

AGENCY POWER AND THE TOBACCO INDUSTRY

Holden and Lee (2009) argue that in countries where public opprobrium has grown and tobacco control regulation has been strengthened, industry ability to accumulate structural power has waned. In the three case study countries, social perceptions of the industry and smoking vary, and development of tobacco control has ranged from Thailand's robust domestic legislation and support for the FCTC, to markedly slower progress both domestically and globally in Cambodia and China. Yet, however gradual and uneven, such shifts have led the tobacco industry to resort to agency power in the form of lobbying, funding of research, and CSR initiatives, among other measures (Holden and Lee 2009).

Cambodia

BATC predictions in the early 1990s that revenues generated by the tobacco industry would delay meaningful tobacco control in Cambodia have proven accurate, but the company also anticipated that legislation adopted by regional neighbours Thailand and Singapore and the growing movement for global tobacco control would have an unwelcome effect on the local situation. BATC efforts to exercise agency power were facilitated by access to key economic and political actors in what has been described as 'Cambodian crony capitalism' (Kheang 2012). BATC chairman Kong Triv, for example, holds 29 percent of company shares, is a CPP senator, has won numerous government contracts for infrastructure development projects, and is involved with manufacturing, distribution, electronics and logging companies (MacKenzie et al. 2004). BATC has also established links to private-sector networks that enjoy access to government agencies, including the International Business Chamber Cambodia, the Cambodian Federation of Employers and Business Associations, and the Cambodian Government Private Sector Forum (MacKenzie and Collin 2015).

Such access has enabled the industry to participate in discussion around regulatory initiatives with government finance and customs officials. In 2007, general manager Arend Ng described amendments to the excise tax system, the result of consultations between the tax department and the tobacco, alcohol and soft drinks industries, as a 'shining example' of industry and government cooperation (BATC 2007). Low tax rates (only Laos has lower levels within the Association of South-East Asian Nations) have meant that cigarettes remain widely affordable to one of the region's poorest populations (Southeast Asia Tobacco Control Alliance 2014b). More controversially, BATC has worked with Cambodian customs authorities to combat smuggling (BATC 2007b), despite evidence of the company's complicity in cigarette smuggling (Collin et al. 2004; MacKenzie et al. 2004).

The importance of CSR is suggested by BATC's description of the company 'as a preferred consultant and partner to the Royal Government, NGOs, and the community in the area of Corporate Social Responsibility, regulatory and excise matters' (BATC 2007a). In 2011, Kun Lim, head of BATC Corporate and Regulatory Affairs, noted the company had 'actively undertaken and embedded CSR objectives into every stage' of its operations, describing how approximately eight hundred families were contracted to grow tobacco based on 'best practice' standards in insect control, irrigation, child labour and environmental health and safety policies (Cambodia Ministry of Finance 2011). Further initiatives include development of tree nurseries in support of government reforestation schemes, establishing work experience programmes, and hosting workshops on agricultural techniques, child labour and gender equality (BATC 2007b).

China

The CNTC's central position within the political and economic system means that it has little need for agency power. As Jin (2014) describes, 'Pro-tobacco policy networks have become the dominant tobacco policy entrepreneurs because of their close connections with government'. The CNTC has used related influence to thwart policy in ways similar to those adopted by TTCs in other markets, ensuring that tobacco control has made limited progress (Redmon et al. 2012). Yet direct access to central and local governments has also enabled the monopoly to pursue some degree of agency power through collaborative philanthropic and CSR projects that have included school construction, infrastructure improvement and social programs. Such initiatives, combined with perceived benefits to the economy, mean that the domestic tobacco industry enjoys a degree of respectability unseen in most other countries (Hu, Lee and Mao 2013).

Agency power has been more important to TTCs seeking to expand their operations into the lucrative Chinese market, and to hinder tobacco control progress. PM's Asian Regional Tobacco Industry Science Team (ARTIST) program was a large-scale regional program that enlisted scientists from tobacco monopolies in China, South Korea, Taiwan and Thailand and enabled PM scientists to communicate with their counterparts, and policy makers, in pursuing collaborations on second-hand smoke (SHS); legal and regulatory initiatives; and the production of findings favourable to the industry (Tong and Glantz 2004; Barnoya and Glantz 2006). For its part, BAT sought to divert attention away from SHS-related health risks, and towards promotion of policies that accommodated smokers and non-smokers. A key element of this strategy were efforts to fund and promote the China-based Beijing Liver Foundation, with the aim of redirecting domestic attention away from the tenth World Conference on Tobacco or Health held in Beijing in 1997, and toward ostensibly more serious issues such as hepatitis. The foundation later evolved into a vehicle for promoting air filtration and ventilation technology and 'resocialisation of smoking' initiatives, and for downplaying the impact of SHS by drawing attention to China's air pollution crisis, with the explicit objective of influencing debate on smoke-free legislation (Muggli et al. 2008).

Another key TTC strategy was support for China's bid to join the WTO, based on the belief that membership would lead to greater access to the domestic cigarette market for overseas manufacturers. BAT efforts on China's behalf included deploying its 'extensive informal links and privileged access to high-level decision-makers' in the European Union and the UK during negotiations (Holden et al. 2010). WTO accession in 2001 did cause the Chinese industry to restructure and consolidate in anticipation of foreign competition, but the market has remained largely closed to TTCs, apart from some degree of relaxation of rules covering retail licensing and licensed manufacture of foreign brands.

Frustrated by restricted market access, evidence suggests that TTCs have engaged in extensive smuggling to get their brands into China. By the late 1990s, an estimated 50 billion illegal cigarettes were entering the market annually, leading the government to implement a crackdown that included increased customs powers, and criminal and administrative penalties aimed at recovering lost annual tax revenue of approximately US$1.8 billion (Lee and Collin 2006). This crackdown forced the industry to reassess its operations, and led to a greater focus on legal operations.

Thailand

Progressive legislation has made Thailand a leader in tobacco control, particularly amongst LMICs. Restrictions on cigarette marketing, typically a significant TTC strategy in new markets, provided the TTM with a competitive advantage over foreign competitors after market opening. This, combined with increasingly determined monitoring and enforcement by the Ministry of Health, and a crucially important civil society sector (Wipfli 2015), prevented TTCs from developing the kinds of structural power accumulated in neighbouring Cambodia.

Agency power has, therefore, gained particular significance for TTCs operating in Thailand. The industry's protracted, and successful, opposition to full public disclosure of cigarette ingredients between 1991 and 1997 is a notable example (MacKenzie et al. 2004). The eventual, diluted requirement for confidential disclosure of ingredients to the Ministry of Health been described as 'useless' by a leading Thai tobacco control advocate (Vateesatokit 2003). Prohibitions on advertising have been challenged by brand-stretching, the use of cigarette brand names on non-tobacco products such as *Camel* clothing, and sports sponsorships, including BAT's staging of an international snooker tournament and the football team Manchester United's visit to Bangkok (MacKenzie et al. 2007).

PMI has tested government commitment to enforcement of bans on promotion through sponsorship of the high-profile ASEAN Art Award program between the mid-1990s and 2006, and funding community organisations, many of which have been involved in tobacco cultivation (MacKenzie and Collin 2008). The strategic value of targeted philanthropy becomes clear when funding recipients, such as the Thai Tobacco Growers Association, lobby to liberalise the domestic tobacco market

(MacKenzie and Collin 2008). The apparent success of PM efforts to influence the discourse around the science on smoking is suggested by the ability of company scientists to build important links with the Chulabhorn Research Institute (CRI), a leading regional research centre in Bangkok and a WHO Collaborating Centre for Capacity Building and Research in Environmental Health Science (MacKenzie and Collin 2008).

As in Cambodia and China, cigarette smuggling has been crucial to TTC agency power in Thailand. Prior to market opening in 1990, complicity in contraband activity enabled TTCs to build consumer demand through a complex network that included local criminal gangs, as well as the police and armed forces (Collin et al. 2004). Once they had achieved market access, TTC management of both legal and illegal operations was strategically important to industry challenges to government policy. In the early 1990s, for example, representatives of BAT, PM and RJR advised the Thai deputy prime minister that proposals for enhanced tobacco control legislation would escalate the contraband trade (Collin et al. 2004), while MacKenzie, Lee and LeGresley (2015) have reported that TTCs set an artificially high price for legal imports, while continuing to supply the contraband market, after the government refused industry requests to lower excise and duty on imports.

Impacts on Global Health Governance: Official Response to the FCTC

Cambodia was part of a regional negotiating bloc that enthusiastically supported the FCTC process, and countries from Southeast Asia and the Western Pacific were among the earliest to ratify the treaty (Wipfli, Fujimoto and Valente 2010). Since ratification in 2005, however, implementation has been limited, arguably due in part to industry input. In 2007, for example, BATC's Arend Ng noted that the company 'had intensified our stakeholder engagement programmes on a number of key issues surrounding the tobacco industry' and had submitted position papers on the FCTC to key government departments and agencies (BATC 2007b). The Cambodian Ministry of Health's 2011 report on FCTC implementation indicated that the country had complied with few of the requirements on taxation, regulation of tobacco product contents and emissions, prohibition of advertising, or measures to combat smuggling. Significantly, there has been no attempt to comply with FCTC Article 5.3, which requires ratifying parties to protect their 'health policies from commercial and other vested interests of the tobacco industry in accordance with national law' (WHO 2015a). The research and advocacy network the Framework Convention Alliance (FCA) noted that far from compliance with Article 5.3, close relations had continued between the industry and Cambodia's political elite (Framework Convention Alliance 2012). Such links may have been relevant to the evolution of requirement for health warnings on cigarette packs. Written warnings adopted in 2010 do not meet FCTC standards, and the Ministry of Health's retreat from its 2008 position that FCTC-compliant graphic warnings would be adopted has not been clarified. Reports of industry participation in talks with the Inter Ministerial Council for Education and Reduction of Tobacco Use on implementation of the health warning (FCA 2012) may provide some explanation.

China was actively unsupportive of a strong treaty during the negotiation process, and pushed for weaker language in the text and limitations in the scope of commitments. Subsequent ratification of the treaty in 2005 came as a surprise to some, but as Jin (2014) argues, China's decision to ratify reflected unrelated objectives, including burnishing its international image following criticism of its handling of the 2003 SARS outbreak, blocking trade liberalisation and combating cigarette smuggling into the country. Limited efforts to implement the FCTC since ratification would seem to support this argument.

Thailand's strong support of the FCTC process, much of it motivated by civil society, (particularly Action on Smoking and Health [ASH] Thailand), included international leadership during negotiations (Wipfli 2015). Subsequent commitment to implementation of treaty articles has been commended by the Head of the Convention Secretariat (WHO 2014a), and has been particularly strong on measures related to taxation, protection from exposure to tobacco smoke, packaging and labelling, promotion and sponsorship, illicit trade and sales to minors (WHO 2014b; WHO 2015b). This stark contrast to Cambodia and China can be linked to the limited structural and agency power available to the industry, including both the TTM and TTCs.

CONCLUSION

Holden and Lee (2009, 349) argue that the FCTC 'represents a turning point in global tobacco control, but it is imperative that it is comprehensively implemented by national governments'. This chapter suggests that analysis of structural and agency power provides a useful framework for understanding the opportunities and obstacles to the FCTC's negotiation and implementation. This requires fuller understanding of both domestic and foreign tobacco industry interests, and their relationship with political and economic elites that shape the policy process. How the industry has accumulated and exercised power in the three cases study countries, and to what degree, has been significantly determined by the distinct political and economic environments it has encountered. Monopolistic and semi-monopolistic markets in China and Thailand, respectively, could be presumed to share some common characteristics in terms of commercial operating space, but the Chinese government's protection of a major state-owned sector has, in fact, more in common with Cambodia's particular blend of free-market principles and concentration of economic and political power.

CNTC structural power continues to slow progress on both domestic tobacco control and implementation of the FCTC (Lv et al. 2011), while also restricting TTC market access, leaving the latter with limited agency power. In Cambodia, BATC's structural power as a major foreign investor, producer and employer has been enhanced through engagement with political and economic elites. This suggests a possible reason for Cambodia's uneven commitment to its FCTC obligations. In Thailand, the TTM's structural power as a state-owned enterprise has been eroded by foreign competition. Efforts to exert agency power, in turn, have been limited by political instability and strong advocacy domestically for stronger public health action. Successive Thai governments have shown generally consistent commitment to tobacco control. Robust legislation, and improving levels of enforcement, appear to have restricted the capacity of both the TTM and TTCs to exert influence over health policy including FCTC negotiation and implementation.

This analysis of the struggle for influence, between public health and tobacco industry interests, in the three countries has relevance for other countries in the region and beyond. Asia-Pacific countries account for over one-half (58 percent) of global cigarette consumption (Euromonitor International 2015a), and the future battle to implement the FCTC is likely to be fiercest in this region. As the tobacco industry continues to globalise, there is a need to better understand how political and economic systems create opportunities and obstacles to its ability to influence policy. Moreover, this chapter argues that opportunities afforded to corporate actors extend beyond their pursuit of new markets, and into the realm of global governance.

NOTE

1. The remainder is split between the Viniton Group (28 percent)—a joint venture between Cambodian Asean International Company and China Tobacco Guangdong Industrial Company—and Huotraco (19 percent), a distributor not involved in cigarette manufacture (Southeast Asia Tobacco Control Alliance 2014a).

REFERENCES

Barnoya, Jaoquin, and Stanton Glantz. 2006. 'The Tobacco Industry's Worldwide ETS Consultants' Project: European and Asian Components'. *European Journal of Public Health* 16: 69–77. doi:http://dx.doi.org/10.1093/eurpub/cki044.
British American Tobacco Cambodia. 2007a. *Excellence*. April. Phnom Penh: BATC.
———. 2007b. *Excellence*. August. Phnom Penh: BATC.
Cambodia Ministry of Finance. 2011. *Corporate Social Responsibility*. British American Tobacco Cambodia. Invest in Cambodia. http://tinyurl.com/pk32csg.

Chaloupka, Frank J., and Adit Laixuthai. 1996. *U.S. Trade Policy and Cigarette Smoking in Asia*. NBER Working Paper No. w5543.Cambridge: National Bureau of Economic Research.

Chantornvong, Sombat, and Duncan McCargo. 2001. 'Political Economy of Tobacco Control in Thailand'. *Tobacco Control* 10 : 48–54 . doi:10.1136/tc.10.1.48.

Chen, Zhengming, Richard Peto, Maigeng Zhou et al. 2015. 'Contrasting Male and Female Trends in Tobacco-Attributed Mortality in China: Evidence from Successive Nationwide Prospective Cohort Studies'. *The Lancet* 386: 1447–56. http://dx.doi.org/10.1016/S0140-6736(15)00340-2.

Collin, Jeff, Eric LeGresley, Ross MacKenzie, Sue Lawrence and Kelley Lee. 2004. 'Complicity in Contraband: British American Tobacco and Cigarette Smuggling in Asia'. *Tobacco Control* 13 : ii104–11. doi:10.1136/tc.2004.009357.

Crotty, James, Gerald Epstein and Patricia Kelly. 1998. 'Multinational Corporations in the Neo Liberal Regime'. In *Globalization and Progressive Economic Policy*, edited by Dean Baker, Gerald Epstein and Robert Pollin. Cambridge: Cambridge University Press.

Du, Ming. 2014. 'China's State Capitalism and World Trade Law'. *International and Comparative Law Quarterly* 63 (2): 409–48.

Euromonitor International. 2015a. *Global Tobacco: Key Findings Part 1; Cigarettes—the Ongoing Quest for Value*. London: Euromonitor International.

———. 2015b. *Cigarettes in China*. London: Euromonitor International.

———. 2015c. *Cigarettes in Thailand*. London: Euromonitor International.

Farnsworth, Kevin, and Chris Holden. 2006. 'The Business-Social Policy Nexus: Corporate Power and Corporate Inputs into Social Policy'. *Journal of Social Policy* 35 (3): 473–94. http://dx.doi.org/10.1017/S0047279406009883.

Framework Convention Alliance. 2012. *Shadow Report. Brief Report on the Implementation of the FCTC's Core Articles in Cambodia up to March 2012*. http://tinyurl.com/lw2vr6j.

Gainsborough, Martin. 2012. 'Elites vs. Reform in Laos, Cambodia, and Vietnam'. *Journal of Democracy* 23: 34–46.

Ghoshal, Baladas. 2015. 'Anatomy of Political Atrophy in Thailand'. *Strategic Analysis* 39 (2): 156–69. doi:10.1080/09700161.2014.1000656.

Gore, Lance L. 2015. 'The Social Transformation of the Chinese Communist Party: Prospects for Authoritarian Accommodation'. *Problems of Post-Communism* 62 (4): 204–16. doi:10.1080/10758216.2015.1037590.

He, Peisen, Takeuchi Takuc and Eiji Yano. 2013. 'An Overview of the China National Tobacco Corporation and State Tobacco Monopoly Administration'. *Environmental Health and Preventive Medicine* 18 (1): 85–90. doi:10.1007/s12199-012-0288-4.

Hogg, Scott L., Sarah E. Hill and Jeff Collin. 2015. 'State-Ownership of Tobacco Industry: A "Fundamental Conflict of Interest" or a "Tremendous Opportunity" for Tobacco Control?' *Tobacco Control*. doi:10.1136/tobaccocontrol-2014-052114.

Holden, Chris, and Kelley Lee. 2009. 'Corporate Power and Social Policy: The Political Economy of Transnational Tobacco Companies'. *Global Social Policy* 9 (3): 328–54. doi:10.1177/1468018109343638.

Holden, Chris, Kelley Lee, Anna Gilmore, Nathaniel Wander and Gary Fooks. 2010. 'Trade Policy, Health and Corporate Influence: British American Tobacco and China's Accession to the WTO'. *International Journal of Health Services* 40 (3): 421–41. doi:10.2190/HS.40.3.c.

Hu, Teh-wei, Anita Lee and Zhengzhong Mao. 2013. 'WHO Framework Convention on Tobacco Control in China: Barriers, Challenges and Recommendations'. *Global Health Promotion* 20 (4): 13–22. doi:10.1177/1757975913501910.

Hu, Teh-wei, Zhengzhong Mao, Jian Shi and Wendong Chen. 2008. *Tobacco Taxation and Potential Impact in China*. Paris: International Union Against Tuberculosis and Lung Disease.

Hughes, Caroline. 2007. 'Transnational Networks, International Organizations and Political Participation in Cambodia: Human Rights, Labour Rights and Common Rights'. *Democratization* 14 (5): 834–52. doi:10.1080/13510340701635688.

Jin, Jiyong. 2014. 'Why FCTC Policies Have Not Been Implemented in China: Domestic Dynamics and Tobacco Governance'. *Journal of Health Politics, Policy and Law* 39 (3): 633–66. doi: 10.1215/03616878-2682630.

John, Glen A . 2000. 'Face to Face with Patrick O'Keefe Chief Executive, British American Tobacco, Southeast Asia'. Tobacco Asia , December 2000–February 2001: 14–22.

Kheang, Un. 2012. 'Cambodia in 2011: A Thin Veneer of Change'. *Asian Survey* 52 (1): 202–9. doi:10.1525/as.2012.52.1.202.

Lee, Kelley, and Jeff Collin. 2006. '"Key to the Future": British American Tobacco and Cigarette Smuggling in China'. *PLoS Medicine* 3 (7): e228. doi:10.1371/journal.pmed.0030228.

Lee, Sungkyu, Pamela Ling and Stanton Glantz. 2012. 'The Vector of the Tobacco Epidemic: Tobacco Industry Practices in Low and Middle-Income Countries'. *Cancer Causes & Control* 23 (1): 117–29. doi: 10.1007/s10552-012-9914-0.

Levitsky, Steven, and Lucan Way. 2010. *Competitive Authoritarianism; Hybrid Regimes after the Cold War*. Cambridge: Cambridge University Press.

Lv, Jun, Meng Su , Zhiheng Hong, Ting Zhang, Xuemei Huang, Bo Wang and Liming Li. 2011. ' Implementation of the WHO Framework Convention on Tobacco Control in Mainland China'. *Tobacco Control*. doi:10.1136/tc.2010.040352.

MacKenzie, Ross, and Jeff Collin. 2008. '"A Good Personal Scientific Relationship": Philip Morris Scientists and the Chulabhorn Research Institute, Bangkok'. *PLoS Medicine* 5 (12): e238. doi:10.1371/journal.pmed.0050238.

———. 2012. '"Trade Policy, Not Morals or Health Policy": The US Trade Representative, Tobacco Companies and Market Liberalization in Thailand'. *Global Social Policy* 12 (2): 149–72.

———. 2016. '"A Preferred Consultant and Partner to the Royal Government, NGOs, and the Community': British American Tobacco's Access to Policymakers in Cambodia'. *Global Public Health*, doi: 10.1050/.17641642.2016.170868.

MacKenzie, Ross, Jeff Collin, Chim Sopharo and Yel Sopheap. 2004. '"Almost a Role Model of What We Would Like to Do Everywhere": British American Tobacco in Cambodia'. *Tobacco Control* 13: ii112–17. doi:10.1136/tc.2004.009381.

MacKenzie, Ross, Jeff Collin and Kopkul Sriwongcharoen. 2007. 'Thailand—Lighting Up a Dark Market': British American Tobacco, Sports Sponsorship and the Circumvention of Legislation'. *Journal of Epidemiology & Community Health* 61 : 28–33. doi: 10.1136/jech.2005.042432.

MacKenzie, Ross, Kelley Lee and Eric LeGresley. 2015. 'To "Enable Our Legal Product to Compete Effectively with the Transit Market": British American Tobacco's Strategies in Thailand following the 1990 GATT Dispute'. *Global Public Health*. doi:10.1080/17441692.2015.1050049.

Manning, Julian C. D. 1991. Visit to Cambodia by JCD Manning in the Company of M/S Tay Choon Hye, GC Reynolds 21–23 November 1991. 26 November 1991 (date on fax). British American Tobacco. Bates No. 301739929/9932.

Muggli, Monique E., Kelley Lee, Quan Gan, Jon Ebbert and Richard D Hurt. 2008. '"Efforts to Reprioritise the Agenda" in China: British American Tobacco's Efforts to Influence Public Policy on Secondhand Smoke in China'. *PLoS Medicine* 5 (12): e251. doi:10.1371/journal.pmed.0050251.

Novotny, Thomas E. 2006. 'The 'Ultimate Prize' for Big Tobacco: Opening the Chinese Cigarette Market by Cigarette Smuggling'. *PLoS Medicine* 3 (7): e279. doi:10.1371/journal.pmed.0030279.

Peou, S. 2011. 'The Challenge for Human Rights in Cambodia'. In *Human Rights in Asia*, edited by Thomas W. D. Davis and Brian Galligan, 123–43. Cheltenham, UK: Edward Elgar.

Redmon, Pamela, Lincoln Chen, Jacob Wood, Shuyang Li and Jeffrey Koplan. 2012. 'Challenges for Philanthropy and Tobacco Control in China (1986–2012). *Tobacco Control*. doi:10.1136/tobaccocontrol-2012-050924.

Southeast Asia Tobacco Control Alliance. 2014a. 'Cigarette Market Shares in Cambodia'. Bangkok: Southeast Asian Tobacco Control Alliance. www.tobaccowatch.seatca.org/market-shares-cambodia.

———. 2014b. 'Southeast Asia Initiative on Tobacco Tax: ASEAN Tobacco Tax Report Card'. http://seatca.org/dmdocuments/ASEANTaxReportCard%20Sep14.pdf.

Thailand Ministry of Finance. 2015. 'State Enterprises. Thailand'. http://dwfoc.mof.go.th/foc_eng/menu5.htm.

Tong, Elisa, Ming Tao, Qiuzhi Xue and Teh-wei Hu. 2008. 'China's Tobacco Industry and the World Trade Organization'. In *Tobacco Control Policy Analysis in China: Economics and Health*, edited by Teh-wei Hu. Singapore: World Scientific Publishing.

Tong, Elisa, and Stanton Glantz. 2004. 'ARTIST (Asian Regional Tobacco Industry Scientist Team): Philip Morris' Attempt to Exert a Scientific and Regulatory Agenda on Asia'. *Tobacco Control* 13: ii118–24. doi:10.1136/tc.2004.009001.

United Nations. 2015. 'Treaty Collection'. https://treaties.un.org/pages/ViewDetails.aspx?src=TREATY&mtdsg_no=IX-4&chapter=9&lang=en.

Vateesatokit, Prakit. 2003. 'Tailoring Tobacco Control Efforts to the Country: The Example of Thailand'. In *Tobacco Control Policy: Strategies, Successes and Setbacks*, edited by Joy de Beyer and Linda Waverley Brigden. Washington, DC: World Bank.

Wan, Xia, Shaojun Ma, Janet Hoek, Jie Yang, Lanyan Wu, Jiushun Zhou and Gonghuan Yang. 2011. 'Conflict of Interest and FCTC Implementation in China'. Tobacco Control. doi:10.1136/tc.2010.041327.

Wipfli, Heather. 2015. *The Global War on Tobacco: Mapping the World's First Public Health Treaty*. Baltimore: Johns Hopkins University Press.

Wipfli, Heather, Kayo Fujimoto and Thomas Valente. 2010. 'Global Tobacco Control Diffusion: The Case of the Framework Convention on Tobacco Control'. *American Journal of Public Health* 100 (7): 1260–66. doi:10.2105/AJPH.2009.167833.

World Health Organization. 2014a. *Thailand: The Secretariat of the WHO FCTC Backs the Public Health Ministry's New Tobacco Control Law*. http://tinyurl.com/pjmkobw.

———. 2014b. *Reporting Instrument of the WHO Framework Convention on Tobacco Control: Thailand*. www.who.int/fctc/reporting/party_reports/thailand_2012_report.pdf.

———. 2015a. 'The WHO Framework Convention on Tobacco Control: An Overview'. www.who.int/fctc/WHO_FCTC_summary_January2015.pdf?ua=1.

———. 2015b. 'Country Office for Thailand'. *Implementation of FCTC*. www.searo.who.int/thailand/areas/fctc/en.

III

Holding Corporations to Account

THIRTEEN

A Proposed Approach to Systematically Identify and Monitor the Corporate Political Activity of the Food Industry with Respect to Public Health Using Publicly Available Information[1]

Melissa Mialon, Boyd Swinburn and Gary Sacks

Unhealthy diets, including high levels of consumption of food products high in saturated fat, sugar and salt, are major risk factors for non-communicable diseases (NCDs) globally (Vartanian, Schwartz and Brownell 2007; Moodie et al. 2013; Stuckler et al. 2012; Swinburn et al. 2011; De Vogli, Kouvonon and Gimeno 2014; Institute for Health Metrics and Evaluation 2013). Correspondingly, the food industry has been identified as a vector of disease, through their supply of unhealthy food products, their marketing strategies, and their corporate political activity (CPA) (a term employed here to refer to 'corporate attempts to shape government policy in ways favourable to the firm' [Baysinger 1984]) (Moodie et al. 2013; Stuckler et al. 2012). As has been recently emphasised by the director-general of the World Health Organization (WHO), Margaret Chan, the CPA of the food industry represents a substantial challenge to NCD prevention efforts (WHO 2013). The dominance, in terms of market share, of prominent food companies in many countries, coupled with their collective efforts as part of trade associations, has meant that a small number of companies have a large degree of economic power, which readily translates to political power (Swinburn et al. 2011; Stuckler and Nestle

2012; Monteiro et al. 2013; ETC Group 2008). Accordingly, there is a heightened risk that food industry profits will be privileged above other considerations, resulting in food governance and public health policy that does not adequately balance public and commercial interests (Moodie et al. 2013).

In their pursuit of ongoing earnings growth, many influential food industry actors may have an inherent conflict of interest with NCD prevention efforts,[2] particularly where company profitability is dependent on the high volume sales of ultra-processed foods that are major contributors to the NCDs epidemic (Moodie et al. 2013). This has led public health experts to propose that the companies producing unhealthy products should not be involved in the development phase of public health policies (Donovan, McHenry and Vines 2014).

Many groups in the public health community have identified the need to increase mechanisms for accountability of the food industry and have called for greater transparency from food companies (Sacks et al. 2013; WHO 2014; Grover 2014; Swinburn et al. 2015). Despite this, there is currently limited monitoring of the CPA of the food industry with respect to public health. At the global level, there are a number of standards that have been developed to guide socially responsible activities of companies, for example, the United Nations (UN) Global Compact, the UN Guiding Principles on Business and Human Rights and the ISO 26 000 standard (UN Global Compact 2013; ISO 2013; UN Human Rights Office of the High Commissioner 2011). However, while anti-corruption measures and political donations are often included in these standards, they do not explicitly include all aspects of CPA, and, unlike with the tobacco industry, they do not explicitly recognise the potential conflict of interest between the food industry and public health (Donovan, McHenry and Vines 2014). The standards are also voluntary with low compliance and have proved ineffective in casting light on the CPA of the food industry (Kraak et al. 2011). When independent bodies have monitored food companies for their policies and actions regarding the NCDs epidemic, results have consistently shown that, despite voluntary engagement, little progress has been observed in terms of public health outcomes (Lang, Rayner and Kaelin 2006; JPMorgan 2008; Kraak, Story et al. 2011; Kleiman, Ng and Popkin 2012). A number of independent organisations regularly identify elements of the CPA of the food industry (The Center for Responsive Politics 2014; The Center for Media and Democracy 2014a, 2014b; Corporate Europe Observatory 2014; The Center for Science in the Public Interest 2014; Corporate Accountability International 2014). Previous approaches to identify and monitor the CPA of the food industry have not been systematic though and many examples have been anecdotal. Most practices have been described in the United States, with little data related to other countries, particularly low- and middle-income countries (LMICs), which the food industry is increasingly penetrating with ultra-processed food products (Monteiro and Cannon 2012; Monteiro, Gomes and Cannon 2010; Igumbor et al. 2012). However, there is a growing interest in CPA in those countries, as illustrated by the recent analysis of the CPA of Coca Cola in China and India over the last decades (Williams 2015). The Access to Nutrition Index (ATNI) is perhaps the most comprehensive monitoring initiative regarding the food industry and public health (Sacks et al. 2013). Nevertheless, ATNI takes CPA into account to a limited extent by measuring self-disclosed formal lobbying as one indicator in its methodology, which represents only one of the many practices identified in the literature on the CPA of the food industry (ATNI 2012).

CPA with respect to public health has been extensively described in other sectors, such as the tobacco, alcohol and pharmaceutical industries (Moodie et al. 2013; Stuckler et al. 2012; Daube 2012; Babor 2000; Hastings 2012; Wiist 2010; Gilmore, Savell and Collin 2011). In particular, the negative influence of the tobacco industry on public health policies and outcomes has been substantially documented, primarily because litigation against the tobacco industry allowed the release of thousands of internal documents that shed light on the practices adopted by the industry (Bero 2013; University of California San Francisco 2013). The CPA of the tobacco industry could help contextualise the CPA of the food industry. However, while the tobacco control community has access to internal documents from the tobacco industry, research on the CPA of the food industry is currently largely limited to publicly available information and key informants (Bero 2013; University of California San Francisco 2013; Saloojee and Dagli 2000; WHO 2000).

The International Network for Food and Obesity/NCD Research, Monitoring and Action Support (INFORMAS) proposes to monitor various aspects of food environments, including the policies and actions of the food industry, with a focus on most prominent food industry actors in a given country, in terms of market share (Swinburn et al. 2013). The systematic identification and monitoring of the CPA of the food industry is part of this project (Sacks et al. 2013). As part of INFORMAS, this chapter aims to (1) propose a framework for classifying the CPA of the food industry with respect to public health and (2) propose an approach to systematically identify and monitor the CPA of the food industry at the country level.

METHODS

A narrative review of the academic literature was conducted to identify previous efforts to describe, identify and monitor the CPA of the food, tobacco, alcohol and other industries with respect to public health. The initial search strategy involved a review of the public health and business literature, including books, scholarly articles and other relevant sources, with the key words *influence* or *tactic* and *industry* or *corporation* and *health*. This was supplemented by snowball searching to identify additional documents in the grey literature. Relevant frameworks for classifying CPA were identified, and these were adapted to the CPA of the food industry based on the findings of the literature review. In parallel, methods for identifying and monitoring the CPA of the tobacco industry, as developed by the WHO and different tobacco control groups, were identified. These were adapted for the purposes of identifying and monitoring the CPA of the food industry.

PROPOSED FRAMEWORK FOR CLASSIFYING THE CORPORATE POLITICAL ACTIVITY OF THE FOOD INDUSTRY WITH RESPECT TO PUBLIC HEALTH

CPA of corporations, in a general sense, has been well documented in the business literature (Hillman and Hitt 1999). From a public health perspective, perhaps the most comprehensive taxonomy of CPA is described by Savell, Gilmore and Fooks (2014), with respect to the tobacco industry. Six long-term strategies have been described: information strategy, financial incentive strategy, constituency building strategy, policy substitution strategy, legal strategy and constituency fragmentation/destabilisation strategy. In order to meet these long-term strategies, the tobacco industry uses different practices in the short term (Hillman and Hitt 1999). The information strategy includes practices through which the industry disseminates information that is beneficial to its activities in order to influence public health policies and outcomes in a way that would favour corporations (Savell, Gilmore and Fooks 2014). Through the financial incentives strategy, the industry provides funds, gifts and other incentives to politicians, political parties and other decision makers (Saloojee and Dagli 2000). The aim of the constituency-building strategy is to gain the favour of public opinion but also of other stakeholders such as the media and the public health community (Bero 2013). When threatened by regulation, the industry proposes alternatives such as voluntary initiatives or self-regulation (Gilmore, Savell and Collin 2011; Fooks et al. 2013; Fooks et al. 2011). The industry also sues its opponents and challenges public policies in courts as part of a legal strategy (Wiist 2010; Union of Concerned Scientists 2012). Finally, the constituency fragmentation/destabilisation strategy refers to the practices employed by the industry to prevent and counteract criticism of a company's products or practices (Savell, Gilmore and Fooks 2014).

Because some tobacco companies shared ownership of a number of alcohol and food firms, documents released after litigation against the tobacco industry (the 'Tobacco Master Settlement Agreement') have been analysed to understand the practices of alcohol and food companies (Bero 2003; State of California 2013). These studies have consistently found that alcohol and food corporations used practices similar to the ones of the tobacco industry to influence public health policies and outcomes (Wiist 2010; Taubes and Couzens 2012; Bond, Daube and Chikritzhs 2010). Where studies have specifically investigated the CPA of the food industry, most focus on isolated practices, and most were published in the last decade (Lumley, Martin and Antonopoulos 2012; Simon 2013; Oshaug 2009; Gomez et al. 2011; Darmon, Fitzpatrick and Bronstein 2008). There are only a small number of publications where multiple practices are described (Nestle 2002; Stuckler and Siegel 2011; Brownell and Warne 2009; Simon 2006; PLoS Medicine Editors 2012). While these authors do not explicitly use the terminology adopted by Savell, Gilmore and Fooks , there is substantial overlap between their description of industry practices and the Savell, Gilmore and Fooks (2014) classification. The exception is that some authors include food industry practices that are directly related to the processing of products, services and marketing in their classifications—whereas, in the broader literature, these are generally considered to be separate from the definition of CPA (Hillman, Keim and Schuler 2004). The strategies described for the tobacco industry appear to encompass all of the practices identified for the food industry.

Based on the various publications on the CPA of the food industry, and on the taxonomy proposed by Savell, Gilmore and Fooks (2014), table 13.1 presents a proposed framework of the CPA of the food industry . Only minor adjustments to the terms used to describe the CPA of the tobacco industry have been made. For example, the term *opposition fragmentation and destabilisation* is preferred to *constituency fragmentation and destabilisation* as it better distinguishes between efforts to build constituency and efforts to disrupt those opposing industry activities.

In proposing the classification of the various strategies and practices, it is recognised that certain practices are likely to relate to multiple different strategies. For example, if the food industry issues a media release to highlight their new policy to reduce the salt content of its products, it could be classified as (1) an information and messaging strategy ('frame the debate on diet- and public health-related issues: emphasise the food industry's actions to address diet- and public health-related issues') or as (2) a policy substitution strategy. In these cases, the practice can be classified as serving both strategies. It is also noted that the proposed framework is not definitive, but should be modified as new findings on the CPA of the food industry emerge.

Table 13.1.   Framework for categorising the CPA of the food industry with respect to public health

Strategies	Practices	Mechanisms
Information and messaging	Lobby policy makers	Lobby directly and indirectly (through third parties) to influence legislation and regulation so that it is favourable to industry
	Stress the economic importance of the industry	Stress the number of jobs supported and the money generated for the economy
	Promote deregulation	Highlight the potential burden associated with regulation (losses of jobs, administrative burden)
		Demonize the 'nanny state'
		Threaten to withdraw investment if new public health policies introduced
	Frame the debate on diet- and public health-related issues	Shift the blame away from the food industry, (e.g., focus on individual responsibility, role of parents, physical inactivity)
		Promote the good intentions and stress the good traits of the food industry
		Emphasise the food industry's actions to address public health-related issues
	Shape the evidence base on diet- and public health-related issues	Fund research, including through academics, ghost writers, own research institutions and front groups
		Pay scientists as advisers, consultants or spokespersons
		Cherry pick data that favours the industry
		Disseminate and use non-peer reviewed or unpublished evidence
		Participate in and host scientific events
		Provide industry-sponsored education materials
		Suppress or influence the dissemination of research
		Emphasise disagreement among scientists and focus on doubt in science
		Criticise evidence and emphasize its complexity and uncertainty

Financial incentive	Fund and provide financial incentives to political parties and policy makers	Provide donations, gifts, entertainment or other financial inducements
Constituency building	Establish relationships with key opinion leaders and health organisations	Promote public-private interactions, including philanthropic, transactional and transformational relationships
		Support professional organisations through funding and/or advertising in their publications
		Establish informal relationships with key opinion leaders
	Seek involvement in the community	Undertake corporate philanthropy
		Support physical activity programs
		Support events (such as for youth or the arts) and community-level initiatives
	Establish relationships with policy-makers	Seek involvement in working groups, technical groups and advisory groups
		Provide technical support and advice to policy-makers
		Use the 'revolving door', (i.e., ex-food industry staff work in government organisations and vice versa)
	Establish relationships with the media	Establish close relationships with media organizations, journalists and bloggers to facilitate media advocacy
Legal	Use legal action (or the threat of) against public policies or opponents	Litigate or threaten to litigate against governments, organisations or individuals
	Influence the development of trade and investment agreements	Influence the development of trade and investment agreements such that clauses favourable to the industry are included (e.g., limited trade restrictions, mechanisms for corporations to sue governments)
Policy substitution	Develop and promote alternatives to policies	Develop and promote voluntary codes, self-regulation and non-regulatory initiatives

Opposition fragmentation and destabilisation	Criticise public health advocates	Criticise public health advocates publicly and personally, (e.g., through the media, blogs)
	Create multiple voices against public health measures	Establish fake grassroots organisations ('astroturfing')
		Procure the support of community and business groups to oppose public health measures
	Infiltrate, monitor and distract public health advocates, groups and organisations	Monitor the operations and advocacy strategies of public health advocates, groups and organisations
		Support the placement of industry-friendly personnel within health organisations

PROPOSED APPROACH TO IMPLEMENT THE FRAMEWORK FOR IDENTIFYING AND MONITORING THE CORPORATE POLITICAL ACTIVITY OF THE FOOD INDUSTRY WITH RESPECT TO PUBLIC HEALTH

In response to the increased political influence of the tobacco industry and because of the major risk to health associated with tobacco consumption, the WHO has recently published a technical guideline for the surveillance of the CPA of the tobacco industry (WHO 2012). This is the fruit of decades of investigation into the tobacco industry documents and of research on the CPA of the tobacco industry. There are a number of tobacco control groups that have contributed to, implemented or refined the recommendations of the WHO for monitoring tobacco industry tactics (WHO 2012; Action on Smoking and Health Australia 2010; Southeast Asia Tobacco Control Alliance 2009; Tobacco Control Research Group 2013). Their approaches have been adapted, based on the literature and on the proposed framework, to identify and monitor the CPA of the food industry.

Figure 13.1 summarises the approach proposed to systematically identify and monitor the CPA of the food industry in a particular country. This proposed approach consists of systematic document analysis, at the country level, using the framework presented in table 13.1. A database can be used to record details about the industry practices identified.

Phase 1: Selection of Food Industry Actors

The sampling of food industry actors is purposive and based on methods recommended by INFORMAS for selecting organisations of interest in a given country (Sacks et al. 2013). Euromonitor is a tool that can be used for this identification (Euromonitor International 2013). An alternative to the use of Euromonitor could be the selection of the most promi-

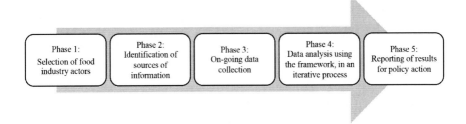

Figure 13.1. **Proposed approach to systematically monitor the CPA of the food industry**

nent food industry actors in a given country based on market surveys (including household expenditure surveys and reports prepared by government trade, industry or agriculture departments) (Sacks et al. 2014). In each country, five to ten food industry actors could initially be selected among:

- the largest processed food manufacturers (including food importers, if applicable) (in terms of market shares);
- the largest non-alcoholic beverage manufacturers (in terms of market shares);
- the largest fast food companies (in terms of market shares);
- the largest food retailers (in terms of market shares);
- the major national trade associations related to food.

Search engines such as Google could be used to retrieve country-specific websites of each food industry actor. The main subsidiaries, as well as the main brands for food and beverage products of processed food and beverage companies, should also be identified (e.g., Milo for Nestle or Gatorade for PepsiCo). Investigators should also keep track of buy-outs and spin-offs of companies over time, including transfers of brands between companies.

Phase 2: Identification of Sources of Information

Based on the recommendations made to identify and monitor the CPA of the tobacco industry, and on the literature on the CPA of the food industry, a number of sources of information were identified and could be targeted for retrieving information related to the CPA of the food industry. Searches would target publicly available information only. These sources are presented in table 13.2. They include industry materials, government materials, such as annual returns of political parties and submissions to public consultations, as well as materials from universities, professional organisations and conferences on diet- and public health–related issues. Sources of information may also include direct requests to government departments, universities and professional bodies, potentially using Freedom of Information (FOI) requests, or equivalent legislation as a basis for the requests. Table 13.2 also presents a number of indirect sources of information, for which no systematic approach to collect data have been developed to date.

As per the principles of INFORMAS, a stepped approach to data collection and analysis is suggested in order to take into account different levels of resources and data availability in different countries. As a 'minimal' step, in any given country, the industry-owned materials, including social media accounts, as well as the media, could be identified and monitored. Government materials and other materials could represent an 'expanded' set of data. Data collection could start at the national level and then move on to sub-national (e.g., state and/or local) levels.

The suggested frequency with which to monitor is annually for most sources of information, and monthly for news or weekly for social media.

Phases 3 and 4: Data Collection and Analysis

It is proposed that these phases involve a thematic qualitative analysis that could be conducted simultaneously to data collection, in an iterative process. For each source of information described in table 13.2, data collection and analysis consists of:

- Reading each document to identify practices that may influence public health policies and outcomes according to the framework of the CPA of the food industry presented in table 13.1 (Hillman and Hitt 1999; Savell, Gilmore and Fooks 2014). The proposed framework should be modified according to the findings.
- Recording the practices in a database and saving evidence (e.g., screenshots, scanned copies of material).
- Where practical, taking notes of negative cases (e.g., documents where no practices related to CPA have been found, e.g., no industry-interests represented on government working groups on diet-related issues).

For some sources of information (e.g., CSR reports or submissions to public consultations), the analysis can be conducted after data collection. In parallel, a database of front groups, as well as a database of individuals with a conflict of interest with the food industry could be created.

Phase 5: Reporting

For this phase, it is proposed that a narrative synthesis is prepared, with illustrative examples of the CPA of the food industry, in a given country. For example, for each food industry actor, strategies that are

Table 13.2. **Sources of information to systematically monitor the CPA of the food industry**

Source of information (general)	Source of information	Organisations or level analysed	Suggested frequency with which to monitor
Industry own materials	Country-specific website of the industry actor: • Composition of diet-related committees • Webpages, reports related to diet-related issues • Voluntary initiatives, commitments and policies related to diet-related issues • Awards to researchers on diet-related issues • Research units or groups on diet-related issues • Submissions to public consultations on diet-related issues • Education material about diet-related issues	Sample of food industry actors, national	Annually (For new projects: 2 years retrospective monitoring for submissions to public consultations)
	Country-specific Corporate Social Responsibility (CSR) webpages/report or website/webpages/information in annual reports of a company's CSR activities (or the company's country-specific activities on its international website)		
	Country-specific website of the industry actor: • News and media releases		Monthly
	Company social media accounts (Twitter, and others where relevant)		Weekly

Government materials	Websites of Ministries (and related agencies) responsible for diet- and public health-related issues:	National	Annually (For new projects: 2 years retrospective monitoring only for FOI requests and submissions to public consultations)
	• Working groups on diet-related issues and conflicts of interest		
	• Public-private initiatives or diet-related issues		
	• Submissions to public consultations from the food industry and its allies (including third parties such as front groups) on diet- and public health-related issues		
	• Freedom of Information (FOI) disclosure log: information on diet-related issue		
	• Minister's diary disclosures: information on diet-related issues		
	• Declarations of interests		
	• Requests, either directly or through FOI legislation for:		
	• A list of meetings of food industry representatives from the selected sample of industry actors, with officials and/or representatives of the government;		
	• Minutes and other reports of these meetings;		
	• All correspondence (including emails) between food industry representatives from the selected sample of industry actors and officials and/or representatives from the government.		
	Websites of Parliament and Senate:	National	
	• Submissions to public consultations from the food industry and its allies (including third parties such as front groups) on diet- and public health-related issues		
	• FOI disclosure logs		
	• Declarations of interests of all members		
	• Requests, either directly or through FOI legislation for:		
	• A list of meetings of food industry representatives from the selected sample of industry actors, with officials and/or representatives of the government;		

	• Minutes and other reports of these meetings; • All correspondence (including emails) between food industry representatives from the selected sample of industry actors, with officials and/or representatives from the government.		
	Register of lobbyists	National	
	Websites of major political parties and websites of commissions in charge of elections: • Donations for elections from the food industry • Political parties annual return: donations from the food industry	National, all parties	
	Website of government • News and media releases on the government's website	National	Monthly
Materials from universities and professional bodies	Websites of a selection of major universities with a school/department of nutrition/dietetics or physical activity: • Research projects, fellowships or grants funded by the selected food industry actors • Prizes or awards offered to students by selected food industry actors • If information is not available online, this information can be directly requested from the universities through an FOI request or a letter to the Vice Chancellor, Deputy Vice Chancellor for research, and research office, including a request for details of relationships or interactions with the food industry, as well as any relevant policies on relationships and funding rules with respect to the industry.	National	Annually (For new projects: 2 years retrospective monitoring for FOI requests only)
	Websites of a selection of major conferences on diet-, public health- or physical activity-related issues: • Sponsors from the food industry • A list of booths, as well as other marketing opportunities paid for	National	Annually

by the food industry
- Education materials and tote bags provided by the food industry
- A list of speakers (including in oral, poster and symposium presentation) who work or receive funds from the food industry and the topic of their presentations
- Awards and prizes from the food industry

Websites of a selection of major professional bodies related to diet-, public health- or physical activity related health issues: • Funds received or sponsors from the food industry • Marketing opportunities paid for by the industry • Awards and prizes granted to professionals or students from the food industry • Professional education resources (including publications or oral presentations) supported by the food industry If information is not available online, it can be directly requested from the organisations, including details of relationships or interactions with the food industry that they think might be helpful, as well as any relevant policies on relationships and funding rules with respect to the industry.	National	
News related to the selected food industry actors and diet-related issues in newspapers, on Google News and through subscriptions to news updates on websites such as Food Navigator or Australian Food News	National	Monthly
Other sources Google Scholar Alert with key words such as: 'influence or tactic and industry or corporation and health and [name of the country]'.	National and international	Indirect data collection, information not monitored *per se*, but recorded if relevant to the framework
Websites of United Nations agencies responsible for diet- related issues, and their regional offices: • Food and Agriculture		

Organization: www.fao.org/
- World Food Programme: www.wfp.org/
- Codex Alimentarius: http://www.codexalimentarius.org/
- World Health Organization: www.who.int/
- United Nations Standing Committee on Nutrition: http://www.unscn.org/
- UNICEF: http://www.unicef.org/
- World Trade Organization: www.wto.org/
- United Nations Industrial Development Organization: http://www.unido.org/

International websites of food industry actors

Websites of international trade associations

Websites of front groups, think tanks working on diet-related issues:
- All webpages with topics related to diet-related health issues
- Twitter pages
- Submissions to public consultations

Websites of conferences on CSR and food industry-related topics

Websites of business journals and other business news platforms

LinkedIn, Viadeo and other professionals social media (for information about the 'revolving door')

Websites of public relations agencies working on behalf of the food industry:
- Submissions to public consultations
- Clients from the food industry

Websites of not-for-profit organisations

Websites of research units, researchers and other scientific organisations conducting research on diet- or physical activity-related health issues

Educational material supplied to
schools and parents by food
companies

Websites of other organisations
working on diet- and public health-
related issues

most commonly used could be identified and described. In addition, case
studies for specific food industry actors could be prepared. This approach has been used for similar reporting of the CPA of other industries
(Fooks et al. 2013; Fooks et al. 2011; Babor 2009; McCambridge, Hawkins
and Holden 2013).

Potential quantitative indicators could include the number of researchers with conflicts of interest in national working groups on diet- or
public health–related issues, the amount received from the food industry
by political parties or the number of food-industry sponsors of national
sporting organisations. This list of indicators could be refined depending
on sources of information and data available in specific countries. As data
for different countries emerge, scorecards illustrating the range of practices used by different companies could be developed.

Given the large amount of data that could potentially be collected
using the proposed approach, the development of a publicly accessible
website could be considered to provide broad access to the data collected.
The tobaccotactics.org website, developed by researchers at the University of Bath (United Kingdom) who monitor the CPA of the tobacco industry, is a model that could be investigated for potential adaption for
use with respect to the food industry (Tobacco Control Research Group
2013). Social media is also likely to be an avenue for highlighting details
of practices used by companies, with a view to exposing these practices
to a broad audience and highlighting the potential risks to public health
from these practices.

DISCUSSION

This paper has proposed a framework for classifying the CPA of the food
industry with respect to public health and an approach to systematically
identify and monitor it based on previous literature in the area and approaches to monitor the CPA of other industries, in particular the tobacco
industry. While previous monitoring efforts with respect to the policies
and practices of the food industry have predominantly focused on the
products and marketing activities of the food industry, the proposed approach aims to capture aspects of CPA that have not previously been
taken into account in a systematic way. The proposed monitoring approach could be used to highlight various aspects of the CPA of the food

industry, with the aim of increasing transparency regarding the potential influence of commercial interests on public health policies and outcomes.

The intention is for the proposed monitoring approach to be implemented at the country level by civil society organisations, including researchers working on CPA and non-government organisations related to public health and/or consumer interests. While it is recognised that the proposed approach may be most suited to high-income countries and in countries with democratic political systems in particular, aspects of the protocol, such as the monitoring of industry-owned materials and of the media, have the potential to be applied more universally. Relevant sources of information may be limited in LMICs, given the limited availability of company websites at the national level, the lack of FOI (or equivalent) legislation in many countries, and less pressure (e.g., from public health advocacy and consumer groups) for companies operating in LMICs to disclose relevant information. For these reasons, the proposed stepped approach could be pilot tested in different countries in order to evaluate its applicability in different contexts. Where monitoring is carried out across multiple countries and over time, it will facilitate comparison of the strategies and practices used by individual companies in different countries, as well as a comparison of in-country and cross-country trends. The proposed monitoring could also be carried out at the global (e.g., UN and its agencies) or regional level (e.g., European Union) to understand the CPA of the food industry more broadly.

The proposed framework is based on various aspects of CPA previously identified in the business and public health literature. While the proposed categorisation of strategies and practices seeks to be comprehensive, the integrated nature of CPA means that the categories are not mutually exclusive. Accordingly, some subjectivity will be needed in order to classify practices that are identified through monitoring activities. Any new practice should be included in the proposed framework. Importantly, the framework is based on the classification of CPA in other industries, most notably the tobacco industry. This will help facilitate comparison of practices used by different industries and it is hoped that the use of common terminology will help bring together different groups that are examining corporate influences on public health.

While the proposed monitoring approach is designed to be relatively inexpensive to conduct, in order to minimise resources needed for monitoring, it is recommended that the focus is only on a prioritised selection of companies in each country. The advantage of this approach is that monitoring is focused on the companies that are likely to have the most influence in each country. However, this approach does not capture the practices of smaller companies in a systematic way. To overcome this limit, a case-study approach could be considered.

A limitation of the proposed monitoring approach is that it will only identify publicly available information, which can be incomplete, is not always representative of all practices, and often lacks detail. CPA is also reflected through personal connections, informal discussions and other activities (e.g., free lunches) that are not going to be captured with the proposed approach. To partially overcome this limitation, the proposed approach could be supplemented with interviews with key stakeholders, such as politicians, civil servants or public health advocates, as well as whistle-blowers from the food industry. The use of stakeholder interviews could be particularly relevant in LMICs where other data sources may be more limited. Methods to gather additional information using crowd-sourcing and social media should also be explored. Timing of data collection is also crucial because the nature of CPA is likely to change over time and the nature and intensity of CPA is likely to vary according to the political climate. For example, the food industry might be more likely to use the policy substitution strategy or the legal strategy in a period when regulation is actively being considered by the government in a given country—whereas when governments that are philosophically less inclined to regulate are in power, other strategies, such as the information and messaging strategy, may be the most prominent. On-going monitoring is therefore recommended in order to track these changes.

It is also noted that the proposed approach does not assess the actual influence of CPA on public health policies and outcomes. This may be the subject of future investigations. For example, tobacco control groups are considering a systematic approach to quantify changes in proposed public health policies after consultation with the tobacco industry (Costa et al. 2014). Regardless of their influence, many of the practices that could be captured through the proposed approach are likely to be legitimate practices of industry (e.g., submissions to public consultations, meetings with politicians). Accordingly, the mere identification of CPA of a particular company is not, in and of itself, an indication of a public health problem. However, these practices may pose a risk to public health policies and outcomes or may simply be perceived as posing a risk, in that there is a likelihood that commercial interests will be privileged above public interest considerations. The rationale behind the proposed approach is that, by monitoring and tracking CPA over time, the transparency and accountability of companies in the food industry can be increased. In addition, implementation of the proposed monitoring approach could help identify mechanisms to better balance public and commercial interests related to public health policy.

CONFLICT OF INTEREST

This chapter was supported by the Australian National Health and Medical Research Council (NHMRC) under grant number APP1041020. The NHMRC had no role in the design, analysis or writing of this chapter.

ACKNOWLEDGEMENTS

The authors would like to their colleague Professor Anna Gilmore, who provided insight and expertise that greatly assisted the development of the proposed framework and approach.

NOTES

1. Mialon, Swinburn and Sacks (2015). Reproduced with permission from Blackwell Publishing Ltd.
2. The term *conflict of interest* is defined here as: 'A conflict of interest can occur when a Partner's ability to exercise judgment in one role is impaired by his or her obligations in another role or by the existence of competing interests. Such situations create a risk of a tendency towards bias in favour of one interest over another or that the individual would not fulfil his or her duties impartially. . . . A conflict of interest may exist even if no unethical or improper act results from it. It can create an appearance of impropriety that can undermine confidence in the individual, his/her constituency or organisation. Both actual and perceived conflicts of interest can undermine the reputation and work of the Partnership' (Roll Back Malaria Partnership 2009).

REFERENCES

ATNI. 2012. *Access to Nutrition Index Methodology Development Report.*

Action on Smoking and Health Australia. 2010. *Countering Tobacco Tactics: A Guide to Identifying, Monitoring and Preventing Tobacco Industry Interference in Public Health.* Australia.

Babor, Thomas F. 2000. 'Partnership, Profits and Public Health'. *Addiction* 95 (2): 193–95.

———. 2009. 'Alcohol Research and the Alcoholic Beverage Industry: Issues, Concerns and Conflicts of Interest'. *Addiction* 104 (1): 34–47.

Baysinger, Barry D. 1984. 'Domain Maintenance as an Objective of Business Political Activity—an Expanded Typology'. *Acad Manage Rev.* 9: 248–58.

Bero, Lisa. 2003. 'Implications of the Tobacco Industry Documents for Public Health and Policy'. *Annual Review of Public Health* 24: 267–88.

Bond, Laura, Mike Daube and Tanya Chikritzhs. 2010. 'Selling Addictions: Similarities in Approaches between Big Tobacco and Big Booze'. *Australasian Medical Journal* 3 (6): 325–32.

Brownell, Kelly D., and Kenneth E. Warne. 2009. 'The Perils of Ignoring History: Big Tobacco Played Dirty and Millions Died. How Similar Is Big Food?' *Milbank Quarterly* 98 (1): 259–94.

Corporate Accountability International. 2014. *Introduction—Corporate Accountability International.* www.stopcorporateabuse.org/campaigns/challenge-corporate-abuse-our-food.

Corporate Europe Observatory. 2014. 'Food and Agriculture'. http://corporateeurope.org/food-and-agriculture.

Costa, Helia, Anna B. Gilmore, Silvy Peeters, Martin McKee and David Stuckler. 2014. 'Quantifying the Influence of Tobacco Industry on EU Governance: Automated Content Analysis of the EU Tobacco Products Directive'. *Tobacco Control.*

Darmon, Keren, Kathy Fitzpatrick and Carolyn Bronstein. 2008. 'Krafting the Obesity Message: A Case Study in Framing and Issues management'. *Public Relations Review* 34 (4): 373–79.

Daube, Mike. 2012. 'Alcohol and Tobacco'. *ANZJPH* 36 (2): 108–10.

De Vogli, Roberto, Anne Kouvonen and David Gimeno. 2014. 'The Influence of Market Deregulation on Fast Food Consumption and Body Mass Index: A Cross-National Time Series Analysis'. *Bulletin of the World Health Organization* 92: 99–107A.

Donovan, Robert J., Julia Anwar McHenry and Anthony J. Vines. 2014. 'Unity of Effort Requires Unity of Object: Why Industry Should Not Be Involved in Formulating Public Health Policy'. *Journal of Public Affairs* 15 (4): 397–403.

ETC Group. 2008. *Who Owns Nature? Corporate Power and the Final Frontier in the Commodification of Life*. ETC Group.

Euromonitor International. 2013. Euromonitor Passport.

Fooks, Gary, Anna Gilmore, Jeff Collin, Chris Holden and Kelley Lee. 2013. 'The Limits of Corporate Social Responsibility: Techniques of Neutralization, Stakeholder Management and Political CSR'. *Journal of Business Ethics* 112: 283–99.

Fooks, Gary, Anna Gilmore, Katherine E. Smith, Jeff Collin, Chris Holden and Kelley Lee. 2011. 'Corporate Social Responsibility and Access to Policy Elites: An Analysis of Tobacco Industry Documents'. *PLoS Medicine* 8: e1001076.

Gilmore, Anna, Emily Savell and Jeff Collin. 2011. 'Public Health, Corporations and the New Responsibility Deal: Promoting Partnerships with Vectors of Disease?' *Journal of Public Health* 33 (1): 2–4.

Gómez, Luis, Enrique Jacoby, Lorena Ibarra, Diego Lucumi and Alexandra Hernandez. 2011. 'Sponsorship of Physical Activity Programs by the Sweetened Beverages Industry: Public Health or Public Relations?' *Rev Saude Publica* 45 (2): 423–27.

Grover, Anand. 2014. *Report to the Human Rights Council (Main Focus: Unhealthy Foods and Non-communicable Diseases)*. New York: United Nations.

Hastings, Gerard. 2012. 'Why Corporate Power Is a Public Health Priority'. *BMJ* 345: e5124.

Hillman, Amy J., and Michael A. Hitt. 1999. 'Corporate Political Strategy Formulation: A Model of Approach, Participation, and Strategy Decisions'. *The Academy of Management Review* 24 (4): 825–42.

Hillman, Amy J., Gerald D. Keim and Douglas Schuler. 2004. 'Corporate Political Activity: A Review and Research Agenda'. *Journal of Management* 30 (6): 837–57.

Igumbor, Ehimario U., David Sanders, Thandi R. Puoane et al. 2012. '"Big Food" the Consumer Food Environment, Health, and the Policy Response in South Africa'. *PLoS Medicine* 9 (7): e1001253.

Institute for Health Metrics and Evaluation. 2013. 'Global Burden of Diseases Visualizations'.

ISO. 2013. 'ISO 26000—Social Responsibility'.

JPMorgan. 2008. *Proof of the Pudding: Benchmarking Ten of the World's Largest Food Companies' Response to Obesity and Related Health Concerns*.

Kleiman, Susan, Shu Wen Ng and Barry Popkin. 2012. 'Drinking to Our Health: Can Beverage Companies Cut Calories while Maintaining Profits?' *Obesity Reviews* 13 (3): 258–74.

Kraak, Vivica, Boyd Swinburn, Mark Lawrence and Paul Harrison. 2011. 'The Accountability of Public-Private Partnerships with Food, Beverage and Quick-Serve Restaurant Companies to Address Global Hunger and the Double Burden of Malnutrition'. *United Nations System Standing Committee on Nutrition: News* 39: 11–24.

Kraak, Vivica, Mary Story, Ellen A. Wartella and Jaya Ginter. 2011. 'Industry Progress to Market a Healthful Diet to American Children and Adolescents'. *American Journal of Preventive Medicine* 41 (3): 322–33.

Lang, Tim, Geof Rayner and Elizabeth Kaelin. 2006. *The Food Industry, Diet, Physical Activity and Health: A Review of Reported Commitments and Practices of 25 of the World's Largest Food Companies*. London: Centre for Food Policy.

Lumley, J., Jane Martin and Nick Antonopoulos. 2012. *Exposing the Charade*. Melbourne: Obesity Policy Coalition.

McCambridge, Jim, Benjamin Hawkins and Chris Holden. 2013. 'Industry Use of Evidence to Influence Alcohol Policy: A Case Study of Submissions to the 2008 Scottish Government Consultation'. *PLoS Medicine* 10 (4): e1001431.

Mialon, Melissa, Boyd Swinburn and Gary Sacks. 2015. 'A Proposed Approach to Systematically Identify and Monitor the Corporate Political Activity of the Food Industry with Respect to Public Health Using Publicly Available Information'. *Obesity Reviews* 16 (7): 519–30.

Monteiro, Carlos A., Fabio S. Gomes and Geoffrey Cannon. 2010. 'The Snack Attack'. *American Journal of Public Health* 100 (6): 975–81.

Monteiro Carlos A., and Geoffrey Cannon. 2012. 'The Impact of Transnational 'Big Food' Companies on the South: A View from Brazil'. *PLoS Medicine* 9 (7): e1001252.

Monteiro Carlos A., Jean-Claude Moubarac, Geoffrey Cannon, Shu Wen Ng and Barry Popkin. 2013. 'Ultra-Processed Products Are Becoming Dominant in the Global Food System'. *Obesity Reviews* 14 (2): 21–38.

Moodie R., David Stuckler, Carlos A. Monteiro et al. 2013. 'Profits and Pandemics: Prevention of Harmful Effects of Tobacco, Alcohol, and Ultra-Processed Food and Drink Industries'. *The Lancet* 381: 670–79.

Nestle, Marion. 2002. *Food Politics: How the Food Industry Influences Nutrition and Health.* Berkeley: University of California Press.

Oshaug, Arne. 2009. 'What Is the Food and Drink Industry Doing in Nutrition Conferences?' *Public Health Nutrition* 12 (7): 1019–20.

PLoS Med. 2012. 'PLoS Medicine Series on Big Food: The Food Industry Is Ripe for Scrutiny'. *PLoS Medicine* 9 (6): e1001246.

Roll Back Malaria Partnership. 2009. *Roll Back Malaria Partnership: Conflict of Interest Policy and Procedure.* Roll Back Malaria Partnership

Sacks, Gary, Boyd Swinburn, Vivica Kraak et al. 2013. 'A Proposed Approach to Monitor Private-Sector Policies and Practices Related to Food Environments, Obesity and Non-communicable Disease Prevention'. *Obesity Reviews* 14 (1): 38–48.

Sacks, Gary, Marion Mialon, Stefanie Vandevijvere et al. 2014. 'Comparison of Food Industry Policies and Commitments on Marketing to Children and Product (Re)formulation in Australia, New Zealand and Fiji'. *Critical Public Health* 25 (3): 1–21.Saloojee, Yussuf, and Elif Dagl. 2000. 'Tobacco Industry Tactics for Resisting Public Policy on Health'. *Bulletin of the World Health Organization* 78 (7): 902–10.

Savell, Emily, Anna B. Gilmore and Gary Fooks. 2014. 'How Does the Tobacco Industry Attempt to Influence Marketing Regulations? A Systematic Review'. *PLoS One* 9: e87389.

Simon, Michele. 2006. *Appetite for Profit: How the Food Industry Undermines our Health and How to Fight Back.* New York: Nation Books.

———. 2013. *Clowning around with Charity: How McDonald's Exploits Philanthropy and Targets Children.* Eat Drink Politics.

Southeast Asia Tobacco Control Alliance. 2009. *Surveillance of Tobacco Industry Activities Toolkit.* Thailand.

State of California—Department of Justice—Office of the Attorney General. 2013. *Master Settlment Agreement.* http://oag.ca.gov/tobacco/msa.

Stuckler, David, and Karen Siegel. 2011. *Sick Societies: Responding to the Global Challenge of Chronic Disease.* Oxford: Oxford University Press.

Stuckler, David, and Marion Nestle. 2012. 'Big Food, Food Systems, and Global Health'. *PLoS Medicine* 9 (6): e1001242.

Stuckler, David, Martin McKee, Shah Ebrahim and Sanjay Basu. 2012. 'Manufacturing Epidemics: The Role of Global Producers in Increased Consumption of Unhealthy Commodities Including Processed Foods, Alcohol, and Tobacco'. *PLoS Medicine* 9 (6): e1001235.

Swinburn, Boyd, Gary Sacks, Kevin D. Hall et al. 2011. 'The Global Obesity Pandemic: Shaped by Global Drivers and Local Environments'. *The Lancet* 378 (9793): 804–14.

Swinburn, Boyd, Gary Sacks, Stefanie Vandevijvere et al. 2013. 'INFORMAS (International Network for Food and Obesity/Non-communicable Diseases Research, Monitoring and Action Support): Overview and Key Principles'. *Obesity Reviews* 14 (1): 1–12.

Swinburn, Boyd, Vivica Kraak, Harry Rutter et al. 2015. 'Strengthening of Account-
ability Systems to Create Healthy Food Environments and Reduce Global Obesity'.
The Lancet 385 (9986): 2534–45.
Taubes, Gary, and Cristin Kearns Couzens. 2012. 'Big Sugar's Sweet Little Lies'. *Moth-
er Jones*.
The Center for Media and Democracy. 2014a. 'PR Watch: Reporting of Spin and Disin-
formation since 1993'. www.prwatch.org.
The Center for Media and Democracy. 2014b. 'SourceWatch'. www.sourcewatch.org/
index.php/SourceWatch.
The Center for Responsive Politics. 2014. 'OpenSecrets.org: Money in Politics—See
Who's Giving & Who's Getting'. www.opensecrets.org.
The Center for Science in the Public Interest. 2014. 'The Integrity in Science Database'.
www.cspinet.org/integrity.
Tobacco Control Research Group. 2013. 'TobaccoTactics'. www.tobaccotactics.org/in-
dex.php/Main_Page.
UN Global Compact. 2013. 'UN Global Compact Overview'. www.unglobalcompact.
org/AboutTheGC/index.html.
Union of Concerned Scientists. 2012. *Heads They Win, Tails We Lose: How Corporations
Corrupt Science at the Public's Expense.* Cambridge, MA: UCS Publications.
United Nations Human Rights Office of the High Commissioner. 2011. *Guiding Princi-
ples on Business and Human Rights.*
University of California San Francisco. 2013. 'Legacy Tobacco Documents Library'.
http://legacy.library.ucsf.edu.
Vartanian, Lenny R., Marlene B. Schwartz and Kelly D. Brownell. 2007. 'Effects of Soft
Drink Consumption on Nutrition and Health: A Systematic Review and Meta-anal-
ysis'. *American Journal of Public Health* 97 (4): 667–75.
WHO. 2000. *Tobacco Industry Strategies to Undermine Tobacco Control Activities at the
World Health Organization.* Geneva: World Health Organization.
———. 2012. *Technical Resource on the Protection of Public Health Policies with Respect to
Tobacco Control from Commercial and Other Vested Interests of the Tobacco Industry for
Country Implementation of WHO Framework Convention on Tobacco Control Article 5.3.*
Geneva: World Health Organization.
———. 2013. *Opening Address at the 8th Global Conference on Health Promotion Helsinki,
Finland—Dr Margaret Chan Director-General of the World Health Organization.* Helsin-
ki: World Health Organization.
———. 2014. *Global Status Report on Noncommunicable Diseases 2014.* Geneva: World
Health Organization.
Wiist, W. H. 2010. *The Bottom Line or Public Health: Tactics Corporations Use to Influence
Health and Health Policy and What We Can Do to Counter Them.* Oxford; New York:
Oxford University Press.
Williams, Simon N. 2015. 'The Incursion of "Big Food" in Middle-Income Countries: A
Qualitative Documentary Case Study Analysis of the Soft Drinks Industry in China
and India'. *Critical Public Health* 25 (4): 1–19.

FOURTEEN

Regulating Baby Food Marketing: Civil Society versus Private Sector Influence

Tracey Wagner-Rizvi

Breastfeeding is essential for reducing infant and child malnutrition, morbidity and mortality. Breastmilk provides protection against illnesses that can interfere with growth, and cause disability or death. More than 800,000 children under five could be saved every year with optimal breastfeeding practices[1] (Black et al. 2013). The risk of a baby becoming ill or undernourished, or dying from diarrhoea, is significantly increased when infant formula or animal milk is prepared or diluted with unsafe water. However, even when artificial feeding is affordable, clean water is available, and good hygienic conditions for preparing and feeding infant formula exist, breastfeeding is the best way of nourishing all infants (United Nations Children's Fund [UNICEF] 2010).

Declining breastfeeding rates were linked with the promotion of infant formula milk for babies as early as 1939 by the paediatrician Dr. Cicely Williams, who described the promotion of sweetened condensed milk for infants as 'misguided propaganda on infant feeding [that] should be punished as the most miserable form of sedition, and that these deaths should be regarded as murder' (Brady and de Oliveira Brady 2004). Concern over links between aggressive promotion of formula milk and declining breastfeeding rates increased during the 1960s and 1970s, as research echoed Williams's observations, leading one doctor to coin the term *commerciogenic malnutrition* to describe the impact of formula on infant health (Jelliffe 1971).

This chapter analyses the on-going efforts of the International Baby Food Action Network (IBFAN) and its member organisations to limit corporate influence over infant and young child feeding. Formed in October 1979, IBFAN has grown from six founding NGOs to a network of 273 groups in 168 countries in both the global North and South and for more than forty years has challenged industry promotion of its products (IBFAN 2015). The chapter specifically studies how IBFAN has been able to counter an industry with far greater resources in order to restrain the industry's promotion of its products.

BACKGROUND

Concerns with the promotion of formula milk and its impact on infant health entered public debate in the early 1970s. In 1973, *New Internationalist* published an interview with two child health specialists with extensive experience in developing countries, who stated that 'vigorous advertising' had created 'serious health problems', and that industry promotional campaigns were irresponsible (Geach 1973). A year later, the development agency War on Want published a report on promotion and sale of powdered milk in developing countries entitled *The Baby Killer* (Muller 1974). Translated into the German by a small Swiss student group, and published under a title that translated into *Nestlé Kills Babies*, the booklet received extensive media coverage in Switzerland, home to Nestlé's corporate headquarters. Nestlé sued the students for libel, earning the company a great deal of negative publicity over the course of the two-year court case. The defendants were eventually found guilty on one count of libel concerning the book's title. Nestlé dropped the three other counts and was advised by the presiding judge to change its marketing tactics if it wanted to be 'spared the accusation of immoral and unethical conduct' (Sokol 2005, 7–8).

At the same time, civil society groups were mobilising to call for an international code of baby food marketing. In 1972, the International Organization of Consumers Unions (IOCU), now Consumers International, proposed to the Codex Alimentarius Commission, founded by the Food and Agriculture Organization (FAO) and the World Health Organization (WHO) in 1963, a draft *Code of Practice for Advertising of Infant Foods*. The Codex Commission, however, decided that the proposal was outside its mandate as a United Nations (UN) agency that dealt with international quality and labelling standards for food products (Chetley 1986, 40–42).

The Nestlé Boycott, organised by civil society groups in 1977, is perhaps the best-known direct action campaign aimed at highlighting the deleterious effects of infant feeding formula. The boycott placed baby food marketing on the global agenda by making clear the link between formula manufacturers, represented by market leader Nestlé, and their impacts on infant health. It symbolically targeted the company's flagship product, Nescafé coffee. Though primarily intended to pressure Nestlé by affecting its bottom line, the boycott also generated negative publicity for the company, thereby undermining its credibility and trustworthiness among the public and policy makers.

The boycott contributed to a broad momentum that compelled the WHO and UNICEF to push in 1979 for an international code to regulate baby food marketing. Joint meetings held in October brought together representatives of the UN, national-level governments, industry, experts from a range of disciplines, and non-governmental organisations (NGOs), including six organisations[2] that would found IBFAN at the meeting (Allain 2005). This marked the first time that NGOs and industry sat as equal participants with government delegates in a UN summit (Chetley 1986, 63–65).

The recommendation for the creation of 'an international code of marketing of infant formula and other products used as breastmilk substitutes' (WHO 1979) was endorsed by the World Health Assembly (WHA), the policy-making body of the WHO, in Resolution 33.32 in May 1980. WHO and UNICEF led the drafting process in consultation with experts, government delegations, NGOs and baby food manufacturers, primarily through the International Council of Infant Food Industries (ICIFI),[3] which had been formed during the Nestlé libel trial in Switzerland. The industry lobbied to minimise restrictions on marketing contained in the proposed Code, while NGOs pushed for it to be as strong and protective as possible (Sokol 2005, 9). The WHA adopted the *International Code of Marketing of Breast-milk Substitutes* (the *Code*) in May 1981 with 118 countries in favour, one against (United States) and three abstentions (Argentina, Japan and Korea) (Chetley 1986, 98). The *Code* was adopted, according to WHA Resolution 34.22, as a 'minimum requirement', and governments were to 'implement it in its entirety' as 'national legislation, regulations or other suitable measures'.

METHODS

This chapter analyses how corporations that produce and promote baby food, with a particular focus on market leader Nestlé, seek to influence the regulation of baby food marketing at the global and domestic levels, and how IBFAN has responded to these actions. This chapter draws on records acquired through work with the IBFAN member organisation in Pakistan from December 1996 to October 2001 and observations of its campaign to enact national legislation to regulate baby food marketing. These records are supplemented and updated with information collected from the websites, publications and archives of WHO, IBFAN and IBFAN member organisations.

In assessing how IBFAN has been able to effectively challenge the baby food industry, despite the seeming imbalance in political power, this analysis applies Fuchs's (2005, 778–79) framework of three dimensions of power: *instrumental, structural* and *discursive power. Instrumental power* is evident in an actor's ability to influence political or policy output, for example, through lobbying or financial support. It depends on actor-specific resources, such as 'financial, organisational, or human resources, as well as access to decision-makers'. *Structural power* 'stresses the importance of the input side of the political process and of the predetermination of the behavioural options of political decision-makers by existing material structures that allocate direct and indirect decision-making power'. From a *discursive* perspective, power is seen to be a function of norms and ideas. Power not only pursues interests, but also creates them: 'Discursive power precedes the formation and articulation of interests due to its role in constituting and framing policies, actors, and broader societal norms and ideas'.

DISCUSSION

Financial Imbalance

Baby food producers, either individually or collectively, and IBFAN and its member organisations have differential access to the types of power described by Fuchs. The baby food industry's main sources of power are its financial resources, and its economic position in the market based on its role as investor, employer and source of tax revenue for government. This affords it considerable instrumental, structural and discursive power, which it uses to try to influence policy, and to protect and advance its interests. Cash-strapped NGOs and networks, meanwhile, rely predominantly on discursive power, which some, including IBFAN, have been able to translate into a degree of instrumental power. The 1979 Nestlé libel trial was a particularly explicit example of how civil society, despite its lesser financial resources and reliance on discursive power, can shape public opinion on an issue, while the industry interest, represented by Nestlé, responds with power rooted in their financial resources.

The baby food industry is able to use instrumental power associated with its financial resources to influence media coverage by threatening legal action or withdrawal of advertisements, which are a powerful source of revenue. In 1999, for example, the IBFAN member organisation in Pakistan published a Nestlé whistle-blower's evidence of the company's strategies and activities related to infant formula in that country. The report contained internal company documentation and the former salesman's account of events surrounding the documents and of their significance. This 'rare insider's view of the hidden but common sales practices' of a large transnational firm revealed 'the systematic and routine manner in which the company buys the loyalty of doctors, persuading them to promote commercial products' rather than breastfeeding (The Network 1999, 6). Among the media that covered the report, Germany's ZDF television network travelled to Pakistan and was scheduled to broadcast its findings on 8 December 1999. Following a meeting between Nestlé's communication's director and a senior ZDF executive, however, the broadcast was cancelled (Baby Milk Action 2000).

Around the same time, a national newspaper in Pakistan refused to publish any further coverage of the Nestlé whistle-blower. With pressure coming from the newspaper's marketing department to pull coverage, the editors implicitly understood that Nestlé had threatened to pull its substantial advertisements from the paper (personal communication by an editor to the author). Such influence represents an example of the company's instrumental power, which increases the entire industry's structural and discursive power by shaping the issues that are included in the public discourse, and by silencing its critics.

The whistle-blower's story, including the cancelled ZDF segment, has since been made into a film called *Tigers* by Academy Award–winning director Danis Tanovic. IBFAN member organisation Baby Milk Action's role as consultant on the film demonstrated its discursive power and related influence on the representation of the issue and the events. Tanovic was set to film in 2006 with funding from British Broadcasting Corporation (BBC), which had sent investigators to Pakistan who confirmed that the activities described in the report were still occurring. The BBC withdrew from the project a month before shooting was to begin for fear of legal action, which delayed production for eight years. Ultimately, however, these obstacles were incorporated into the final version of the film as a meta-story in which the filmmakers filmed characters based on themselves trying to convince a potential insurer and lawyer that their project was legally viable even if Nestlé was named. When the legal risks are deemed too acute, the film-within-a-film falls through. This account reveals the extent of Nestlé's influence and extensive efforts to silence its critics, casting doubt on the company's claims of responsible conduct and trustworthiness.

Nestlé has denied the allegations in the report and the events in the film, describing them as 'not at all consistent with our policy and practices on the responsible marketing of breast milk substitutes' (Newbould 2014). However, perhaps having learned from the public relations disaster of the 1979 Swiss libel trial, the company has not initiated legal proceedings against the filmmakers, whose work premiered at the 2014 Toronto International Film Festival.

Capital mobility is another source of structural power for the baby food industry. As Fuchs suggests, corporations need not declare the pos-

sibility of moving investments and jobs for a government to realise that
such actions may be taken in response to unfavourable policy (2005, 776).
Nestlé, however, expressed precisely this possibility to the government of
Zimbabwe in 1998 when it threatened to pull its factories out of the
country if legislation based on the *Code* was enacted. The country's Minister of Health described the move, an economic blackmail of sorts, as an
'idle threat' (Baby Milk Action 1999). Zimbabwe called the company's
bluff by enacting the law, and Nestlé backed down from its threatened
withdrawal (Allain 2005, 81). It is less certain in the current global economic environment, however, that governments of low- and middle-income countries (LMICs) would be prepared to challenge transnational
corporations in this way.

Self-Regulation: Source and Product of Corporate Power

The trend in global governance toward self-regulation and self-moni-
toring is both a source and a product of corporate structural power.
Codes of conduct represent an important source of discursive power that
is used to support the company's political legitimacy, and of instrumental power that can be utilised to counter calls for binding national legislation, thereby increasing its structural power. Critics argue that multinational corporations introduce voluntary codes of conduct when seeking
to stall or pre-empt more stringent and legally binding regulation by
public actors (Vogel 2005, 10; Fuchs 2005, 788) and question whether 'the
very corporations accused and indicted of some of the worst excesses . . .
[can] be—voluntarily—part of a solution' (Pearson and Seyfang 2001, 72).

Certainly, the baby food industry has been lobbying against government regulation and in favour of voluntary codes of conduct since the
1970s when the ICIFI circulated a *Code of Ethics* within two days of the
conclusion of the first hearing of the Nestlé libel trial. The proposed code
was intended to counter negative publicity associated with the trial, and
to demonstrate industry commitment to finding a solution to the problem. ICIFI self-regulation, however, failed to satisfy activist calls for more
stringent regulation of baby food marketing contained in the *Code*, which
the WHA adopted in 1981. Nestlé's own corporate codes of conduct,
most recently its *Policy and Instructions for Implementation of the WHO
International Code of Marketing of Breastmilk Substitutes* (Nestec Ltd. 2010),
are cited as evidence of its responsible and ethical business operations
independent of binding national legislation.

As market leader, Nestlé has spearheaded efforts to prevent formal
regulation either independently, or as part of industry associations such
as the ICIFI and the International Association of Infant Food Manufacturers (IFM).[4] In a leaked memo to Nestlé's CEO Arthur Furer when the
Code was being drafted, the company's vice president, Ernest W.
Saunders, described the need for an effective 'counter-propaganda opera-

tion' against the *Code* as 'urgent' (Ratner 1981). However, still stinging from the libel trial and conscious that trust was important for discursive power, Saunders recommended that because of the 'lack of credibility for any company to overtly sell itself when it has been attacked', the company should promote 'third party rebuttals of the activists' case'. The result was that the ICIFI was at the forefront of industry efforts to counter the *Code*, although Nestlé called the shots from behind the scenes (Ratner 1981). The IFM, described on its website as a 'non-profit organization founded in 1984 to protect and promote infant and young child nutrition around the globe' (International Association of Infant Food Manufacturers 2015), continues to represent industry's interests globally, including at the WHO, the FAO, the Codex Alimentarius Commission, and UNICEF.

Corporate Social Responsibility

Fuchs's (2005, 773) argument that 'acceptance of a growing political role for business in the end depends on the public perception of its legitimacy' has clear relevance to the baby food industry's dependence on positive public perceptions of its responsibility and trustworthiness in relation to its ability to self-regulate. Nestlé has worked to gain public trust through its inclusion in various voluntary initiatives to demonstrate its corporate social responsibility (CSR) credentials such as joining the United Nations Global Compact in 2002, two years after it was launched. Corporations subscribing to the Compact pledge to implement ten principles relating to human rights, labour standards, environmental sustainability and anti-corruption measures. Participation by baby food corporations, however, does not depend upon or reflect their compliance with the *Code*. Critics of Nestlé's inclusion argue that it has provided the company with a new platform from which to establish political legitimacy, and shape norms and ideas in favour of self-regulation, and that it facilitates closer ties with top political officials (Richter 2004).

The FTSE4Good, a series of indices to measure companies' environmental, social and governance practices, represents a similar opportunity. Unlike the Global Compact, however, FTSE4Good *does* consider the marketing practices of baby food companies, albeit with diminishing standards. Baby food manufacturers were initially obliged to demonstrate compliance with the *Code* in order to be included in the FTSE4Good index, but new criteria adopted in 2003 required only that they demonstrate that policies and systems are in place to achieve *Code* compliance eventually (Save the Children 2007). Yet no manufacturers were able to meet even this reduced standard. FTSE4Good revised the criteria again in September 2010, maintaining that it was not able to engage with companies that were excluded from the index, and that it was better to introduce requirements that companies were able to meet and gradually raise the standards over time (FTSE 2011; Makepeace 2011).

In March 2011, Nestlé became the first baby food manufacturer included in the FTSE4Good index (FTSE 2011). This provided the company with opportunity to exercise discursive influence to protect its instrumental and structural power, by suggesting that that their marketing practices complied with the *Code,* and to undermine efforts to hold it accountable. In January 2014, for instance, *The Guardian* quoted Nestlé chairman Peter Brabeck-Letmathé describing the company as

> the only infant formula producer which is part of FTSE4Good. We are being checked and controlled by FTSE4Good. They make their audits in different parts of the world and we have to prove that we are complying with the WHO Code and up to now we can prove that in everything we are. (Confino 2014)

FTSE has written to Nestlé to clarify that their assessment is based on the FTSE4Good criteria and does not reflect compliance with the *Code* and the two should not be conflated (Makepeace 2011). This clarification, however, was not reported in *The Guardian* or other media, leaving readers with the impression that the company is meeting international baby food marketing standards.

Formal Regulation: The Need, the Challenges

Irrespective of corporate or industry voluntary codes of conduct and CSR initiatives, IBFAN maintains that legislation is necessary to regulate baby food marketing and give legal weight to the *Code's* provisions. To this end, it employs its discursive power to discredit the industry's arguments for self-regulation, and its claim to a role in the regulatory process. The *Code* assigns NGOs a watchdog role in Article 11.4 (WHO 1981) and IBFAN seeks to demonstrate that self-regulation is inadequate by monitoring company compliance with the *Code* and publicising violations. The International Code Documentation Centre (ICDC), an IBFAN Specialist Office, serves as the focal point for global monitoring of *Code* compliance. Every three years it coordinates systematic exercises to collect evidence of manufacturer violations in various countries in all regions of the world (IBFAN 2014a), also noting new marketing trends that 'stretch' the *Code,* to demonstrate the need for the enactment and enforcement of formal regulation.

The ICDC provides training for governments on *Code* implementation in national legislation, and on other appropriate measures to protect breastfeeding from corporate influence. Between 1991 and December 2014, the ICDC conducted fifty-seven training courses that were attended by 1,604 government officials from 146 countries. The training course has had positive impacts in seventy-five of those 146 countries (51 percent), with forty-six enacting relevant laws, fifteen enforcing/monitoring laws, eleven drafting laws, and three introducing policies concerning the commercial pressures on breastfeeding (ICDC 2015). Finally, the ICDC also summarises each company's level of compliance with the *Code* (IBFAN 2009), and assesses each country's efforts to implement the *Code* as legislation or other measures (see, for example, IBFAN 2014b).

The industry meanwhile works to influence national infant feeding policy during the drafting process. When a draft law to regulate the marketing of baby food was being developed in Pakistan, for example, the industry presented its feedback directly to the Ministry of Health through meetings and letters in an attempt to pressure the government to weaken the proposed provisions. On 27 November 1997, for example, the chairman of Nestlé Milkpak, the Pakistan subsidiary, wrote to the secretary of health, saying the draft law, if enacted, would be 'impractical and not workable and therefore bereft of any support from either the industry or the paediatric community in the country'. He also referred to the proposed law's 'draconian provisions' and expressed his concern that it was the most extreme such law found anywhere in the world (Ali 1997). The proposed legislation went through at least twelve drafts, as health officials and NGO and industry representatives grappled over its provisions, before it was finally adopted in 2002.

In cases where baby food companies have been charged for violations under national legislation, they have mounted retaliatory challenges to the laws themselves. In India, for example, a gazetted NGO filed a complaint in 1994 against Nestlé under the Infant Milk Substitutes Act of 1992. In response, the company in 1995 challenged several provisions of the act, especially those that allow NGOs to bring cases against corporations, and requirements that labels state that the product is to be used only on the advice of a health professional (Brady and de Oliveira Brady 2004, 25). The case was drawn out over decades, with Nestlé eventually restricting the scope of the petition to challenging specific provisions under which the complaint had been filed and the company had been formally charged in 2012. The High Court of Delhi in 2013 agreed with Nestlé that it could not have been expected during the period between enactment of the law and the NGO's complaint to comply with these provisions due to their inconsistencies with another law, which were removed only in 1997 (High Court of Delhi 2013).

In the Philippines in 2006, baby food manufacturers challenged the constitutionality of revised rules for implementing the 1986 Milk Code. In this case, the U.S. Chamber of Commerce also intervened, writing a 'scathing letter' to the country's president that argued that new rules would put 'at risk' the country's 'reputation as a stable and viable destination for investment' which, they continued, 'we know you would want to avoid such a situation occurring'. The government was requested to 're-examine' the regulation and offered its help in drafting new rules for the industry (Jimenez 2007). In October 2007, the Supreme Court lifted its restraining order on implementation of the new rules, and upheld nearly all provisions of the Milk Code and rules (Supreme Court of the Philippines 2007). In both these cases, and in others, IBFAN's NGO membership has been able to support governments with evidence that legislation is necessary, and an appropriate governance response. These challenges to national efforts to regulate the industry reveal the importance of non-legislative measures by NGOs to complement formal regulation.

Norms Surrounding Infant Feeding and Baby Food Regulation

As key actors in governance of the industry, IBFAN and baby food manufacturers are able to use their discursive power to shape norms and values, but must do so within existing norms and ideologies. Keck and Sikkink (1998) note the importance of framing issues to resonate with existing belief systems:

> Both [Nestlé] and the Boycott tried to capitalise on the transcultural desire to do the best thing for one's baby. The baby food companies tried to convince mothers that infant formula was a modern healthy way to feed their babies, but the baby food network mobilised information and testimony strategically to convert the bottle from a symbol of modernity and health into a potentially dangerous threat to infant health in the third world (205).

Fuchs maintains that 'the dominance of certain norms and ideas is at once the product of and grounds for business's discursive power' (2005, 794). The baby food industry uses this power to frame the negative impacts of formula promotion as a problem that affects only LIMCs and therefore not warranting *Code* compliance or formal restrictions on product promotion in high income countries. Nestlé, for example, creates a false distinction between 'lower-risk countries' and 'higher-risk countries' based on levels of mortality, morbidity and acute malnutrition among children under five years of age, and says it 'adheres to the WHO Code as a minimum requirement in [developing] countries' (Nestec Ltd. 2010). The *Code*, and subsequent WHA resolutions, however, apply equally to *all* countries, and make no distinction based on national income. Manufacturers continue to violate the *Code*, even in LMICs, where they claim to abide by it, often by at once relying on and reinforcing popular ideas about infant feeding. Product promotion emphasises mothers' rights to choose how to feed their babies, but simultaneously undermines their ability to make fully informed decisions. The industry seeks to position its product as a close replica of mother's milk, claiming in some cases that it is 'closer than ever to mother's milk', 'inspired by mother's milk' or 'patterned after breastmilk' (IBFAN 2014a). Product labels prescribe their use 'when breastfeeding is not possible', creating the impression that breastfeeding is difficult to the point of being impossible. Companies stress that baby milks fill a legitimate need; however, the extent of the 'need' has been, at least in part, manufactured by misleading information and unethical marketing practices.

The challenge for IBFAN is to establish that breastfeeding is valuable and worth protecting against corporate pressures—by using its discursive power to re-establish breastfeeding as a norm that is widely supported by society. It must confront the discursive power of the baby food industry, which attempts to frame infant feeding as a matter of personal choice while creating the impression that many women are unable to breastfeed their babies, and promoting their products as a safe and healthy breastmilk substitute. IBFAN and other civil society organisations do this by highlighting the many health benefits of breastfeeding for babies and mothers, and the number of babies whose lives could be saved and illnesses that could be prevented if they were breastfed.

CONCLUSION

This analysis of civil society efforts to hold corporations to account with respect to the marketing of breastmilk substitutes demonstrates that different types of power are accessible to civil society in order to influence health policy at the global and national levels. Although the baby food industry seemingly has a greater ability to accumulate and exercise power, especially because of its financial resources, IBFAN and its member organisations have been able to use their own discursive and institutional power to create greater public awareness and regulatory measures to effectively challenge the impact of Nestlé and other baby food manufacturers.

Fuchs (2005, 795) argues that, although the political power of corporations and industries has increased with growing globalisation, this same power and the ability to exercise it face limits and challenges. In part, this is the result of corporate power becoming increasingly discursive in nature, making it more vulnerable to bad publicity such as that surrounding the Nestlé libel trial and the Nestlé Boycott campaign. It is also vulnerable to other non-state actors such as NGOs and advocacy networks like IBFAN that use discursive power to hold corporations accountable, shape public values and draw attention to key issues.

The analysis in this chapter argues that voluntary self-regulation initiatives like company codes of conduct, the UN Global Compact and FTSE4Good are not a sufficient means of holding corporations accountable with respect to public health. Rather, the state remains an important actor in terms of introducing enforceable mechanisms such as national legislation that protects the public's well-being. Despite their relatively limited financial resources, NGOs and networks like IBFAN provide evidence that formal regulation is necessary. In the absence of, and complementary to, national legislation, they are able to use their discursive power to keep corporations in check and hold them to account with respect to public health.

NOTES

1. WHO recommends initiation of breastfeeding within one hour after birth, exclusive breastfeeding (no other food or drink) for six months, followed by continued breastfeeding along with complementary foods for another eighteen months or longer (WHO 2015).
2. International Organization of Consumers Unions (IOCU) (now called Consumers International), Interfaith Center on Corporate Responsibility (ICCR), Infant Formula Action Coalition (INFACT), OXFAM, War on Want, Déclaration de Berne.
3. Initial members were Cow & Gate, Dumex, Meiji, Morinaga, Nestlé, Snow Brand, Wakado and Wyeth.
4. Currently comprised of Abbott, Danone Nutricia, Fonterra, Friesland Campina, Mead Johnson Nutrition and Perrigo.

REFERENCES

Ali, Syed Yawar. 1997. Letter to secretary of health, Pakistan. 27 November.
Allain, Annelies. 2005. *Fighting an Old Battle in a New World: How IBFAN Monitors the Baby Food Market*. Development Dialogue Offprint. Uppsala, Sweden: Dag Hammarskjöld Foundation.
Baby Milk Action. 1999. Boycott News. Issue 26, December. http://archive.baby milkaction.org/boycott/boyct26.html#2.
Baby Milk Action. 2000. 'Nestlé Under Investigation by Pakistan Anti-Corruption Body in Raza Case'. Press Release, 28 March.
Black, Robert E., Cesar G. Victora, Susan P. Walker et al. 2013. 'Maternal and Child Undernutrition and Overweight in Low-Income and Middle-Income Countries'. *Lancet* 382: 427–51.
Brady, Mike, and Sonia de Oliveira Brady, eds. 2004. *Using International Tools to Stop Corporate Malpractice—Does It Work? Checks and Balances in the Global Economy*. Cambridge: Baby Milk Action.
Chetley, Andrew. 1986. *The Politics of Baby Foods: Successful Challenges to an International Marketing Strategy*. New York: St. Martin's Press.
Confino, Jo. 2014. 'Nestlé Chairman Warns against Playing God over Climate Change'. *The Guardian*, 31 January. www.theguardian.com/sustainable-business/blog/nestle-chairman-climate-change-controversy-peter-brabeck.
FTSE. 2011. *A Note on the New FTSE4Good Breast Milk Substitute (BMS) Marketing Criteria and Its Impact on the FTSE4Good March 2011 Review*. 11 March. www.ftse.com/products/downloads/FTSE4Good_Web_Update_March_2011.pdf.
Fuchs, Doris. 2005. 'The Commanding Heights? The Strength and Fragility of Business Power in World Politics'. *Millennium* 33 (3): 771–802.
Geach, Hugh. 1973. 'The Baby Food Tragedy'. *New Internationalist*. August.
High Court of Delhi. 2013. *Nestlé India Limited & ANR vs Union of India and ORS*. High Court of Delhi decision. 31 May. http://lobis.nic.in/ddir/dhc/SID/judgement/06-06-2013/SID31052013CW48321995.pdf.
IBFAN. 2009. *State of the Code by Company 2009*. Penang, Malaysia: International Baby Food Action Network-International Code Documentation Centre.
———. 2014a. *Breaking the Rules 2014: BTR in Brief*. Penang, Malaysia: International Baby Food Action Network-International Code Documentation Centre.
———. 2014b. *State of the Code by Country 2014*. Penang, Malaysia: International Baby Food Action Network-International Code Documentation Centre.

———. 2015. *About IBFAN*. http://ibfan.org/about-ibfan.

ICDC. 2015. *Educating Government Officials to Stop the Promotion of Breastmilk Substitutes*. www.ibfan-icdc.org/index.php/results.

International Association of Infant Food Manufacturers. 2015. *International Association of Infant Food Manufacturers*. www.ifm.net.

Jelliffe, D. B. 1971. 'Commerciogenic Malnutrition?' *Food Technology* 25: 153–54.

Jimenez, Cher S. 2007. 'Spilled Corporate Milk in the Philippines'. *Asia Times Online*, 25 July. www.atimes.com/atimes/Southeast_Asia/IG25Ae01.html.

Keck, Margaret E., and Kathryn Sikkink. 1998. *Activists Without Borders: Advocacy Networks in International Politics*. Ithaca, NY: Cornell University Press.

Makepeace, Mark. 2011. 'Letter to IBFAN'. 17 June. www.ftse.com/products/downloads/Letter_to_IBFAN.pdf.

Muller, Mike. 1974. *The Baby Killer*. London: War on Want, March.

Nestec Ltd. 2010. *Nestlé Policy and Instructions for Implementation of the WHO International Code of Marketing of Breastmilk Substitutes*. Vevey, Switzerland: Nestec Ltd.

Newbould, Chris. 2014. 'Danis Tanovic's Tigers Offers Thought-Provoking Look into Pakistani Food Companies'. *The National*, 21 December. www.thenational.ae/arts-lifestyle/dubai-international-film-festival/danis-tanovics-tigers-offers-thought-provoking-look-into-pakistani-food-companies.

Pearson, Ruth, and Gill Seyfang. 2001. 'New Hope or False Dawn? Voluntary Codes of Conduct, Labour Regulation and Social Policy in a Globalizing World'. *Global Social Policy* 1 (1): 49–78.

Ratner, Jonathan. 1981. 'Influence Peddling, Nestlé Style'. *Multinational Monitor* 2 (2).

Richter, Judith. 2004. *Building on Quicksand: The Global Compact, Democratic Governance and Nestlé*. 2nd ed. Geneva: CETIM, IBFAN/GIFA, Berne Declaration.

Save the Children. 2007. *A Generation On: Baby Milk Marketing Still Putting Children's Lives at Risk*. London: Save the Children.

Sokol, Ellen. 2005. *The International Code Handbook: A Guide to Implementing the International Code of Marketing of Breastmilk Substitutes*, 2nd ed. Penang, Malaysia: IBFAN-ICDC.

Supreme Court of the Philippines. 2007. *Pharmaceutical and Health Care Association of the Philippines vs. Health Secretary Franciso Duque III*. Supreme Court decision, 9 October. http://sc.judiciary.gov.ph/jurisprudence/2007/october2007/173034.htm.

The Network (Association for Rational Use of Medication in Pakistan). 1999. *Milking Profits: How Nestlé Puts Sales Ahead of Infant Health*. Islamabad: The Network.

UNICEF. 2010. *Facts of Life*, 4th ed. New York: United Nations Children's Fund.

Vogel, David. 2005. *The Market for Virtue: The Potential and Limits of Corporate Social Responsibility*. Cambridge: Harvard University Press.

WHO. 1979. *Joint WHO/UNICEF Meeting on Infant and Young Child Feeding: Statement and Recommendations*. Geneva: World Health Organisation.

———. 1981. *International Code of Marketing of Breast-milk Substitutes*. Geneva: World Health Organization.

———. 2015. 'Infant and Young Child Feeding (Fact Sheet N°342)'. www.who.int/mediacentre/factsheets/fs342/en.

FIFTEEN

Epidemiology in the Struggle over Contamination of the Ecuadorian Amazon

Communities, Controversy and Chevron

Ben Brisbois

Recent decades have seen increasing conflict between local communities and extractive industry[1] around the world, often involving Indigenous and other marginalised groups (People's Health Movement, Global Equity Gauge Alliance and MedAct 2015). Health researchers can become involved in conflicts when communities seek to demonstrate the effects of resource extraction on their health, often in connection with court cases or government decisions. Such partnerships between communities and health researchers represent one potential avenue for holding extractive sector corporations to account for the effects of their actions. Some potential risks of this strategy, however, are suggested by internal tensions within the discipline of epidemiology, a central science in public health. These tensions involve the appropriate balance between scientific 'objectivity' and 'advocacy' for real-world improvements in population health (Krieger 1999; Savitz, Poole and Miller 1999; Brisbois 2014). This chapter explores the controversy that arose after researchers from the London School of Hygiene and Tropical Medicine (LSHTM) carried out an environmental epidemiology study in support of the legal battle of Ecuadorian Amazonian communities against Texaco (now Chevron)—a legal battle that would eventually see an Ecuadorian court order Chevron to pay over USD 19 billion in damages in 2011, subsequently reduced on appeal to approximately $9 billion (Kimerling 2013).

At the centre of this controversy were questions about the role of public health science as it relates to the public good and corporate power. In describing such 'epidemiology wars', Shim and Thomson (2010) point out that related methodological debates typically correspond to differing visions of the social role of epidemiology: as a source of objective information to feed into more or less functional public health policy processes, or as a resource in struggles to improve the health of groups marginalised by existing social structures. Partnerships between epidemiologists and communities challenging the extractive sector would appear to fall squarely within a more politically engaged vision of public health, raising the prospect that the resulting research will be viewed by disciplinary peers as 'biased' or 'unscientific'.

In addition to such disagreements within the discipline, more profound challenges relate to the process of confronting corporations through legal processes in inequitable state structures. Foucault (1980, 1) has argued that the form and functioning of a typical court embodies and reinforces the discursive underpinnings of hierarchical nation-states. Indigenous communities and other groups can be further marginalized by inequitable state structures when challenging extractive sector activities. Foucault further argues that biomedical ways of knowing, such as epidemiologic surveillance, similarly perform disciplining functions on unruly bodies in the service of (unfair) social orders (166). Thus, marginalised communities seeking justice by using epidemiology studies to support legal action may find themselves disciplined twice over, by both the public health *and* judicial arms of state power.

At the very least, these potential obstacles suggest a need to understand how such partnerships generate or fail to generate influential scientific evidence, and challenge or subtly reinforce inequitable social structures. In response, this chapter examines epidemiologic writing in connection with the Ecuador Chevron lawsuit. Focusing on the epidemiologic studies featured in the lawsuit and the controversy they sparked among public health scientists provides a window into the internal social dynamics of the discipline of epidemiology vis-à-vis communities and corporate actors. This chapter examines these studies using discourse analysis, informed by scholarship on social studies of science, and provides an illustrative case study to inform future collaborations between health researchers and communities in the face of extractive sector activity.

BACKGROUND

Oil and Health (Research) in the Ecuadorian Amazon

In 1967, a consortium of foreign companies struck oil in Ecuador's Oriente region, which lies within the Amazon watershed and is known for its biological and cultural diversity (Rochlin 2011). A wholly owned subsidiary of Texaco then carried out exploration and extraction until Ecuador's state-run petroleum company took over operations in 1990. Over this period, the Oriente's physical and social geographies were profoundly transformed by a combination of oil extraction and land reform encouraging occupation by highland and Pacific-coast Ecuadorian migrants (*colonos*) of so-called 'empty' lands in the Oriente—notwithstanding the pre-existing presence in the region of numerous Indigenous groups (Larrea 2006).

In 1993, an Ecuadorian-born lawyer launched a class-action lawsuit in New York on behalf of a somewhat-unlikely coalition of *colono* and Indigenous plaintiffs, brought together in their shared experience of Texaco's decades of oil extraction (Sawyer 2002). A key contention in the lawsuit was that Texaco failed to meet industry-standard environmental practices in its Ecuadorian operations, resulting in decades of massive releases of oil and other contaminants into the Amazonian environment— and into its human and non-human inhabitants. Chevron (with which Texaco merged in 2001[2]) successfully fought to have the New York lawsuit dismissed in 2002 on the grounds that it was essentially an Ecuadorian matter, and another lawsuit opened in Lago Agrio, Ecuador, in 2003.

Prominent claims presented by plaintiffs in the lawsuits, both in New York and in Lago Agrio, drew on epidemiologic studies published in international public health journals (Loue 2013; Rochlin 2011). These papers originated in a partnership between the Frente para la Defensa de Amazonia (FDA: Front for the Defence of Amazonia)—an Oriente organization formed in response to the lawsuit—and a local community health institute (San Sebastián and Hurtig 2005). A Spanish (Basque) physician named Miguel San Sebastián had been working in the Oriente since 1990, and subsequently carried out a community-based study of the health impacts of petroleum extraction in the region, thereby earning a PhD at the LSHTM (San Sebastián 2001).

San Sebastián's study was framed as a developing-country application of 'popular epidemiology' (San Sebastián and Hurtig 2005), a term that describes situations in which community concerns—parental concern over childhood leukaemia cases, for example—motivate partnerships with epidemiologists in opposition to industry, often involving legal action (Brown 1987). As is commonly the case in popular epidemiology projects, the Ecuadorian study had a shoestring budget and involved community members as research assistants, while attempting to maintain epidemiologic rigour (San Sebastián and Hurtig 2005). Articles based on the research included one paper that reported increased cancer incidence in a community situated close to oil fields (San Sebastián et al. 2001), and cross-sectional analyses that found increased levels of skin infections, and nasal and throat irritation (San Sebastián, Armstrong and Stephens 2001), and increased odds of spontaneous abortion (San Sebastián, Armstrong and Stephens 2002) in communities located close to oil fields.

While courtroom debates have revolved around the validity of the Ecuadorian petroleum health studies (Loue 2013), parallel debates took place in the pages of public health journals. In 2002, a cancer-focused analysis based on data from Ecuador's national cancer registry (Hurtig and San Sebastián 2002) was published in the *International Journal of Epidemiology* (*IJE*). Its lead author, another LSHTM graduate named Anna-Karin Hurtig, would subsequently help San Sebastián to document the Oriente popular epidemiology process (San Sebastián and Hurtig 2005). While the cancer analysis did not employ data collected through this popular epidemiology study, the cancer study similarly showed increased health impacts in communities located close to oilfields. As described below, this study triggered a debate in the pages of the *IJE* that involved epidemiologists from around the world, bringing to the fore prominent questions about the tension between 'objectivity' and 'advocacy' in epidemiology. A related debate occurred in the pages of the *International Journal of Occupational and Environmental Health* (*IJOEH*) after Chevron held a press conference on 2 February 2005 to present reports it had commissioned from well-known epidemiologists. These reports cast doubt on the validity of research showing health effects of Texaco's activities, including Hurtig and San Sebastián's cancer study. Shortly after the press conference, Chevron ran full-page ads in major Ecuadorian newspapers featuring quotes from the consultant reports. In response, an open letter with sixty-one signatories from around the world, mostly researchers with public health and medical institutional affiliations, took issue with the conduct of 'Texaco and its consultants' (Breilh et al. 2005, 217). Briefly, the letter encouraged their 'colleagues' (i.e., the consultants in question) not to submit critiques of published studies to 'industries that may be assumed to have vested interests in gainsaying inconvenient scientific evidence, such as Texaco's apparent interest in protecting itself by undermining the Amazonian people's quest for environmental justice' (218). Subsequent letters and commentaries in the *IJOEH* explored many of the same themes as the *IJE* debate. Together, these exchanges illustrate epidemiology's fault lines as they relate to community-involved studies on resource extraction.

METHODS

This controversy was examined using discourse analysis of peer-reviewed articles, drawing on observations from 'science studies' scholarship, a broad, interdisciplinary field that seeks to understand the social dynamics of scientific knowledge production. A key premise of science studies scholarship is that science is not a simple depiction of nature and its properties, but rather reflects the institutions, relationships and power dynamics involved in scientific research (Jasanoff 2001; Latour 1987). Much science studies research therefore seeks to understand how scientific knowledge is 'socially constructed', especially within social groupings such as academic disciplines.

Ethnographic studies of how scientists work have demonstrated the intimate relationship between the social dynamics of science and the production of journal articles and other texts (Atkinson 1999; Latour 1987; Callon, Law and Rip 1986; Myers 1990). This has led to substantial work in science studies relying upon *discourse analysis* of scientific writing (Ashmore, Myers and Potter 1995). Discourse analysis relates writing to accompanying social processes, analysing features of texts such as genre conventions, word choices, portrayals of people and places, and linkages to prior texts (Johnstone 2007). It also seeks to identify the explicit and implicit assumptions underlying texts, which can express and naturalize power relations (Fairclough 2003).

The first stage of analysis identified scientific journal articles dealing with the health effects of oil development in the Ecuadorian Amazon, using searches in Medline, Web of Science and Google Scholar with combinations of the following keywords: *oil, petroleum, Amazon, Ecuador, epidemiology, health, cancer, dermatologic, reproductive* and *death*. The resulting eighteen inclusions were read in depth with special attention to disciplinary identity in epidemiology, based on the observation that patterns of evaluation (expressions of approval or disapproval) and other 'metadiscourse' (authorial presence in the text) in scientific writing reflect shared disciplinary assumptions (Hyland 1998; Hunston 1993).

Analysis of these articles made it clear that the contentious exchanges in the *IJE* and *IJOEH* merited in-depth examination. Studies of scientific controversies show them to vividly illustrate disciplinary norms as scientists argue over what those norms are and how they should be interpreted (Pinch 1990). In particular, controversies often involve significant 'boundary work', or rhetorical manoeuvres by which scientists within a given discipline attempt to exclude outsiders or rivals and shore up the discipline's core subject matter, methods and standards for evaluating good research (Gieryn 1983). The analysis therefore narrowed to a total of eleven texts: one epidemiology research report, three related commentaries, and three related letters to the editor in the *IJE*; and one open letter and three responses to it in the *IJOEH*. The following section discusses the results of this analysis using specific passages to illustrate the social dynamics of this controversy. All emphasis (i.e., italics) in these passages has been added to illustrate specific discursive points.

DISCUSSION

IJE: Angels, People and 'Epidemiology versus Epidemiology'

As previously mentioned, the paper that began the exchange in the *IJE* is a study of cancer incidence in communities located close to, and farther from, oil extraction activities (Hurtig and San Sebastián 2002). Aside from an introduction that describes a history of oil extraction and related pollution in the Oriente, there is little in the body of the paper belying Hurtig and San Sebastián's 'popular' objectives: it employs conventional scientific passive voice ('Incidence rates for overall and specific sites *were calculated*', 1023), for example, and follows epidemiologic conventions for reporting relative risks and confidence intervals. Previous discourse analysis of the genre of the epidemiology journal article, however, has identified its final paragraph as one of its few sites allowing expression of individuality in the form of policy recommendations (Skelton and Edwards 2000; Brisbois 2014). Hurtig and San Sebastián (2002, 1025) take advantage of this space in a way that appears consistent with their self-defined role as popular epidemiologists:

> Further research is necessary to determine if the observed associations do reflect an underlying causal relationship. . . . Meanwhile, an environmental monitoring system to assess, control and assist in elimination of sources of pollution in the area, and a surveillance system to gain knowledge of the evolution of cancer incidence and distribution in the area, *are urgently recommended*.

As an accompanying commentary by one of the paper's anonymous reviewers explains (Siemiatycki 2002), this policy recommendation responding to past injustices (as described in the paper's introduction) fits squarely in the more socially engaged vision of epidemiology to which popular epidemiology belongs. Siemiatycki (2002, 1028) outlines the limitations of Hurtig and San Sebastián's analysis before concluding that their final recommendation 'does not flow as a consequence of this study'. He specifically invokes the tension between 'scientific' and 'activist' visions of public health and characterizes Hurtig and San Sebastián's concluding paragraph as an illustration of the perils of the latter: 'Epidemiological research is sometimes used as a cover of scientific legitimacy in calling for sensible public health precautions. While this definitely puts epidemiologists "on the side of the angels", it also *risks compromising the scientific credibility of epidemiology*' (Siemiatycki 2002, 1028).

This attempt to preserve the scientific integrity of epidemiology is consistent with classic definitions of boundary work as attempts by scientists to set limits on what is considered legitimate work within their disciplines. Its 'helpful' tone is also a common boundary work rhetorical strategy emphasizing the expertise of disciplinary insiders (Gieryn 1983), as in another passage from Siemiatycki's (2002, 1029) commentary:

> In assessing methodological quality, *we must make allowances* for the resources and local conditions in which the investigators find themselves. . . . The study by Hurtig and San Sebastián represents a *bold* attempt to use imperfect data to derive scientific knowledge; it is *useful* in highlighting the issue and drawing attention to the limitations of the data. But it does not provide *strong* evidence in favour of the hypothesis. *Nevertheless*, given the complexity of disease aetiology, and the need to discover both universal and local facets of disease aetiology, *we should* encourage the conduct of research such as this.

The use of first-person voice (*we*) suggests that Siemiatycki considers himself to be addressing fellow epidemiologists, while the pattern of usage of modals (*must/should*), evaluative language (*bold/strong*) and other metadiscourse (*nevertheless*) suggests that he feels himself to be speaking to shared disciplinary assumptions in epidemiology. Hurtig and San Sebastián's (2003) provocatively titled reply to the editor, 'Epidemiology on the Side of the Angels . . . or the People?', disputes Siemiatycki's conclusions on the appropriateness of their recommendations. His response in a subsequent letter is less diplomatic. He states that 'the strength of evidence in their study was *weak*' (Siemiatycki 2003, 659), but allows that it 'raises important questions' concerning etiological reasoning in epidemiology, especially in resource-poor settings such as the Ecuadorian Amazon. In giving this as the reason why he 'recommended the publication of this report', (659) Siemiatycki characterizes the study as essentially unworthy of publication except as a useful conversation starter. He also, intentionally or otherwise, affirms his own intellectual authority over Hurtig and San Sebastián as the expert whose discretion allowed publication of their article. Such rhetorical strategies are recognizable as boundary work, additionally applying familiar recognizable 'epidemiology wars' arguments to Hurtig and San Sebastián's alliance with marginalised communities facing Chevron.

IJOEH: Texaco, Its Consultants, and 'Elevating the Level of Scientific Discourse'

Beginning with Breilh et al.'s (2005) letter, another illustrative exchange over oil and health in the Ecuadorian Amazon took place in the *IJOEH*. Hurtig, San Sebastián and Siemiatycki would not be involved this time, but themes from their *IJE* exchange over Hurtig and San Sebastián's cancer study figure prominently. Like Siemiatycki, Breilh et al. position themselves as defending 'scientific integrity', but their critique is targeted at six consultants 'retained by Texaco' (217) to critically appraise studies showing health impacts of Texaco's activities. This letter clearly indicates that the consultants belong to Texaco (they are 'its consultants'), and that this belonging, rather than any incautious recommendations made by Hurtig and San Sebastián, represents the real threat to science. The letter does devote two paragraphs to discussing the relationship between epidemiology, the settings in which it takes place, and public health policy recommendations based on preliminary or incomplete evidence. It reframes the issues raised by Siemiatycki, however, by asserting that 'the onus cannot be put on scientists to ensure that data are available to evaluate adverse health effects' (217). The signatories recommend instead that 'a company extracting minerals or biological raw materials [be required to] accept responsibility, as good corporate citizens, for determining what protective measures it would be prudent to impose, and to monitor its success in controlling potential adverse human health and environmental effects' (217).

In response to Breilh et al.'s call for scientists to be cautious when consulting for industry, a *very* epidemiologically interesting reply from two of the consultants in question presents them as 'elevating the level of scientific discourse' (Rothman and Arellano 2005, 327). Kenneth Rothman is a well-known epidemiologist whose epidemiology textbook is widely used in graduate public health programs. While it is obvious why Chevron would want a scientist of his stature to question links between their activities and health outcomes, it is not obvious why he would take time away from his prolific research activities to carry out critical appraisal—a basic skill taught in introductory epidemiology classes. Rothman's (1998) published criticisms of the tendency of epidemiologists to make public health recommendations in their articles and his insistence that epidemiology can (and should) take place free of social influences (Rothman, Adami and Trichopoulos 1998), however, suggest that the *IJE* debate would have presented him an inviting target.

Rothman and Arellano (2005, 327) state that Breilh et al.'s letter 'suggests that reviewing a scientific study is itself a sociopolitical statement', indicating that these authors believe it is *not*. Consistent with this view that epidemiologic methods can be applied in a social vacuum, the reply carefully avoids important social dimensions of the Chevron-Amazon affair. In contrast to, or perhaps in intentional avoidance of, Breilh et al.'s reference to environmental justice, they suggest common ground with the sixty-one signatories in that they 'support fully the preservation of the Amazon forests', but see this as unrelated to the results of the epidemiology study in question (327). Portraying Breilh et al. as being motivated by environmental concern could conceivably represent boundary work, analogous to attempts by nineteenth-century scientists to characterize their rivals as hysterical or motivated by religion (Gieryn 1983).

More obviously, however, framing the dispute as one over environmental conservation of a forest, and not as an environmental justice issue involving marginalised communities and large transnational corporate actors, allows Rothman and Arellano to steer clear of any messy 'sociopolitical' discussion that might cast doubt on the position that they are blameless in carrying out consulting work for Chevron:

> Breilh et al. contend that Chevron-Texaco should not be allowed to request an expert evaluation of scientific work that bears on a dispute to which it is a party. They also imply that it is inappropriate to review scientific studies for corporations embroiled in legal concerns. Apparently, in their view, *one side in a dispute* can obtain advice but the other side may not. (Rothman and Arellano 2005, 328)

Portraying Chevron as simply 'one side in a dispute' is an extraordinary statement that essentially puts a coalition of Amazonian peasants and Indigenous peoples on equal footing with one of the world's largest transnational corporations, ignoring the enormous imbalance in power. Sawyer (2001) has documented Chevron's complicated status as a corporate 'person' attempting to disavow its connection to its Ecuadorian subsidiary. Sawyer (2002) also describes the complex process by which some Indigenous and *colono* plaintiffs forged a common 'class' to pursue the initial lawsuit against Texaco. These complexities, not to mention the 'history of environmental pollution and human rights violations' in the Oriente described by Hurtig and San Sebastián (2005, 1172), are conspicuously absent from Rothman and Arellano's simplistic characterization of the situation.

The neat dismissal of the dispute as being about preservation of the Amazon rainforest therefore allows Rothman and Arellano to remain confident that it is unproblematic for epidemiologists to carry out work for industries in conflict with marginalised communities. When the issue is one of 'environmental justice' (Breilh et al. 2005, 218), in contrast, the appropriate response of epidemiologists appears very different. The linkage of Rothman and Arellano's espousal of supposedly neutral 'objectivity' with ahistorical contextual descriptions is consistent with work showing the intimate relationship between the framing of health problems and the ways in which epidemiologists respond to them (Brisbois 2014). Viewed in this light, the obstacles faced by communities facing the extractive sector, and health researchers allied with them, include persistent ways of thinking in the discipline of epidemiology as expressed and reinforced by discursive strategies such as those documented in the *IJE* and *IJOEH* exchanges.

CONCLUSION

The multi-billion-dollar decision against Chevron suggests that the Oriente popular epidemiology study may have achieved its goal of supporting the FDA's struggle. This decision remains in place at the time of writing, even after Chevron commissioned a re-analysis of Hurtig and San Sebastián's data (Arana and Arellano 2007) and two additional studies on cancer in the Oriente (Kelsh, Morimoto and Lau 2009; Moolgavkar et al. 2014). Recent developments include a (disputed) finding by a New York court of fraud against the plaintiffs' lawyers, blocking seizure of Chevron's assets in the United States, and the commencement of lawsuits in Canada and Brazil attempting to seize Chevron's assets in those countries, after Chevron removed its assets from Ecuador (Kimerling 2013). The likelihood that the plaintiffs will ever collect on the settlement is unclear, however, and Chevron has vowed to continue fighting the decision indefinitely, financed with its essentially unlimited resources.

If one were to state, echoing Foucault, that the reproduction of inequities is in some way 'built in' to modern courts and public health institutions, the Amazon-Chevron affair might therefore provide some corroboration. While the letter responding to Texaco's consultants (Breilh et al. 2005) suggests a homogenous 'Amazonian people', San Sebastián and Hurtig (2005) raise the possibility that lawsuit participants such as the Front for the Defence of Amazonia might have interests different than those of 'the community' (804)—but provide no substantiation of this point from their own experience in the Oriente. A U.S. lawyer who conducted a study that informed the initial lawsuit observes that the plaintiffs' legal team and NGO supporters opportunistically misrepresented the lawsuit as being primarily about Indigenous concerns in their public relations efforts (Kimerling 2013). Consistent with this apparent strategic appropriation of Indigenous suffering, the plaintiffs' lawyers successfully named FDA as the sole administrator of funds in the settlement. While overcoming historical animosities between certain Indigenous and *colono* groups in the lawsuit was somewhat unexpected (Sawyer 2002), Kimerling (2005) also documents resistance to meaningful engagement by FDA with some of the Indigenous groups most affected by oil-related health and social effects. As Kimerling (2008, 270) states, 'It remains to be seen whether a victory in court, or settlement through plaintiffs' counsel, will obtain meaningful remedies for affected populations and the environment, or simply empower and enrich a new layer of elites, and set back grassroots struggles for corporate accountability and environmental justice by promoting conflict, corruption and cynicism'.

Rather than adopting a romantic view of 'communities' as homogenous, therefore, health researchers attempting to support grassroots struggles against extractive industry should be attentive to internal power dynamics within those struggles. The controversy documented in this chapter also illustrates several additional obstacles communities and health researchers may encounter when working together to hold corporations to account. Practical, logistical issues such as a scarcity of resources and data to do proper epidemiology are compounded by resistance based on long-standing fault lines in public health. The initial study on health effects of Chevron's activities was explicitly framed as a challenge to conventions in epidemiology, while subsequent debates employed recognizable arguments from objectivity/advocacy tensions in the discipline. The rhetorical 'boundary work' strategies used to make these arguments by established epidemiologists simultaneously erased residents of the Oriente from the debate, and damaged the reputations of those researchers working with them.[3]

While Chevron's ability to hire world-renowned epidemiologists is the most obvious manifestation of corporate power in this debate, these disciplinary dynamics indicate that it is not the full story. The participation of Kenneth Rothman is particularly suggestive in that his subsequent defence of his actions resonates strongly with disciplinary debates he had previously engaged in. Indeed, the exchange between Siemiatycki and Hurtig and San Sebastián appears to have created a perfect (paid) opportunity for Rothman to denounce trends in epidemiology he had been decrying for years. The fate of the people living with toxic contamination in the Oriente appears to have been secondary to—or conveniently overlooked in—Rothman's desire to 'elevate the level of scientific discourse'. The interaction of corporate funding with disciplinary identity therefore appears to be an important topic for further study, as well as a factor to consider in community-university partnerships dealing with extractive sector impacts on health.

Finally, in an episode featuring an extractive-sector multinational, the issue of 'extraction' by outsiders is also important for global health researchers to consider. A growing body of scholarship points to the problematic dependency of global health research (and the careers it helps to build) on the existence of huge North-South inequities (Crane 2013; Janes and Corbett 2009). It is worth noting that the vast majority of participants in the controversy described in this chapter were linked to academic institutions in the global North, with a handful also listing institutional affiliations in Quito and other metropolitan centres in Latin America. San Sebastián and Hurtig, researchers with long-term commitments to the Oriente, nevertheless moved on to academic positions in Sweden. Even critical social science scholarship on the Chevron lawsuit (including the present chapter) advances the careers of Northern researchers, with unclear benefits for peasant and Indigenous residents of the Oriente. This suggests that efforts by public health researchers to partner with communities facing the extractive sector, in addition to taking strategic guidance from case studies such as this chapter, should not stop at challenging specific corporations. Reflexive examination of the power structures creating both environmental injustices, and health researchers seeking to address such injustices, is a challenging but necessary long-term goal.

NOTES

1. For the purposes of this chapter, *extractive industry* refers to companies engaged in removal of materials from the earth's crust, such as oil and gas or mining companies.
2. After the merger, the new company was known as ChevronTexaco until 2008, when it removed Texaco from its name and became simply Chevron.
3. Thanks to Nora Kenworthy for this observation.

REFERENCES

Arana, Alejandro, and Felix Arellano. 2007. 'Cancer Incidence Near Oilfields in the Amazon Basin of Ecuador Revisited'. *Occupational and Environmental Medicine* 64 (7): 490.

Ashmore, M., G. Myers and J. Potter. 1995. 'Discourse, Rhetoric and Reflexivity: Seven Days in the Library'. In *Handbook of Science and Technology Studies*, edited by S. Jasanoff, G. Markle, T. Pinch and J. Petersen, 321–42. London: Sage.

Atkinson, D. 1999. *Scientific Discourse in Sociohistorical Context: The Philosophical Transactions of the Royal Society of London, 1675-1975*. Mahwah, NJ: Lawrence Erlbaum Associates.

Breilh, J., J. C. Branco, B. I. Castleman, M. Cherniack, D. C. Christiani, A. Cicolella, E. Cifuentes et al. 2005. 'Texaco and Its Consultants'. *International Journal of Occupational and Environmental Health* 11 (2): 217–20.

Brisbois, Ben W. 2014. 'Epidemiology and "Developing Countries": Writing Pesticides, Poverty and Political Engagement in Latin America'. *Social Studies of Science* 44 (4): 600–24. doi:10.1177/0306312714523514.

Brown, P. 1987. 'Popular Epidemiology—Community Response to Toxic-Waste Induced Disease in Woburn, Massachusetts'. *Science Technology & Human Values* 12 (3–4): 78–85.

Callon, Michel, John Law and Arie Rip. 1986. 'How to Study the Force of Science'. In *Mapping the Dynamics of Science and Technology*, 3–15. London: MacMillan.

Crane, Johanna Tayloe. 2013. *Scrambling for Africa: AIDS, Expertise, and the Rise of American Global Health Science*. Ithaca, NY: Cornell University Press.

Fairclough, Norman. 2003. *Analysing Discourse: Textual Analysis for Social Research*. New York: Routledge.

Foucault, Michel. 1980. *Power/Knowledge: Selected Interviews and Other Writings, 1972-1977*. Toronto: Random House.

Gieryn, T. F. 1983. 'Boundary-Work and the Demarcation of Science from Non-Science—Strains and Interests in Professional Ideologies of Scientists'. *American Sociological Review* 48 (6): 781–95.

Hunston, Susan. 1993. 'Evaluation and Ideology in Scientific Writing'. In *Register Analysis: Theory and Practice*, edited by Mohsen Ghadessy, 57–73. New York: Pinter Publishers.

Hurtig, A. K., and Miguel San Sebastián. 2002. 'Geographical Differences in Cancer Incidence in the Amazon Basin of Ecuador in Relation to Residence near Oil Fields'. *International Journal of Epidemiology* 31 (5): 1021–27.

———. 2003. 'Epidemiology on the Side of the Angels . . . or the People?' *International Journal of Epidemiology* 32 (4): 658–59. doi:10.1093/ije/dyg210.

————. 2005. 'Epidemiology vs Epidemiology: The Case of Oil Exploitation in the Amazon Basin of Ecuador'. *International Journal of Epidemiology* 34 (5): 1170–72. doi:10.1093/ije/dyi151.

Hyland, Ken. 1998. 'Persuasion and Context: The Pragmatics of Academic Metadiscourse'. *Journal of Pragmatics* 30 (4): 437–55.

Janes, Craig R., and Kitty K. Corbett. 2009. 'Anthropology and Global Health'. *Annual Review of Anthropology* 38: 167–83. doi:10.1146/annurev-anthro-091908-164314.

Jasanoff, Sheila. 2001. *Handbook of Science and Technology Studies*. Thousand Oaks, CA: Sage Publications.

Johnstone, B. 2007. *Discourse Analysis*, volume 2. Malden, MA: Blackwell.

Kelsh, Michael A., Libby Morimoto and Edmund Lau. 2009. 'Cancer Mortality and Oil Production in the Amazon Region of Ecuador, 1990-2005'. *International Archives of Occupational and Environmental Health* 82 (3): 381–95. doi:10.1007/s00420-008-0345-x.

Kimerling, Judith. 2005. 'Indigenous Peoples and the Oil Frontier in Amazonia: The Case of Ecuador, ChevronTexaco, and Aguinda v. Texaco'. *New York University Journal of International Law and Politics* 38: 413.

————. 2008. 'Transnational Operations, Bi-National Injustice: Indigenous Amazonian Peoples and Ecuador, ChevronTexaco, and Aguinda v. Texaco'. *L'observateur Des Nations Unis* 24: 207–74.

————. 2013. 'Oil, Contact, and Conservation in the Amazon: Indigenous Huaorani, Chevron, and Yasuni'. *Colorado Journal of International Environmental Law and Policy* 24 (1): 43–114.

Krieger, N. 1999. 'Questioning Epidemiology: Objectivity, Advocacy, and Socially Responsible Science'. *American Journal of Public Health* 89 (8): 1151–53.

Larrea, Carlos. 2006. *Hacia una historia ecológica del Ecuador: Propuestas para el debate*. Quito: Corporación Editora Nacional.

Latour, Bruno. 1987. *Science in Action: How to Follow Scientists and Engineers through Society*. Cambridge, MA: Harvard University Press.

Loue, Sana. 2013. 'Forensic Epidemiology and Environmental Justice'. In *Forensic Epidemiology in the Global Context*, edited by Sana Loue, 99–119. New York: Springer.

Moolgavkar, Suresh H., Ellen T. Chang, Heather Watson and Edmund C. Lau. 2014. 'Cancer Mortality and Quantitative Oil Production in the Amazon Region of Ecuador, 1990–2010'. *Cancer Causes & Control* 25 (1): 59–72. doi:10.1007/s10552-013-0308-8.

Myers, Greg. 1990. *Writing Biology: Texts in the Social Construction of Scientific Knowledge*. Madison: University of Wisconsin Press.

People's Health Movement, Global Equity Gauge Alliance and MedAct. 2015. 'Extractive Industries and Health'. In *Global Health Watch 4*, 229–44. London: Zed Books.

Pinch, Trevor. 1990. 'The Culture of Scientists and Disciplinary Rhetoric'. *European Journal of Education* 25 (3): 295–304.

Rochlin, James. 2011. 'Development, the Environment and Ecuador's Oil Patch: The Context and Nuances of the Case against Texaco'. *Journal of Third World Studies* 28 (2): 11–39.

Rothman, Kenneth J. 1998. 'Writing for Epidemiology'. *Epidemiology* 9 (3): 333–37.

Rothman, Kenneth J., and F. Arellano. 2005. 'Responses to "Texaco and Its Consultants": Elevating the Level of Scientific Discourse'. *International Journal of Occupational and Environmental Health* 11 (3): 327–28.

Rothman, Kenneth J., H. O. Adami and D. Trichopoulos. 1998. 'Should the Mission of Epidemiology Include the Eradication of Poverty?' *Lancet* 352 (9130): 810–13.

San Sebastián, Miguel. 2001. 'Oil Development in the Amazon Basin of Ecuador: The Popular Epidemiology Process'. London: London School of Hygiene & Tropical Medicine. http://researchonline.lshtm.ac.uk/682309.

San Sebastián, Miguel, and Anna Karin Hurtig. 2005. 'Oil Development and Health in the Amazon Basin of Ecuador: The Popular Epidemiology Process'. *Social Science & Medicine* 60 (4): 799–807. doi:10.1016/j.socscimed.2004.06.016.

San Sebastián, Miguel, B. Armstrong and C. Stephens. 2001. 'La salud de mujeres que viven cerca de pozos y estaciones de petroleo en la Amazonia Ecuatoriana'. *Revista Panamericana de Salud Pública* 9 (6): 375–84.

———. 2002. 'Outcomes of Pregnancy among Women Living in the Proximity of Oil Fields in the Amazon Basin of Ecuador'. *International Journal of Occupational and Environmental Health* 8 (4): 312–19.

San Sebastián, Miguel., B. Armstrong, J. A. Cordoba and C. Stephens. 2001. 'Exposures and Cancer Incidence Near Oil Fields in the Amazon Basin of Ecuador'. *Occupational and Environment al Medicine* 58 (8): 517–22.

Savitz, D. A., C. Poole and W. C. Miller. 1999. 'Reassessing the Role of Epidemiology in Public Health'. *American Journal of Public Health* 89 (8): 1158–61. doi:10.2105/AJPH.89.8.1158.

Sawyer, Suzana. 2001. 'Fictions of Sovereignty: Of Prosthetic Petro-Capitalism, Neoliberal States, and Phantom-Like Citizens in Ecuador'. *Journal of Latin American Anthropology* 6 (1): 156–97. doi:10.1525/jlca.2001.6.1.156.

———. 2002. 'Bobbittizing Texaco: Dis-Membering Corporate Capital and Re-Membering the Nation in Ecuador'. *Cultural Anthropology* 17 (2): 150–80. doi:10.1525/can.2002.17.2.150.

Shim, Janet K., and L. Katherine Thomson. 2010. 'The End of the Epidemiology Wars? Epidemiological "Ethics" and the Challenge of Translation'. *BioSocieties* 5 (2): 159–79.

Siemiatycki, J. 2002. 'Commentary: Epidemiology on the Side of the Angels'. *International Journal of Epidemiology* 31 (5): 1027–29.

———. 2003. 'Epidemiology on the Side of the Angels . . . or the People? Response'. *International Journal of Epidemiology* 32 (4): 658–59. doi:10.1093/ije/dyg211.

Skelton, John R., and Sarah J. L. Edwards. 2000. 'The Function of the Discussion Section in Academic Medical Writing'. *BMJ: British Medical Journal* 320 (7244): 1269.

SIXTEEN

Citizens United, Public Health and Democracy

The Supreme Court Ruling, Its Implications and Proposed Action[1]

William H. Wiist

PUBLIC HEALTH AND CORPORATIONS

Public health has a long history of research, advocacy and policy related to health risks from corporate products and practices. Public health has focused on the tobacco industry (Novotny and Mamudu 2008), the pharmaceutical industry (Brody 2007), firearms manufacturers and sellers (Wintermute 1996; Hemenway 2004), the alcohol industry (Barbor 2009), the food and agriculture industry (Nestle 2002; Friedman 2008), the lead industry (Rabin 2008), motor vehicle manufacturers (Lee 1998) and others, as well as the deceptive strategies of corporations (Michaels 2008).

The American Public Health Association has official policies related to corporate products and practices to guide research, advocacy and programs. Examples of policies posted on the association's website (www.apha.org) concern asbestos (policy 20096), toxic chemicals (policy 20077), safety and effectiveness of drugs (policy 20613), food products and antibiotics (policy 2004–13), infant formula (200714), silica (policy 9512), tobacco and alcohol advertising (policy 1992–9213) and food advertising directed at children (policy 20317). The association's Trade and Health Forum and its occupational health and safety, medical care, and international health sections address corporate-related health issues such

as trade policies, worker rights, occupational safety and access to pharmaceuticals. The *Citizens United* decision may turn out to be a pivotal
point in the ability of public health to address such concerns.

THE *CITIZENS UNITED* CASE

Citizens United, a nonprofit corporation that received some funding from
for-profit corporations, released a film about 2008 presidential candidate
Hillary Clinton that it considered to be a documentary, although it was
critical of the senator. Citizens United wanted to broadcast the film on a
video-on-demand channel within thirty days of the primary election and
wanted to advertise the film on broadcast and cable stations. Federal
election laws prohibited communications funded from a corporate treasury that advocated for or against a candidate during that time period.

Believing that sections of the federal elections campaign laws were
unconstitutionally applied to the film, Citizens United filed a suit against
the Federal Elections Commission that went to the U.S. Supreme Court.
Interest in the case was keen prior to oral arguments: the Supreme Court
received fifty-three amicus briefs for the case, totalling two thousand
pages (Carney 2009). On 21 January 2010, the Court announced its split
(5–4) ruling (*Citizens United v. Federal Elections Commission*), agreeing with
a lower court position that the film advocated voting against Senator
Clinton but ruling that laws that prohibit campaign independent expenditures (advocacy for or against a candidate's election that is not coordinated with the candidate or the candidate's party or agents [Nonprofit
Electoral Advocacy after *Citizens United*]) by corporations constitute a
ban on free speech. Before *Citizens United*, only certain nonprofit corporations that did not accept corporate or labour contributions could use
independent expenditures for or against candidates.

The ruling allows corporations and labour unions to expend funds
directly from their general treasury for advocacy advertising for or
against candidates for federal office. The Court did not distinguish
among political speech via different communications media. The Court
overruled an earlier decision (*Austin v. Michigan State Chamber of Commerce*, 494 US 652 [1990]) that restricted corporations' independent expenditures, but other Court rulings were unchanged (Rutkow, Vernick and
Teret 2010). The ruling invalidated portions of the Bipartisan Campaign
Reform Act of 2002 (known as the McCain–Feingold Act). The Court
neither eliminated nor expanded the limitations on corporations' contributions to a candidate's election campaign fund or the prohibitions on
corporate coordination with a candidate's campaign, and upheld earlier
rulings on Federal Election Commission requirements for disclosure and
disclaimers (the name and address of the organization that funded an
advertisement, whether the advertisement was authorized by the candi-

date or the candidate's political committee or agent, and who was responsible for the content).

PUBLIC HEALTH AND *CITIZENS UNITED*

Concerns about the disproportionate influence of corporate wealth on elections apply equally to support of or opposition to public health measures and to candidates across the political spectrum. The ruling could exacerbate—or create new—challenges for public health through more election campaign funding, front groups, political appointments of corporate officials or lobbyists to government positions ('revolving door'), and research or program funding streams.

The *Citizens United* decision may inhibit or influence individuals campaigning for political office because of corporate pressure applied through advocacy advertising for or against them or promotion of positions during the critical weeks just prior to an election. Candidates who might otherwise publicly espouse a public health position on personal health risks, environmental hazards, or occupational safety issues could choose to remain silent or align themselves with corporations that oppose health protections. A candidate could be particularly vulnerable if an industry within the candidate's district is responsible for a health hazard and the candidate supports public health measures. Incumbents' voting records could make them especially vulnerable.

Although not all corporations or industries oppose public health measures or candidates who favour public health positions, *Citizens United* expands the means for them to exert such influence. Tobacco industry documents show that the industry's campaign contributions influenced individual legislators to be more favourable toward their industry (Dearlove and Glantz 2000; Monardi and Glantz 1998). Corporate contributions to elections could similarly influence proposed or existing health policies concerning restrictions on taxation of unhealthful foods and beverages; advertising of unhealthful products such as sugar-sweetened drinks, high-fat foods or alcohol to children or vulnerable communities; requirements for restaurant menu labelling; or issues of reproductive rights, air quality standards, global climate change, comprehensive school health education, worker health and safety, gun show background checks and others.

Expanded corporate campaign advertisement funding could exert greater influence on government research funding streams. In the past political pressure was used to try to end funding for the Centers for Disease Control and Prevention's National Center for Injury Prevention and Control to stop its firearm-related injury research (Kassirer 1995). The tobacco industry tried to stop federal funding for tobacco policy research (Landman and Glantz 2009). Increased corporate election campaign funding could also lead to public health advocacy groups competing for corporate financial contributions and to conflicts of interest and co-optation of public health organizations.

Expanded corporate campaign advertising funding could increase pressure on candidates to make political appointments of corporate or industry officials or lobbyists to decision-making positions in regulatory agencies, advisory boards or committees, with authority over their own industry and with consequences for health (Brody 2007; Nestle 2002). For example, a corporate vice president, a member of a family that contributes to political causes, received a 2004 presidential appointment to the Cancer Advisory Board of the National Cancer Institute (Schor 2010; Mayer 2010). One of the family's companies produces formaldehyde and lobbied against its classification as a carcinogen by a federal agency (Mayer 2010).

Debates about public issues can be influenced during election campaigns by corporate contributions to front groups, which purport to take one position but actually have a different agenda not apparent from their name (Landman 2009). The Coalition to Protect Patients' Rights opposed the health care reform legislation of 2010 (SourceWatch). These groups may be nonprofit 501(c)(4) social welfare or 501(c)(6) business league organizations under Internal Revenue Service regulations; these classifications differ in permissible political activities and reporting requirements. Since *Citizens United*, front groups have proliferated, and they played a large role in the 2010 election campaign. Contributions to such groups are growing, with much of the money coming from corporations; there is little federal agency oversight (Luo and Strom 2010), and fewer groups are reporting donors' identities than in past elections ('Public Citizen Fading Disclosure').

Corporate campaign contributions related to the health insurance reform debate of 2009 to 2010 illustrated some types of corporate influence on health policy (box 16.1). Corporate campaign contributions targeted members of Congress who had direct influence over health care legislation, and health industries may have received special consideration of their positions and access to policy makers (Kirckpatrick 2009; Perdomo 2009).

Box 16.1: Corporate Campaign Contributions Related to U.S. Health Care Reform Debate, 2009–2010

- During the 111th Congress's 2010 election cycle (as of October 2009), the health care industry sector was the third largest contributor to members of the Senate Finance Committee (whose bill served as the basis for the new law): political action committees gave $7,832,512 and individuals gave $6,643 626 (Open Secrets, Top 5 industries).

- From 2005 to 2010, the chairman of the Finance Committee (at the time bill became law) received $390,500 from health professions political action committees (Open Secretes, Senate Finance Committee).
- During the 2008 election cycle, the president received $18–$20 million from the health care industry, including more than $700,000 from the insurance industry (Johnson 2010; Mayer, Beckel & Kiersh 2009).
- House of Representative opponents of the reform bill received 15 percent more in contributions from the health and insurance industries during the past twenty years than did supporters (Beckel, 2009).
- Pharmaceutical manufacturer's organization contributed $2,553,986 to the two major parties and their candidates in federal and state campaigns (Open Secrets, Pharmaceutical Research and Manufacturers of America).

DEMOCRACY AND *CITIZENS UNITED*

Public health policy is founded on the role of government in protecting and promoting the health of the population when individuals acting alone cannot (Gostin 2000). At issue here is whether the electoral process primarily represents citizens or corporations and therefore whether government will give precedence to public health or corporate interests. Comparison of the Court's arguments about corporate influence on democratic processes with information about citizens' influence is pertinent to public health.

Burdensome Election Campaign Regulations

The Court's position in *Citizens United* is that the Federal Election Commission's regulations on advocacy and their enforcement, particularly regarding political action committees (PACs), were so burdensome, expensive and restrictive as to restrain corporate political speech and that limiting corporate political speech to PACs was a ban on speech. A PAC is an organization set up by, but separate from, an organization (e.g., a corporation or labour union) to collect money to distribute to election campaigns.

Corporate PACs—a specific type of PAC with separate, segregated funds—can only solicit contributions from individuals associated with the corporation, such as officers, employees and stockholders. The corporation must file with the Federal Election Commission within ten days after setting up the PAC, and the group must have a separate account and a treasurer. Limitations on fundraising and types of expenditures, as well as record-keeping and reporting requirements, apply. By contrast to the effect of *Citizens United*, the regulations governing PACs restrain the disproportionate influence of corporations because contributions are limited to $5,000 per candidate per election, $15,000 annually to a national party committee, and $5,000 annually to another PAC (FEC 2007).

Silencing Voices

The Court expressed concern that under previous rulings the government could silence particular voices and that the government should not be able to determine which speakers are worthy. The Court emphasized that the right of citizens to speak is a precondition to, and a necessity of, self-government, particularly in political campaigns. The corporation's role in democratic processes flows from the constitutional rights that persons hold; these rights have been extended to corporations over the past hundred years (Nace 2003) (box 16.2). The Court's rationale was that despite not being 'natural persons', corporations are associations of citizens entitled to First Amendment rights.

Box 16.2: Rights of Corporations
  Commercial and political speech
  Unlimited life span
  Sue and be sued
  Own other corporations and property
  Diversified mission and products
  Integrate with other corporations
  Limited liability for shareholders, board, and management
  Right to initiate and sign contracts

The Court thus ignored historical analyses of some Supreme Court cases, particularly *Santa Clara County v. Southern Pacific Railway* (118 US 394 [1886]), sometimes cited as the source decision giving corporations personhood (Nace 2003; Kaplan 2003). The analysis of *Santa Clara* showed that later courts' presumption that corporations have personhood rights misapplied the *Santa Clara* Court's reporter's notes, which carry no legal authority, but which stated that corporations are persons. In *Santa Clara*, the Court did not rule on, hear arguments for or discuss the issue of corporate personhood. The reporter's statement may have been based on a railroad employee's fraudulent testimony in another case, the influence of a justice with ties to railroads or the reporter's own connections to railroad companies.

MONEY AND POLITICAL INFLUENCE

Scholars and politicians disagree about the effects of money on elections and on the votes of elected officials, and about the likely effects of the *Citizens United* decision. However, some analysts and elected officials called the Court's decision 'disastrous', 'radical' and 'lawless' in publicly denouncing the ruling, predicting it would open the flood gates of corporate (and even foreign corporate) influence on elections ('The Court's Blow to Democracy'; Obama 2010; Rothschild 2010). Although public opinion polls can be subject to methodological issues and biases, if they are conducted by independent organizations with rigorous methods and full reporting, they can provide timely information about issues. A poll taken shortly after the *Citizens United* ruling found that 80 percent of respondents disagreed with the Court (Langer 2010; Eggen 2010).

Effects on Campaign Spending

Some concerns about the Court's decision are related to the large amounts of money required for political campaigns, particularly for television advertising, which could enable large corporate contributions to disproportionately influence the outcome.

In the 2008 federal election cycle, the average cost to win a U.S. Senate campaign was more than $8.5 million dollars and to win a House campaign, $1.4 million (Open Secrets, Centre for Responsive Politics 2008). A candidate seeking a Senate seat needed to raise more than $23,000 every day for a year (or to retain that seat, $3,881 each day of a six-year Senate term). A candidate for the House of Representatives needed to raise almost $4,000 each day for a year (for reelection, $1,880 each day over a two-year House term).

In 2000, the television industry sold 1.2 million political advertisements for $771 million in sales in the top seventy-five media markets (Alliance for Better Campaigns n.d.). During the 2008 election year, spending by candidates and interest groups on media reached $2.8 billion: approximately $2 billion on local broadcast television, $400 million for radio and local cable and $200 million for national cable and networks (Seelye 2008). During the week of 28 September–4 October 2008, the campaigns of presidential candidates Barack Obama and John McCain spent $28 million on television advertisements, approximately $10 million more than the two top candidates spent in the same period of the 2004 presidential campaign (Rabinowitz 2008).

The Court said its ruling applied to labour unions and that the imbalance between the wealth of corporations and labour unions was irrelevant. If the entire U.S. labour movement spent all of its assets on a campaign, however, it would not equal 0.10 percent of the assets of the four largest banks in the United States (Nichols 2010). Some research showed that business PAC contributions influenced congressional roll call voting patterns but that labour's did not (Peoples 2009). Business PACs out-spend labour PACs four to one (Krumholz 2010).

Effects on the Political Process

The Court rejected the argument that financial contributions to candidates have a corrupting influence or create a perception of corruption, with contributors receiving a quid pro quo of favourable votes. Corporate contributions may go only to those whose position or philosophy already aligns with the corporation's, and corporations sometimes contribute about equally to the major political parties. But at least one study showed that tobacco industry campaign contributions influenced legislators (Dearlove and Glantz 2000).

The Court argued that an appearance of corporate influence and access would not cause the electorate to lose faith in democracy. Although public opinion polls need to be interpreted cautiously, recent surveys found that a large majority of respondents believed Congress is dysfunctional, corrupt and selfish (Pew Research Center 2010); few wanted current members of Congress reelected; and a large majority thought that Congress is more interested in serving special interests than the electorate (Salant 2010).

The Court's majority also contended that corporate contributions would not result in a decrease in the electorate's participation in the democratic process. Justice John Paul Stevens's dissenting opinion argued that corporate advertising could lead citizens to lose faith in their ability to influence policy and decrease participation. Until the 2008 election, voter participation had generally declined from 1960 to 2004 (Peters and Wolley n.d.). Owners and managers of the largest U.S. corporations are among the small proportion of the population in which wealth is concentrated; they exert the most powerful political and foreign policy influence (Winters and Page 2009). Hypothetically, an expansion of such influence under *Citizens United* could exacerbate voters' feelings of powerlessness and lead to a less mobilized (Southwell 2008), more passive and demoralized (LaBranche 2007) citizenry.

Corporate Power and Influence

Recent polls showed that 86 percent of respondents believed that big companies have too much power and influence in Washington (Corso 2008). A large majority thought that corporations don't balance profit with public interest, and the proportion who believed too much power is concentrated in corporations was larger than in previous surveys (Pew Research Center 2003). The power corporations exert on democratic processes through various tactics, including political campaign contributions and lobbying, has been shown to influence health and health policy (Wiist 2010a). A large majority of respondents recently told pollsters that the amount corporations can contribute to election campaigns should be limited, that they should obtain shareholder approval to support candidates, that Congress has done too little to regulate corporations and that Congress should be able to limit the amount corporations can contribute to elections (Survey USA 2010).

Reports of effects of the *Citizens United* ruling came swiftly. Target contributed to the election campaign of a candidate with a history of antigay positions (Overby 2010). News Corporation, parent of Fox News and the *Wall Street Journal*, contributed $1 million to a governors association's election campaign fund (Lichtblau and Stelter 2010). The U.S. Chamber of Commerce, a group funded by business, used contributions to try to defeat members of Congress who supported health care reform ('The Secret Election'). The amount of independent expenditures on election campaigns increased (Farnam and Eggen 2010).

PUBLIC HEALTH AND AMELIORATING *CITIZENS UNITED*

The *Citizens United* decision galvanized citizens groups and some members of Congress to try to ameliorate the ruling's expansion of corporate financial influence on election campaigns. Congresspersons and organizations such as Move to Amend, Free Speech for People and Public Citizens Don't Get Rolled are advocating a range of strategies to redress the effects of the *Citizens United* ruling (box 16.3) (Krumholz 2010; Korten 2010; Public Citizen n.d.). Corporate funding of election campaigns and corporate lobbying are major obstacles to the passage of any of the proposals.

Box 16.3: Propo sed Actions to Ameliorate the Effects of the *Citizens United* Ruling

- Require shareholders to approve political spending by their corporations.
- Pass the Fair Elections Now Act, which would create a voluntary public financing system for congressional elections in which candidates would qualify for federal matching funds ($4/$1 donated) by raising a large number of small donations (≤ $100) from individuals in their community.
- Give qualified candidates equal amounts of free broadcast air time for political messages.
- Ban political advertising by corporations that receive government money, hire lobbyists, or collect most of their revenue abroad.

- Impose an excise tax on corporations' contributions to political committees and their expenditures on political advocacy.
- Prohibit companies that make political contributions and expenditures from trading their stock on national exchanges.
- Require corporations to disclose money used to influence public opinion (other than product promotions) in their required filings with the Securities and Exchange Commission.
- Require the chief executive officer of a corporation that pays for a political commercial to appear as the sponsor.
- Limit the election-related spending of foreign-owned corporations and corporations with federal contracts.
- Require companies to inform shareholders about political spending.
- Require corporations, unions, and advocacy groups to have designated accounts for political activities.
- Tighten rules against coordination between political campaigns and other groups (e.g., prohibit hiring the same advertising firms or consultants).
- Strengthen Federal Election Commission regulations to increase transparency and disclosure.

A constitutional amendment that eliminates corporate political speech or personhood would address the most fundamental level of the issue, but amending the Constitution is a lengthy and difficult process, and few proposed amendments have been enacted. Funding election campaigns entirely through public money would decrease candidates' dependence on corporate funding, and free broadcast, cable and Internet advertising for qualified candidates could reduce the size of the campaign chests successful politicians now require. At the time of writing, some of the legislative proposals shown in box 16.3, such as the Fair Elections Now Act (S 752; HR 6116) and the Democracy Is Strengthened by Casting Light on Spending in Elections Act (HR 5175; S 3628), were under consideration by Congress.

The field of public health has a role in corporate reform efforts, including election campaign finance reform. A primary preventive focus on the corporation as a fundamental distal factor in health is consistent with the public health code of ethics (APHA 2002). Some public health professionals have emphasized public health research and advocacy related to disease-promoting corporate products (Freudenberg 2005). Viewing the corporation as an institution (Wiist 2006) that uses a repertoire of tactics (Wiist 2010b) to influence health and policy broadens the scope of public health to include working toward election campaign finance reform.

Public health professionals have expertise regarding the health effects of corporate products and operations and are skilled in policy development, advocacy and coalition building. Public health practitioners can use this expertise to collaborate with other organizations around the globe (Hawken 2007) through a variety of methods (Starr 2005) to reform corporations and related economic policies. The influence of global trade policy (Blouin, Chopra and van der Hoeven 2009) and the growing number of transnational corporations (Progressive Policy Institute 2005) illustrate the challenge and underscore the need for such coordinated efforts. In the United States, public health professionals can use their advocacy and coalition-building skills to work with other organizations toward passage of the proposals in box 16.3 and of democratic measures at the local level (Community Environmental Legal Defense Fund n.d.; Yesfor-Portland n.d.) that will protect public health.

Public health researchers could examine whether election campaign contributions influence votes by members of Congress on positions taken by the American Public Health Association (APHA 2010). Research is needed on the influence of campaign contributions to elected judges who rule on environmental laws and regulations, worker safety and health. The influence of lobbying, the revolving door between industry and government, and front groups on legislation, regulations, public opinion and voting patterns also warrant study.

Corporate political speech directed against the interests of public health may be the most important challenge the field of public health faces. The citizenry that public health serves—and many elected officials—want reform of corporate influence on elections. To remain a viable endeavour with hope of having a significant influence on the health of the public, the profession must respond. *Citizens United* is a call for public health to refocus its efforts on fundamental reform of the corporation, particularly corporations' right to political speech.

ACKNOWLEDGEMENTS

I thank the anonymous reviewers and the journal editors for their helpful suggestions and comments.

NOTE

1. Wiist (2011). Reproduced with permission from the Sheridan Press.

REFERENCES

Alliance for Better Campaigns. 'Gouging Democracy: How the Television Industry Profiteered on Campaign 2000'. www.campaignlegalcenter.org/attachments/1712.pdf.

American Public Health Association. 2002. 'Principles of Ethical Practice of Public Health'. www.apha.org/NR/rdonlyres/1CED3CEA-287E-4185-9CBD-BD405FC6085 6/0/ethicsbrochure.pdf.

———. 2010. ' APHA Annual Congressional Record: How Members of Congress Supported Public Health '. *Nations Health* 40 : 5–10

Barbor, Thomas F. 2009. 'Alcohol Research and the Alcoholic Beverage Industry: Issues, Concerns and Conflicts of Interest '. *Addiction* 104 (1) : 34–47

Beckel, Michael. 2009. ' Opponents of House Health Reform Bill Received 15 Percent More in Health Industry Contributions Than Supporters'. *Open Secrets, Centre for Responsive Politics* , 8 November. www.opensecrets.org/news/2009/11/opponents-of-house-health-refo.html.

Blouin, Chantal, Mickey Chopra and Rolph van der Hoeven. 2009. ' Trade and Social Determinants of Health '. *Lancet* 373 (9662) : 502–7

Brody, Howard. 2007. *Hooked: Ethics, the Medical Profession, and the Pharmaceutical Industry* . Lanham, MD: Rowman and Littlefield Publishers.

Carney, E. N. 2009. 'Citizens United Sparks Pitched Battle: Outside Groups Are Straining the Court System in Their Attempts to Influence What Could Be a Landmark Campaign Finance Case'. *National Journal,* 31 August. www.nationaljournal.com/njonline/no_20090831_2098.php.

Citizens United v. Federal Elections Commission. 130 US 876 (2010).

Community Environmental Legal Defense Fund . n.d. http://celdf.org.

Corso, Regina A. 2008. ' Very Large Majorities of Americans Believe Big Companies, PACs, Political Lobbyists and the News Media Have Too Much Power and Influence in D.C.'. *Harris Interactive* , 11 March. www.harrisinteractive.com/vault/Harris-Interactive-Poll-Research-Very-Large-Majorities-Of-Americans-Believe-Big-Com-2008-03.pdf.

Dearlove, Joanna, and Stanton Glantz. 2000. *Tobacco Industry Political Influence and Tobacco Policy Making in New York 1983–1999* . San Francisco: Institute for Health Policy Studies, University of California, San Francisco. http://escholarship.org/uc/item/2t45x412.

'Democracy, Inc.'. [editorial] *Nation* , 28 January 2010. www.thenation.com/article/democracy-inc.

Eggen, D. 2010. 'Poll: Large Majority Opposes Supreme Court's Decision on Campaign Financing'. Washington Post , 17 February. www.washingtonpost.com/wpdyn/content/article/2010/02/17/AR2010021701151.html.

Farnam, T. W., and Dan Eggen. 2010. 'Interest Group Spending for Mid-Term Up Five-Fold from 2006; Many Sources Secret'. *Washington Post,* 4 October. www.washingtonpost.com/wp-dyn/content/article/2010/10/03/AR2010100303664.htm.

Federal Election Commission. 2007. 'Federal Election Commission Campaign Guide: Corporations and Labour Organizations'. www.fec.gov/pdf/colagui.pdf.

Freudenberg, Nicholas. 2005. ' Public Health Education Advocacy to Change Corporate Practices: Implications for Health Education Practice and Research '. *Health Educ Behav* 32 (3) : 298–319; discussion 355–62.

Friedman, Roberta R. 2008. *Menu Labelling in Chain Restaurants: Opportunities for Public Policy* . New Haven, CT: Rudd Centre for Food Policy and Obesity, Yale University.

Gostin, Lawrence O. 2000. *Public Health Law: Power, Duty, Restraint.* Berkeley: University of California Press.

Hartmann, Thom. 2002. *Unequal Protection: The Rise of Corporate Dominance and the Theft of Human Rights.* San Francisco, CA: Berrett-Koehler Publishers.

Hawken, Paul. 2007. *Blessed Unrest: How the Largest Movement in the World Came into Being and Why No One Saw It Coming* . New York: Penguin.

Hemenway, David. 2004. *Private Guns, Public Health.* Ann Arbour: University of Michigan Press.

Jacobson, Brad. 2010. 'Obama Received $20 Million from Healthcare Industry in 2008 Campaign'. *The Raw Story,* 12 January. http://rawstory.com/2010/01/obama-received-20-million-healthcare-industry-money-2008.

Kaplan, Jeffrey. 2003. 'The Birth of the White Corporation'. Reprinted from By What Authority. Spring. Women's International League for Peace and Freedom. www.wilpf.org/docs/ccp/CPOWER_whitecorps.htm.

Kassirer, Jerome P. 1995. 'A Partisan Assault on Science—the Threat to the CDC'. *N Engl J Med* 333 (12) : 793–94.

Kelly, Marjorie, and Allen White. 2007. *Corporate Design: The Missing Business and Public Policy Issue of Our Time* . Boston: Tellus Institute.

Kirkpatrick, David D. 2009. 'Obama Is Taking an Active Role in Talks on Health Care Plan'. *New York Times*, 12 August. www.nytimes.com/2009/08/13/health/policy/13health.html?pagewanted=1&_r=1.

———. 2010. 'Lobbyists Get Potent Weapon in Campaign Ruling '. *New York Times*, 21 January. www.nytimes.com/2010/01/22/us/politics/22donate.html?fta=y.

Korten, Fran. 2010. '10 Ways to Stop Corporate Dominance of Politics'. *Yes! Magazine*, 28 January. www.alternet.org/rights/145441/10_ways_to_stop_corporate_dominance_of_politics.

Krumholz, Sheila. 2010. 'Statement on Campaign Finance to US Senate Committee'. *Open Secrets, Centre for Responsive Politics*, 2 February. www.opensecrets.org/news/2010/02/center-for-responsive-politics-9.html.

LaBranche, Stephane. 2005. 'Abuse and Westernization: Reflections on Strategies of Power'. *J Peace Res*. 42 (2) : 219–35.

Landman, Anne. 2009. 'Attack of the Living Front Groups: PR Watch Offers Help to Unmask Corporate Tricksters'. *PR Watch*, 28 August. www.prwatch.org/help+unmask+propagandists.

Landman, Anne, and Stanton A. Glantz. 2009. 'Tobacco Industry Efforts to Undermine Policy-Relevant Research'. *Am J Public Health* 99 (1) : 45–58.

Langer, Gary. 2010. 'In Supreme Court Ruling on Campaign Finance, the Public Dissents'. *ABC News*, 17 February. http://blogs.abcnews.com/thenumbers/2010/02/in-supreme-court-ruling-on-campaign-finance-the-public-dissents.html.

Lee, Matthew T. 1998. 'The Ford Pinto Case and the Development of Auto Safety Regulations, 1893–1978'. *Bus Econ Hist*. 27 (2) : 390–401.

Lichtblau, Eric, and Brian Stelter. 2010. 'News Corp. Gives G.O.P. $1 million'. *New York Times*, 17 August. www.nytimes.com/2010/08/18/us/politics/18donate.html?_r=1&hp.

Luo, Michael, and Stephanie Strom. 2010. 'Donor Names Remain Secret as Rules Shift'. *New York Times*, 20 September. www.nytimes.com/2010/09/21/us/politics/21money.html?pagewanted=1&_r=1&sq=front groups&st=cse&scp=1.

Marx, Michael, Mari Margil, John Cavanagh, Sarah Anderson, Chuck Collins, Charlie Cray and Marjorie Kelley. 2007. 'Strategic Corporate Initiative: Toward a Global Citizen's Movement to Bring Corporations Back under Control'. *Corporate Ethics International*. www.corpethics.org/downloads/SCI_Report_September_2007.pdf.

Mayer, Jane. 2010. 'The Billionaire Brothers Who Are Waging a War against Obama'. *New Yorker*, 30 August. www.newyorker.com/reporting/2010/08/30/100830fa_fact_mayer.

Mayer, Lindsay R., Michael Beckel and Aaron Kiersh. 2009. 'Diagnosis: Reform'. *Open Secrets, Centre for Responsive Politics*, 17 June. www.opensecrets.org/news/2009/06/diagnosis-reform.html.

Michaels, David. 2008. *Doubt Is Their Product: How Industry's Assault on Science Threatens Your Health*. New York: Oxford University Press.

Monardi, Fred, and Stanton A. Glantz. 1998. 'Are Tobacco Industry Campaign Contributions Influencing State Legislative Behaviour?' *Am J Public Health* 88 (6) : 918–23.

Nace, Ted. 2003. *Gangs of America: The Rise of Corporate Power and the Disabling of Democracy*. San Francisco, CA: Berrett-Koehler Publishers.

Nestle, Marion. 2002. *Food Politics: How the Food Industry Influences Nutrition and Health*. Berkeley: University of California Press.

Nichols, John. 2010. 'Unions Can't Compete with Corporate Campaign Cash'. *Nation* [blog], 24 January. www.thenation.com/blogs/thebeat/521020/unions_can_t_comp

ete_with_corporate_campaign_cash.

Nonprofit Electoral Advocacy After Citizens United. Washington, DC: Alliance for Justice. www.afj.org/assets/resources/citizens_united_fact_sheet.pdf.

Novotny, Thomas E., and Hadii M. Mamudu. 2008. 'Progression of Tobacco Control Policies: Lessons from the United States and Implications for Global Action'. Health, Nutrition and Population Discussion Paper. Washington, DC: International Bank for Reconstruction and Development.

Obama, Barack H. 2010. State of the Union Address. Delivered 27 January. www.whitehouse.gov/the-press-office/remarks-president-state-union-address.

Open Secrets, Centre for Responsive Politics. 2008. 'Election Stats. Election Cycle 2008'. www.opensecrets.org/bigpicture/elec_stats.php?cycle=2008.

———. 2009. 'Pharmaceutical Research and Manufacturers of America'. www.opensecrets.org/orgs/all_summary.php?id=D000000504&nid=4265.

———. 2013. 'Max Baucus. Top 5 Industries, 2005–2010, Campaign Committee'. www.opensecrets.org/politicians/summary.php?cycle=2010&type=I&cid=N00004643.

———. 2015. 'Senate Finance Committee 111th Congress (2010 Cycle): Overview'. www.opensecrets.org/cmteprofiles/overview.php?cmte=SFIN&cmteid=S12&cycle=2010.

Overby, Peter. 2010. 'The Real Lesson in Target's Campaign Cash Trouble'. *National Public Radio*, 16 August. www.npr.org/templates/story/story.php?storyId=129236311.

Peoples, Clayton D. 2009. 'Revising Power Structure Research: Present Problems, Their Solutions, and Future Directions '. *Polit Power Soc Theory* 20 : 3–38.

Perdomo, Daniella. 2009. 'White House's Ties to Health Care Industry Deeper Than Visitor Records Show'. *AlterNet* , 26 November. www.alternet.org/news/144209/white_house's_ties_to_health_care_industry_deeper_than_visitor_records_show?page=entire.

Peters, Gerhard, and John T. Wooley. n.d. 'Voter Turnout in Presidential Elections'. *American Presidency Project*. www.presidency.ucsb.edu/data/turnout.php.

Pew Research Center for People and the Press. 2003. 'The 2004 Political Landscape. Part 7. Business, Government, Regulation and Labour'. 5 November. http://people-press.org/report/?pageid=756.

———. 2010. 'Congress in a Wordle'. 22 March. http://pewresearch.org/pubs/1533/congress-in-a-word-cloud-dysfunctional-corrupt-selfish.

Progressive Policy Institute. 2005. 'The World Has over 60,000 Multinational Companies. Trade Fact of the Week'. 27 April. www.ppionline.org/ppi_ci.cfm?knlgAreaID=108&subsecID=900003&contentID=253303.

Public Citizen. n.d. 'FENA Short Summary'. http://citizen.org/Page.aspx?pid=2325.

'Public Citizen Fading Disclosure: Increasing Number of Electioneering Groups Keep Donors' Identities Secret'. 15 September 2010. www.citizen.org/document/Disclosure-report-final.pdf.

Rabin, Richard. 2008. 'The Lead Industry and Lead Water Pipes "A Modest Campaign"'. *Am J Public Health* 98 (9): 1584–92.

Rabinowitz, Steve. 2008. 'TV Advertising Spending Continues to Grow; over $28 Million Spent from September 28–October 4'. Rabinowitz/Dorf Communications. *Wisconsin Advertising Project*, 8 October. http://wiscadproject.wisc.edu/wiscads_release_100808.pdf.

Richey, Warren, and Linda Feldman. 2010. ' Supreme Court's Campaign Finance Ruling: Just the Facts '. *Christian Science Monitor*, 2 February. http://news.yahoo.com/s/csm/20100202/ts_csm/276880.

Rothschild, Matthew. 2010. 'Feingold Slams Supreme Court over "Citizens United", Implies Roberts and Alito Lied under Oath'. *Progressive*, 17 September. www.progressive.org/wx091710.html.

Rutkow, Lainie, Jon S. Vernick and Stephen P. Teret. 2010. 'The Potential Health Effects of Citizens United'. *N Engl J Med* 362 (15) : 1356–58.

Salant, Jonathan D. 2010. 'Few Americans Want Members of Congress Re-elected, Poll Finds'. 12 February. http://news.yahoo.com/s/bloomberg/20100212/pl_bloomberg/aesowriv31_g.

Schor, Elana. 2010. 'Koch Leaves Federal Cancer Panel as Groups Urge Ethics Probe'. *New York Times*, 27 October. www.nytimes.com/gwire/2010/10/27/27greenwire-koch-leaves-federal-cancer-panel-as-groups-urg-61710.html.

Seelye, Katharine Q. 2008. 'About $2.6 billion Spent on Political Ads in 2008'. *New York Times*, 2 December. http://thecaucus.blogs.nytimes.com/2008/12/02/about-26-billion-spent-on-political-ads-in-2008.

SourceWatch. 'Coalition to Protect Patients' Rights'. www.sourcewatch.org/index.php/Coalition_to_Protect_Patients%27_Rights.

Southwell, Priscilla L. 2008. 'The Effect of Political Alienation on Voter Turnout, 1964–2000'. *J Polit Mil Sociol* 36 (1) : 131–45.

Starr, Amory. 2005. *Global Revolt: A Guide to the Movements against Globalization*. New York: Zed Books.

Survey USA. 2010. 'Results of Survey. USA News Poll #16270. Americans Broadly in Favor of Limiting What Corporations Can Spend to Influence U.S. Elections'. 10 February. www.surveyusa.com/client/PollPrint.aspx?g=05cabb5f-599f-47a8-98fb-e3e254e425e4&d=0.

'The Court's Blow to Democracy'. [editorial] *New York Times*, 21 January 2010. www.nytimes.com/2010/01/22/opinion/22fri1.html?scp=7&sq=citizens%20united%20supreme%20court&st=cse.

'The Secret Election'. [editorial] *New York Times*, 18 September 2010. www.nytimes.com/2010/09/19/opinion/19sun1.html?_r=1.

Wiist, William H. 2006. 'Public Health and the Anticorporate Movement: Rationale and Recommendations'. *Am J Public Health* 96 (8) : 1370–75.

———, ed. 2010a. *The Bottom Line or Public Health: Tactics Corporations Use to Influence Health and Health Policy and What We Can Do to Counter Them*. New York: Oxford University Press.

———. 2010b. 'The Corporation: An Overview of What It Is, Its Tactics, and What Public Health Can Do.' In *The Bottom Line or Public Health: Tactics Corporations Use to Influence Health and Health Policy and What We Can Do to Counter Them*, edited by W. H. Wiist, 3–72. New York: Oxford University Press.

———. 2011. 'Citizens United, Public Health and Democracy: The Supreme Court Ruling, Its Implications and Proposed Action'. *AJPH* 101 (7): 1172–79.

Wintemute, Garen J. 1996. 'The Relationship between Firearm Design and Firearm Violence: Handguns in the 1990s'. *JAMA* 275 (22) : 1749–53.

Winters, Jeffrey A., and Benjamin I. Page. 2009. 'Oligarchy in the United States?' *Perspect Polit* 7 (4) : 731–51.

YesForPortland. n.d. 'Answers '. http://yesforportland.org/faq/#4.

SEVENTEEN
Conclusion

Nora Kenworthy, Ross MacKenzie and Kelley Lee

The term *industrial epidemics* was coined by Slade (1989) to describe the commodification of dangerous goods and services, and their consequent impacts on population health. First used with reference to the tobacco industry, the concept has been extended to the consumption of alcohol, food, automobiles and other products that can create an inherent dichotomy between the interests of public health and commercialized economic activity (Majnoni d'Intignano 1998). Jahiel and Babor (2007, 1335) broadened the concept further to include 'diseases of consumers, workers and community residents caused by industrial promotion of consumable products, job conditions and environmental pollution'.

As well as confirming the acute relevance of industrial epidemics to the global economy of the early twenty-first century, this collection of case studies further demonstrates that the health implications of corporations are the result, not 'simply of their core business activities, but also their ability to influence the political environment in which they operate' (Hawkins and Roemer-Mahler 2013). We begin by recognising that there is a complex relationship between corporations and global health arising from the transformation of social and environmental health determinants by economic globalisation. The impacts are evidenced by distinct shifts in the occurrence and spread of many communicable diseases, such as HIV/AIDS, tuberculosis and pandemic influenza, as well as non-communicable diseases (NCDs) such as cardiovascular and respiratory diseases, cancers and diabetes. Not only are emerging epidemiological patterns suggesting an exacerbation of existing health disparities (Friel and Marmot 2011), but also there is growing evidence of novel spatial and temporal (transboundary) disease patterns (Pearce 2011). It is widely agreed

243

that collective action through global health governance (GHG), to manage and redress these impacts, is urgently needed.

This collection of case studies examines the relationship between corporations and GHG, defined as collective action (in the form of agreed rules, processes and institutional arrangements) by public and private actors to address global health challenges. Our particular focus on corporations stems from their prominence as key actors in an increasingly globalised world economy, and the extent of their impacts on health. Our aim has been to empirically document the myriad forms of influence and impact corporations have in GHG, and to identify avenues to better hold corporations to account for their roles and impacts. Below, we highlight some of the many insights yielded by the case studies in this volume.

CORPORATE IMPACTS ON PUBLIC HEALTH IN A GLOBALISING WORLD

First, as described above, a world economy and global governance system dominated by large corporations are resulting in profound impacts on public health worldwide. The first four case studies in the book illustrate these impacts in relation to the garment, tobacco, asbestos and lead industries. In addition to describing the direct effects on public health of these industries, in terms of both what they produce and their methods of production, these chapters extend their analyses to how corporations influence the global governance of those industries. Kenworthy examines how public-private partnerships in the garment industry 'produce specific and varying health outcomes in populations, and manufacture certain notions of responsibility for population health'. MacKenzie and Hawkins argue that pharmaceutical corporations manufacturing cessation aids have 'successfully shaped the discourse around how smokers quit' including the 'framing of e-cigarettes as harm reduction products', while Scott and colleagues examine the major role of unhealthy diets in the rise of NCDs and, in particular, the processed food industry's use of political tactics in Mexico and California 'to shape relevant policies in its favour'. In their analysis of extractive resource operations, Taylor and George show that decades of ineffective government action on lead exposure in a small Australian town have been the result of powerful vested interests involved in the 'production of knowledge about environmental contamination problems'.

THE SCOPE OF CORPORATE INFLUENCE IN GHG

The case studies in part 2 delve deeper into the corporate influence of GHG in different geographical, political, economic and social settings. We argue that corporations have capitalised on the changing architecture of global governance. While many decisions impacting global health are made at transnational levels, they are enforced, contested, given meaning and implemented at national and subnational levels. Much of this influence specifically derives from global economic instruments such as bilateral, regional and multilateral trade and investment agreements that challenge traditional state-based authority. Such agreements have been particularly instrumental in creating a 'governance gap' between corporations and the institutions and processes intended to regulate their social and environmental impacts. Rather than the 'eclipse of the state' (Evans 1997) predicted by many observers of globalisation, the national arena survives but has been joined by a proliferation of new governance 've-nues' in which corporations wield growing political power.

New governance venues include an increasingly multifaceted transnational sphere, in which corporations have substantial resources and power to manage relationships and influence policymaking, as described in the case studies by Moon and Suzuki, and Wagner-Rizvi. Holden and Hawkins emphasise the importance of 'multi-level governance' structures, which have proliferated in the wake of neoliberal reforms, and span regional, national and subnational venues for policy making and implementation. Corporations strategically seek policy-making forums where they are most able to exert influence and have the scope and resources necessary to engage in what is described as 'venue-shifting' by Holden and Hawkins and 'forum shopping' by Schram and Labonte. This capacity sheds further light on Calvert's analysis of how the asbestos industry has 'persuaded governments in both producing and consuming LMICs to ignore the regulations now in place in industrialized countries'. Weak global asbestos governance, amid the transition of production and consumption from high- to low- and middle-income countries (LMICs), can also be explained in terms of venue shifting. Corporations thrive globally by operating in jurisdictions unwilling or unable to regulate their activities.

Notwithstanding such direct impacts on GHG, a striking feature of several case studies is the observation that patterns of corporate influence rely not only on structural exploitation or strategic institutional circumvention, but also on more informal avenues of influence. Corporate activities in this domain go beyond simple public relations exercises and instead represent far-reaching efforts to reframe public discourses about corporate goods and industry harms. Ideational power enables corporations to shape publicly accepted norms about behaviours, responsibilities, and the social and political roles of the corporation, and to influence or discredit research, expert opinions and scientific evidence. Moon and Suzuki describe corporations' use of lobbying, public communication and financial support of non-profit organisations, in addition to their manipulation of scientific research, as 'indirect or informal channels' of influence used across four health-related industries: tobacco, alcohol, food and non-alcoholic beverages, and pharmaceuticals. Scott et al. document the use of a number of these strategies in their analysis of soda tax initiatives in two California towns by both corporate interests and civil society. The variable success of these initiatives was due, in part, to efforts by both sides to frame the debates around values that resonated with vastly different communities. Their findings appear to indicate that lower-income, less well-financed communities are more susceptible to beverage industry messaging than those that are more affluent. Scott et al. and Moon and Suzuki also document the extensive use of front groups posing as grassroots organisations to carry out such discursive campaigning.

Corporate efforts to shape public discourse span many industries, and often involve strategies aimed at 'reframing' debates about corporate harm. These can include renaming harmful products and rephrasing messages about consumer behaviours, as well as broader discursive strategies to influence cultural perceptions of corporate actors. Such power extends to influence over how harms (and potential strategies for averting harms) are portrayed, most obviously in what has been described as the medicalisation of global health, that is, the redefinition of human or social problems as treatable medical conditions requiring technological solutions that align with the economic interests of pharmaceutical corporations and other related industries (Clark 2014). Examples from the case studies include Cassidy's assessment of corporate pathologising of gambling addiction to support the push for unrestricted gambling access, and MacKenzie and Hawkins's analysis of how the medicalisation of smoking cessation provides corporations further room to market cessation as a project of consumption.

Corporations can also exert normative influence. The extraordinary expansion of corporate social responsibility (CSR) efforts in recent years demonstrates the extent to which corporations are concerned not only with their public image, but also with influencing the public's ideas about what it means to 'do good'. CSR initiatives that range from providing community services to self-regulatory business behaviour (Frynas and Stephens 2014) allow corporations to strengthen their influence over global health discourse, while providing new opportunities to portray themselves as beneficent and moral leaders (Dolan and Rajak 2011). Being perceived as a responsible actor allows corporations to inhabit new roles as moral arbiters, upstanding corporate citizens and global health leaders. But as Wagner-Rizvi argues in her assessment of baby food marketing, corporate self-regulation offers insufficient protection for public health. Many corporations attempt to influence norms about consumer exposures to harm, deploying dialogues about individual responsibility and behavioural choices to distance themselves from public health issues inherent to their products. For instance, Cassidy explores the efforts of the gambling industry in many different countries to create a bifurcated notion of their consumer: the 'responsible gambler' is made normative while the addicted gambler is portrayed as weak, 'vulnerable' and a source of multiple health problems.

One of the most important normative shifts with regard to corporate actors, is the increase in claims of personhood, citizenship and partnership. As Wiist notes, the *Citizens United* decision in the United States has potentially 'catastrophic' public health impacts, in part because it enshrines corporations' rights to spend unparalleled amounts of money on campaigns for candidates who will support their policy positions. Stevenson's case study, which details the rise of public-private partnerships (PPPs) as a paradigm for global health collaboration, makes clear that 'partnership' is another means by which corporations secure publicly legitimate roles. This echoes Kenworthy's analysis of the closure of a previously successful PPP that had provided HIV services in Lesotho's garment industry, which provides rare insight into what happens to those who rely on PPP and CSR arrangements when they close down. This case raises broader questions about the challenges PPPs pose to equitable global health care, their production of specific and varying health outcomes in populations, and the manufacture of notions of responsibility for population health.

Finally, corporate involvement in the production of knowledge and expertise has far-reaching effects at multiple levels. As the case studies by Cassidy, Moon and Suzuki, MacKenzie and Hawkins, and MacKenzie and Lee document, corporate investment in researchers and research trials is widespread across industries, as are corporate efforts to discredit independent research findings, as described in Brisbois's chapter. Such efforts represent a conflict of interest for researchers, but are also indicative of corporations' extensive efforts to influence the public's access to information, and the credibility of certain forms of knowledge and knowledge production. Additionally, corporations may be involved in so-called 'boundary work'. In contrast with discursive efforts to shift or reframe debates, boundary work involves efforts to exclude outsiders from a discourse or reinforce the boundaries of a discipline. As Brisbois notes in his detailed analysis of corporate influence in a scientific debate over the epidemiological impact of Chevron's activities in the Amazon, scientists themselves engage in boundary work that questions the credibility of more 'popular' epidemiologic studies of corporate harm.

HOLDING CORPORATIONS TO FULLER ACCOUNT THROUGH GHG

The case studies in part 3 consider not only the impacts arising from, and forms of influence exerted by corporations, but also the potential to hold corporations to fuller account through GHG. Given the evidence of the range and depth of corporate power presented in the preceding case studies, this seems a daunting task. Arguably, the most successful effort to date to achieve collective action to address a global health problem created and sustained by corporate actors has been the Framework Convention on Tobacco Control (FCTC). The international treaty has been heralded as the first negotiated under the auspices of the World Health Organization (WHO), and many have called for similar instruments to be agreed for alcohol, food and global health as a whole (Gostin et al. 2013). However, the FCTC experience shows that international agreements do not necessarily translate into effective regulation of corporations in national or local contexts. MacKenzie and Lee describe how negotiation and implementation of the FCTC has been challenged by the tobacco industry's dizzying array of options for subverting and circumventing regulation in three Asian countries. The chapter draws attention to the particular political and economic conditions that have shaped the FCTC's success. Article 5.3 of the FCTC sets out measures to limit industry influence over tobacco control policy, including implementation of the FCTC, and its effectiveness will benefit from an understanding of the broad range of impacts and influence described in this book.

Nevertheless, recent crises in the world economy have raised concerns about the corporation as a particular form of business organization, and renewed debates about new approaches to effective regulation through global governance. For example, the UN System Task Team on the Post-2015 UN Development Agenda (2013) draws attention to 'increased coherence, coordination and collective decision-making at the global level' amid 'deepening economic globalization, and increasing migration, trade and capital flows, and climate change and increased activities in the global commons'. The report concludes that, to 'achieve coherence in global governance, all three dimensions of sustainable development—sustainable economic growth, social inclusion and protection of the environment and the global commons—need to be integrated at the global level'.

In this book, Wagner-Rizvi presents compelling evidence that, despite a significant imbalance in resources, civil society organisations, such as the International Baby Food Action Network in Pakistan, can utilise discursive and agency power to raise public awareness and campaign for meaningful regulation. Mialon et al. put forth a framework for categorising the corporate political activity of the food industry with respect to public health focused on systematically identifying and monitoring six industry strategies. This represents a shift, from core narratives focused on deregulation and the health responsibilities of individuals, to quasi-regulation of corporate actors through improved transparency and accountability. Wiist goes further, arguing that the time has arrived to move beyond the repetitive and resource-consuming model of mounting campaigns against single products, companies or even industries. Instead, he calls for engagement in more fundamental, upstream actions, including contesting the legal rights of corporations.

Progress on these and other approaches for regulating the public health impacts and influence of corporations more effectively, is supported by Bakan's (2004) reminder that political organisation remains just as important, if not more so, as economic organisation. Indeed, despite the worldwide spread and intensification of globalisation, the state retains significant formal power over corporate actors. Corporations ultimately depend on effective state institutions for their continued existence and functioning in societies. If state power has shifted in recent decades to explicitly protect the corporation, so too can it be brought back to better serve the public interest. A critical impediment to such restructuring, however, is the widespread misperception that the corporation exists beyond state control—an assessment fuelled by extensive corporate engagement in non-state and transnational governance structures. Furthermore, as Wiist notes, recent recognition of corporate 'citizenship' radically expands corporate capacity to oppose and undermine efforts to restructure power.

Events in early 2016 highlighted the urgent need for, and value of, efforts to hold corporations to account. The poisoning of Flint, Michigan's water supply beginning in 2014 resulted in extensive health problems, and highlighted the importance of citizens and researchers in bringing attention to government responsibility. Lesser known are two other legacies of corporate involvement in the crisis: General Motors, Flint's largest employer and a primary polluter of the Flint river, was removed from the water supply because the contaminated water was corroding engine parts, 'an option that was not afforded other Flint residents and businesses' (Colias 2016). Nestlé, the largest owner of private water in the state as a source of supply for its brand of bottled water, has reported ties to Governor Snyder's administration and stands to profit from the crisis due to Flint's reliance on bottled water (O'Connell 2016). Meanwhile, ongoing legal action against DuPont alleges 'decades-long' chemical pollution in West Virginia (Rich 2016). These events underscore the pragmatic and political value of case study research in uncovering corporate harms, and the need to create accountability mechanisms that require that corporations are held responsible for the social and environmental effects of their operations.

The task of holding corporations to account will require a range of fundamental changes to our political systems that include strengthening political democracy by regulating political campaign financing, overturning the legal standing of corporate personhood and eliminating corporate welfare, among others (Bakan 2004; Korten 2000; Wilkinson and Pickett 2010). Such dramatic change will be achieved neither quickly nor easily. The challenge now, as many of these chapters make clear, is for citizens, civil society groups and governments themselves to recognise, document and rein in the influence corporations wield over numerous venues and scales of GHG.

REFERENCES

Bakan, Joel. 2004. *The Corporation*. New York: Penguin.
Clark, Jocelyn. 2014. 'Medicalization of Global Health 1: Has the Global Health Agenda Become Too Medicalized?' *Global Health Action* 7: 23998. doi: 10.3402/gha.v7.23998.
Colias, Mike. 2016. 'How GM Saved Itself from Flint Water Crisis'. *Automotive News*, 31 January.
Dolan, Catherine, and Dinah Rajak. 2011. 'Introduction: Ethnographies of Corporate Ethicizing'. *Focaal* 60: 3–8.
Evans, Peter. 1997. 'The Eclipse of the State? Reflections on Stateness in an Era of Globalization'. *World Politics* 50 (1): 62–87.
Friel, Sharon, and Michael G. Marmot. 2011. 'Action on the Social Determinants of Health and Health Inequities Goes Global'. *Annual Review of Public Health* 32: 225–36.
Frynas, Jędrzej, and Siân Stephens. 2014. 'Political Corporate Social Responsibility: Reviewing Theories and Setting New Agendas'. *International Journal of Management Reviews* 17: 483–509.
Gostin, L., E. Friedman, K. Buse, A. Waris, M. Mulumba, M. Joel, L. Dare, A. Dhai and D. Sridhar. 2013. 'Towards a Framework Convention on Global Health'. *Bulletin of the World Health Organization* 91: 790–93.
Hawkins, Benjamin, and Anne Roemer-Mahler. 2013. 'Corporations as Political Actors: New Perspectives for Health Policy Research'. In *Social Policy Review 25: Analysis and Debate in Social Policy*, edited by Gary Ramia, Kevin Farnsworth and Zoe Irving, 113–28. Bristol: Policy Press.
Jahiel, René, and Thomas F. Babor. 2007. 'Industrial Epidemics, Public Health Advocacy and the Alcohol Industry: Lessons from Other Fields'. *Addiction* 102 (9):1335–39.
Korten, David. 2000. *The Post-Corporate World: Life After Capitalism*. Sydney: Pluto Press.
Majnoni d'Intignano, Beatrice. 1998. 'Industrial Epidemics'. In *Governments and Health Systems: Implications of Differing Involvements*, edited by David Chinitz and Joshua Cohen, 585–96. Chichester: John Wiley & Sons.
O'Connell, Kit. 2016. 'After Bottling Michigan's Clean Water, Nestle Comes under Fire for Ties to Snyder Admin'. *Mint Press News*, 3 February. Accessed 3 February 2016. www.mintpressnews.com/nestle-guzzles-michigans-clean-water-donates-bottled-water-to-flint-water-crisis-victims/213360.
Pearce, Neil. 2011. 'Epidemiology in a Changing World: Variation, Causation and Ubiquitous Risk Factors'. *International Journal of Epidemiology* 40: 503–12.
Rich, Nathaniel. 2016. 'The Lawyer Who Became DuPont's Worst Nightmare' *New York Times Magazine*, 6 January.
Slade, J. 1989. 'The Tobacco Epidemic: Lessons from Psychoactive Drugs'. *Journal of Psychoactive Drugs* 21: 282–91.
UN System Task Team on the Post-2015 UN Development Agenda. 2013. *Global Governance and Governance of the Global Commons in the Global Partnership for Development beyond 2015*. New York: OHCHR, OHRLLS, UNDESA, UNEP and UNFPA.
Wilkinson, Richard, and Kate Pickett. 2010. *The Spirit Level: Why Equality Is Better for Everyone*. London: Penguin.

Index

LMICs. *See* low- and middle-income countries

London School of Hygiene & Tropical Medicine, 213, 215, 216

low and middle income countries, 29, 48, 76, 79, 80, 83, 120, 121, 125, 126, 139, 159, 167, 179, 193, 194, 204, 208, 245; markets for asbestos in, 103–104, 105, 105–111, 111–112; marketing of pharmacotherapy in, 32; marketing of smoking cessation in, 29, 32; non-communicable diseases in, 126; public-private partnerships and, 120, 125, 126; tobacco industry strategies in, 132, 159–170

LSHTM. *See* London School of Hygiene & Tropical Medicine

malaria, 122, 124, 125. *See also* Roll Back Malaria Partnership

Malawi, 77

Malaysia, 112

'Mamohato hospital. *See* Queen 'Mamohato Memorial Hospital

marginalised communities, 120, 213, 219, 221

Master Tobacco Settlement Agreement, 107, 181

McDonald, Corbett, 108

McGill University, 108

MDG. *See* Millennium Development Goals

medicalisation, 28–36, 246; benefit to corporations, 246; and global health, 246; of gambling, 90–91, 246; of smoking cessation, 28–36, 244, 246

Mexico, 41–45, 45, 112, 244

MGM Resorts International, 93

Millennium Development Goals, 122, 124, 126

Minimum Unit Pricing, 152–155

MLG. *See* Multi-level governance

Model List of Essential Medicines, 74

Mount Isa Mines Limited Agreement Act 1985, 1997, 66

MSPs. *See* Scotland, Members of the Scottish parliament

multi-level governance, 145–155, 245; concept of 145–146, 146–147, 149; corporate adaptation to 147–148, 149, 153, 155; impact on policy-making, 154–155

MUP. *See* Minimum Unit Pricing

NAFTA. *See* North American Free Trade Agreement

Namibia, 139

nanny state. *See* paternalism, corporate critiques of government

narrative review, 28, 133, 179

National Centre for Responsible Gaming, 91, 93, 96

National Environmental Protection Measures, Australia, 54, 57, 58, 63

National Gambling Impact Commission, 90

National Institute of Public Health, Mexico, 42

National Smokers' Alliance, 79

NCD. *See* non-communicable diseases

NCRG. *See* National Centre for Responsible Gaming

neoliberalism, 121, 127, 245; economic policies, 121, 133; ideologies of, 90; reforms, 245

NEPM. *See* National Environmental Protection Measures, Australia

Nestlé, 200, 200–201, 201, 202–204, 206, 207, 208, 209, 249; challenges to The International Code of Marketing of Breast-milk Substitutes by, 201, 203, 204, 205–206, 206; corporate social responsibility by, 205–206, 206; FTSE4Good and, 206; India, 207; International Council of Infant Food Industries, formation of, 201, 204; instrumental power, use of, 202, 202–203, 204, 206; legal action regarding *The Baby Killer*, 202; media coverage of, 200, 202, 206; Nescafé boycott, 200–201; Pakistan, 202–203, 207; Philippines, 207; self-regulation by, 204–205; structural power, use of, 200, 202, 203, 204, 206; whistle-blower 202–203; Zimbabwe 204

About the Contributors

CO-EDITORS

Nora J. Kenworthy is an assistant professor in the School of Nursing and Health Studies at the University of Washington Bothell. Her research focuses on global health governance, public-private partnerships and corporate social responsibility for HIV treatment in southern Africa. She is the author of a forthcoming book on the impacts of HIV treatment programs on democratic governance in Lesotho (Vanderbilt University Press), and co-editor, with Richard Parker, of *HIV Scale-Up and the Politics of Global Health* (Routledge, 2014).

Kelley Lee is Tier 1 Canada Research Chair in global health governance in the Faculty of Health Sciences, Simon Fraser University. She is a fellow of the UK Faculty of Public Health and Canadian Academy of Health Sciences. Her research focuses on the need for collective action to address the public health impacts of globalisation. Her research funding includes major grants from the U.S. National Institutes of Health, European Research Council, Economic and Social Research Council, Rockefeller Foundation and Wellcome Trust. She has written extensively on global health governance, including *Global Health and International Relations* (Polity Press, 2012) and *Transformations in Global Health Governance* (Palgrave Macmillan, 2014).

Ross MacKenzie received his PhD from the London School of Hygiene and Tropical Medicine and is a lecturer in the Department of Psychology at Macquarie University in Sydney, Australia. His research interests include the implications of global expansion of the tobacco industry, global health governance and medicalisation of smoking cessation. He has previously worked at the Centre for Global Change and Health at the London School of Hygiene and Tropical Medicine; School of Public Health, University of Sydney; and Action on Smoking and Health (ASH) Thailand.

CONTRIBUTORS

Ben Brisbois is a postdoctoral fellow in the Healthier Cities and Communities Hub of the Dalla Lana School of Public Health, University of Toronto. His research interests include occupational and environmental health hazards in Ecuador's banana industry, discursive aspects of global health research, and community-based climate change adaptation. His professional experience includes working for Health Canada and Environment Canada and in Guyana for a Canadian youth development NGO.

John Calvert is a political scientist teaching in the Faculty of Health Sciences at Simon Fraser University with a PhD from the London School of Economics. He specializes on the public policy aspects of international trade agreements, climate change, occupational health and safety and disability issues. He is associate director of the SSHRC-funded research project Adapting Canadian Work and Workplaces to Climate Change and BC co-chair of an SSHRC-funded project assessing Canada's disability system. He is on the editorial board of the *Canadian Foreign Policy Journal*.

A. Ángela Carriedo (MPH, RD, RNut) is a PhD student in public health and policy at the London School of Hygiene and Tropical Medicine. She obtained a master's in public health nutrition at the LSHTM. Her research interests are on governance and policy process for the Mexican obesity regulations. She has worked as a researcher at the National Institute of Public Health in Mexico for the past seven years and as a lecturer of food and nutrition policies at Universidad Iberoamericana, Mexico City, for five years. Her research focus includes the use of evidence and policy actions involved on the design and evaluation of food and nutrition policies, including soda tax, food labelling and dietary guidelines.

Rebecca Cassidy is professor of anthropology at Goldsmith College, University of London. She has written on kinship, class and thoroughbred breeding in the horseracing industries of Newmarket and Kentucky. She has conducted fieldwork in the UK with gamblers and members of the gambling industries since 1996. Her recent work, supported by the European Research Council, focuses on the production and circulation of knowledge about gambling.

Steven George is an environmental scientist and consultant with a strong interest in the causes and impacts of environmental pollution on society and human health. He has worked on projects in mining communities such as Broken Hill, Townsville and Port Pirie and has carried out extensive work in identifying the extent and degree of metal and metalloid contamination of urban soils across Australia. He has investigated and published findings on the impacts of industrialisation and urbanization on the state of Australian cities.

Dr. Benjamin Hawkins is a lecturer in global health policy at the London School of Hygiene and Tropical Medicine, teaching global health policy. His current research focuses on the role of research evidence and corporate actors in health policy making at the national and global levels. In particular his work focuses on the global alcohol and tobacco industries. Prior to entering academia he worked in sales and marketing for the alcohol producer Diageo.

Christopher Holden is a reader in international social policy at the University of York, UK. He has published widely on the relationships between the global economy, transnational corporations and health and social policy. He has been a member of the editorial board of the *Journal of Social Policy* and of the international advisory board of the journal *Global Social Policy*. He co-edited *The Global Social Policy Reader* (2009) and *Social Policy Review* (2009–2011).

Cécile Knai, PhD, MPH, RNut (public health) is a senior lecturer in public health policy in the Policy Innovation Research Unit, London School of Hygiene and Tropical Medicine. She obtained a master's in public health from the University of California at Berkeley and a PhD from the LSHTM. She previously worked at the World Health Organization Regional Office for Europe in the food and nutrition unit. Current research interests include the evaluation of local and national public health-related voluntary agreements with the private sector, analysis of industry-funded education campaigns and evaluation of food- and nutrition-related legislation on public health.

Ronald Labonté holds a Canada research chair in globalization and health equity and is a professor in the Faculty of Medicine, University of Ottawa; and in the Faculty of Health Sciences, Flinders University of South Australia. His work focuses on the health equity impacts of contemporary globalization, on which he has published extensively. Present research interests include health equity impacts of comprehensive primary health care reforms; health worker migration; medical tourism; global health diplomacy; globalization, trade and tobacco control; and trade and food security.

Melissa Mialon is a PhD candidate at the World Health Organization Collaborating Centre for obesity prevention, Deakin University, in Australia. Melissa has developed and implemented an approach to monitor the corporate political activity of the food industry. Before joining Deakin University, Melissa completed an MSc in food science and engineering at

Agrosup Dijon in France. Melissa also completed a placement at the United Nations Standing Committee on Nutrition in Geneva.

Suerie Moon, MPA, PhD is a lecturer on global health at the Harvard T.H. Chan School of Public Health, and research director and co-chair of the Forum on Global Governance for Health at the Harvard Global Health Institute. Her work focuses on the intersection of global governance and public health, and has examined the global response to the 2013–2015 Ebola outbreak, trade and investment regimes, intellectual property rules, policies to enhance innovation and access to medicines in low- and middle-income countries, global health financing and the functioning of the global health system.

Gary Sacks is a senior research fellow at the World Health Organization (WHO) Collaborating Centre for Obesity Prevention at Deakin University. Gary's research focuses on policies for the prevention of obesity and related non-communicable diseases, with a focus on strengthening accountability of governments and the food industry.

Ashley Schram is a PhD candidate in population health at the University of Ottawa. Her area of work centres on the critical political economy of trade and health, investigating pathways between international trade and investment agreements, and non-communicable diseases, with a focus on the role of private actors and investor-state dispute-settlement mechanisms in national regulatory policy space and the role of the food industry in creating obesogenic food environments.

Courtney Scott is a PhD candidate in public health and policy at the London School of Hygiene and Tropical Medicine, studying the politics of product reformulation efforts to reduce sugar consumption in the United States. She previously worked in nutrition policy advocacy in California, focusing on anti-sugary drink policies, and international non-communicable disease advocacy in Brussels. She is a registered dietitian (United States) and earned her master's in public health nutrition from the University of California–Berkeley.

Michael Stevenson is a lecturer at the University of Waterloo, and a research fellow at the Balsillie School of International Affairs. His current work relates to governance innovation focused on meeting the health needs of marginalized populations, and the implications of the rise of private authority in domains long associated exclusively with state stewardship.

Elina Suzuki is a consultant at SEEK Development in Berlin, where she works on projects related to global governance, global health financing, maternal and child health, and education. She was previously a research assistant at the Harvard Global Health Institute. Elina graduated from McGill University and received a master's of science degree from the Harvard School of Public Health.

Boyd Swinburn is a professor of population nutrition and global health at the University of Auckland and Alfred Deakin professor and director of the WHO Collaborating Centre for Obesity Prevention at Deakin University in Melbourne. His major research interests are on community and policy actions to prevent childhood and adolescent obesity, and reduce the 'obesogenic' food environment. He has contributed to over thirty WHO consultations and reports on obesity, authored over three hundred publications and given over four hundred presentations.

Mark Patrick Taylor is a professor of environmental science at Macquarie University Sydney, Australia. His main research, teaching and consulting interests are in environmental health. His research program investigates environmental pollution and risks to human health from aerosols, dusts, sediments, soil and water. He has published more than two hundred research papers and reports. He provides expert evidence and advice to government, industry, lawyers and community on a range of environmental matters, particularly environmental pollution. In October 2015, he was appointed by the NSW environment minister to review NSW EPA's management of contaminated sites.

Tracey Wagner-Rizvi is a PhD candidate in global governance at the Balsillie School of International Affairs, University of Waterloo. Her research looks at how civil society and corporate actors influence global health policy making, and how global health governance is changing in response to such influence.

William H. Wiist holds a courtesy faculty appointment in international health at Oregon State University. Prior to retirement he was professor and senior scientist at Northern Arizona University. He edited and co-authored *The Bottom Line or Public Health* (Oxford University Press, 2010). He conducted community-based research on the prevention of heart disease, cancer and violence in African American, Latino and Native American communities. His course teaching included corporations and health, and economic globalization and health. His recent policy publications focus on public health's role in the prevention of war.